K

Palliative Care
For Non-Cancer
Patients

Palliative Care for Non-Cancer Patients

Edited by

Julia M. Addington-Hall

Department of Palliative Care & Policy,
Guy's, King's & St Thomas' School of Medicine
St Christopher's Hospice
London

and

Irene J. Higginson

Professor and Head of Department of
Palliative Care and Policy
Guy's, King's & St Thomas' School of Medicine
St Christopher's Hospice
London

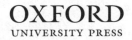

OXFORD
UNIVERSITY PRESS

OXFORD

UNIVERSITY PRESS

Great Clarendon Street, Oxford OX2 6DP

Oxford University Press is a department of the University of Oxford.
It furthers the University's objective of excellence in research, scholarship,
and education by publishing worldwide in

Oxford New York

Auckland Bangkok Buenos Aires Cape Town Chennai
Dar es Salaam Delhi Hong Kong Istanbul Karachi Kolkata
Kuala Lumpur Madrid Melbourne Mexico City Mumbai Nairobi
São Paulo Shanghai Singapore Taipei Tokyo Toronto

Oxford is a registered trade mark of Oxford University Press
in the UK and in certain other countries

Published in the United States
by Oxford University Press Inc., New York

First published 2001
Reprinted 2002

British Library Cataloguing in Publication Data
Data available

Library of Congress Cataloging in Publication Data
Palliative care for non-cancer patients/edited by Julia Addington-Hall and
Irene J. Higginson.
p. cm.
Includes bibliographical references.
1. Palliative treatment. I. Addington-Hall, Julia. II. Higginson, Irene.
R726.8.P3428 2001 616'.029—dc21 00-054848
ISBN 0-19-262960-3 (Hbk)

10 9 8 7 6 5 4 3 2 1

Typeset in Minion by
J&L Composition Ltd, Filey, North Yorkshire
Printed in Great Britain on acid-free paper by
Biddles Ltd, Guildford and King's Lynn

Foreword

Dame Cicely Saunders, OM

The dissatisfied dead cannot noise abroad the negligence they have experienced.

(Hinton 1967)

Hinton's book, *Dying*, published nearly 20 years after the launch of the National Health Service, was based not only on a detailed study of patients dying in the wards of a teaching hospital (Hinton 1963) but also on a wide survey of people in other situations. It amply illustrated the truth, summarised in his telling indictment of the lack of provision and practice in this area of widespread need. This new book, *Palliative Care for Non-cancer Patients*, illustrates not only the many challenges that still remain to be taken up but points to some of the ways forward in both research and therapy.

The hospice movement, which also dates from 1967 with the opening of St Christopher's Hospice, was only the beginning of an adequate response that had been prepared for by many years of experience, research, and consultation (Clarke 1998). It has since shown that its basic principles and practice can be interpreted across different cultures and developed with widely different resources. An essential founding concept was termed 'total pain'.

Patients attempting to describe pain use such phrases as 'it seemed as if all of me was wrong' and speak not only of [pain and] other symptoms, but also include descriptions of their mental distress or their social and spiritual problems.

(Saunders 1964)

The original focus on patients with malignant disease enabled some ground-breaking research with which the myths inhibiting the adequate use of opiate drugs were addressed and confuted (Wall 1997). However, it is time for this full account of similar challenges presented by the care of people facing persistent distress among often more disadvantaged groups. The original concept of total pain, which was such a catalyst, may prove to be equally stimulating here. Skills, and even more importantly, attitudes, are gradually being interpreted and finding response in new therapeutic developments.

Initially, that first research and teaching hospice provided in-patient care for cancer patients. After 1969 it moved out into home care in the community and has since developed to meet the needs of people for most of the period of persistent disease, although full implementation is still too patchy for any complacency. Such care will surely be the major way of approaching the problems of the even larger groups described here. The major differences in prognostic accuracy possible and the challenges of when to change gear will undoubtedly present new difficulties in developing positive attitudes to palliation in place of inappropriate attempts towards cure or the prolongation of life. It will call for the same multi-professional approach that has distinguished palliative care so far. Lessons from those who face the crises of death from malignant disease have had much to teach the living. The long haul of some other diseases may be less dramatic and stimulate less compelling reading but are part of the reality of our existence and have other important pointers to pass on. Isolation makes suffering much harder to endure and overcome and is a social as well as a medical challenge.

The lessons learned so far in the now world-wide field of palliative care were never meant to be confined to one group of patients and families. Carers struggling to cope over long periods of stress are equally deserving of support and understanding and their voices are too often unheard. Their burdens are eloquently documented by Seale and Cartwright. They conclude their important book *The Year before Death* by looking at those, on the whole, older people associated with 'long term restrictions and less help available from relatives'. They end with the demands presented in this timely book. 'The development of adequate services to meet the needs of this group presents an even greater challenge than that initially taken on by the hospice movement' (Seale and Cartwright 1994). There could hardly be a better incentive than that presented in the following pages.

References

Clarke, D. (1998). Originating a movement: Cicely Saunders and the development of St Christopher's Hospice, 1957–1967. *Mortality* **3**(1): 43–63.

Hinton, J.M. (1963). The physical and mental distress of the dying. *Quart J Med NS* **32**: 1–20.

Hinton, J.M. (1967). *Dying.* Harmondsworth: Penguin Books.

Saunders, C. (1964). The symptomatic treatment of incurable malignant disease. *Prescribers' Journal* **4**(4): 68–73.

Seale, C. and Cartwright, A. (1994). *The Year before Death.* Aldershot: Avebury Press.

Wall, P.D. (1997). The generation of yet another myth on the use of narcotics. *Pain* **73**: 121–2.

Preface

The development of medical treatments and the extension of life expectancy during much of the last century left much suffering un-addressed. The development of the modern hospice movement, in the UK and the US, challenged conventional thinking that symptoms could not be controlled and that death was failure. Although a small number of hospices had existed for many years, the development by Dame Cicely Saunders of St Christopher's Hospice in South London in 1967, marks for many the beginning of a modern hospice movement, concerned not only with the best in care, but also research into improving practice and education. In the intervening thirty or so years the principles and philosophy of hospice care have spread world-wide. They have been adapted to the needs of patients and families living in different societies, and modified to work within and alongside a wide range of health care systems. Many people with cancer have been enabled to maintain a good quality of life, to die well, and to know that their families are supported after their deaths. There is much to celebrate. But sadly there are still patients who even today miss out on the best in care, still die in pain, without appropriate physical, psychological and spiritual support.

While some cancer patients do miss out on care, cancer accounts for only one in four deaths, and far fewer patients with non-malignant diseases seem to receive appropriate care. And there is a lack of knowledge of what is to be done for the best. It is this lack of knowledge that drove us to prepare this book.

Since the inception of modern hospice care, it has been recognized, that the principles of hospice care might apply to other patients with progressive life-threatening or advanced diseases. But the focus of hospice and palliative care has remained on cancer. This has enabled the rapid progress we have seen in symptom control and in the development of appropriate services. But the question remains of whether other people would also benefit from the principles and practice of hospice and palliative care. The gaps in what we know means that it is often not possible to provide definitive answers to questions such as *which* other patients, and *when*. We hope, however, that readers will—like us—be stimulated, provoked, informed and challenged by the material presented here, and that this volume will therefore play an important role for those who wish to seek ways to improve care, and those who wish to furthering our understanding of the needs of patients with progressive non-malignant disease. In the future, just as research into the management of problems and into providing care improved the lot of patients with cancer, circumstances for those with non-cancer diseases will be improved.

We are indebted to the authors of each chapter in the volume. They have risen magnificently to the challenge of being requested to produce evidence-based chapters in areas with often limited evidence. It has been a great privilege to work with them, during the time consuming and complex area to producing a book of this scale and scope. We would thank Bimpe Akinwunmi, who provided secretarial support to us during the production of the volume. She has, as always, been professional, patient and supportive—even when vexed by our administrative abilities.

Each of us also have people to whom we are indebted. JAH is grateful for the forbearance and encouragement of Keith, and for the diversions provided by Jonathan and Edward. IJH is grateful to the friends, family and colleagues who endured her during the preparations for the book.

Contents

List of Contributors

Julia M. Addington-Hall
Senior Lecturer/Deputy Head
Dept of Palliative Care & Policy
Guy's, King's & St Thomas' School of Medicine
London, UK

Stephen Barclay
General Practictioner and Health Services
Research Training Fellow
Department of Public Health and Primary Care
Cambridge University, Cambridge, UK

Cynthia Benz
Person with MS
Berkshire, UK

Gabi Brogan
Specialist registrar in Palliative Medicine
St Joseph's Hospice
London, UK

Eduardo Bruera
Director of Symptom Control & Palliative Care
MD Anderson Cancer Center
Texas, USA

Lewis M. Cohen
Director of the Renal Palliative Care Initiative
Baystate Medical Center, Springfield
Massachusetts, USA

Carol Davis
Consultant and Senior Lecturer in Palliative
Medicine
Hospital Palliative Care Team
Southampton General Hospital
Southampton, UK

Robert Dunlop
Hon. Senior Lecturer
Dept of Palliative Care & Policy
Guy's, King's & St Thomas' School of Medicine
London, UK

Polly Edmonds
Clinical Senior Lecturer
Dept. of Palliative Care & Policy
Guy's, King's & St Thomas' School of Medicine
London, UK

Rob George
Consultant in Palliative Medicine
Middlesex Hospital
London, UK

Michael J. Germain
Medical Director, Renal Transplantation
Tufts University School of Medicine, USA

J. Simon. R. Gibbs
Senior Lecturer in Cardiology
National Heart & Lung Institute
London, UK

Ann Goldman
CLIC Consultant in Palliative Care
Department of Haematology and Oncology
Great Ormond Street Hospital
London, UK

Patricia Hanrahan
Assistant Professor/Research Associate
Department of Psychiatry
University of Chicago, USA

M.A. Henegham
Duke University Medical Center
Durham
North Carolina, USA

Irene J. Higginson
Professor of Palliative Care & Policy
Dept. of Palliative Care & Policy
Guy's, King's & St Thomas' School of Medicine
London, UK

John H. James
Chief Executive, Kensington &
Chelsea and Westminster Health Authority
London, UK

Jonathan Koffman
Lecturer in Palliative Care
Dept. of Palliative Care & Policy
Guy's, King's & St Thomas' School of Medicine
London, UK

Daniel J. Luchins
Department of Psychiatry
University of Chicago, USA

Joanne Lynn
Director, RAND Center to Improve Care of the
Dying
Arlington, USA

Ian Maddocks
Professor Emeritus
Flinders University of South Australia

Kathleen Murphy
Department of Psychiatry
University of Chicago, USA

Catherine M. Neumann
Teaching Assistant
Div. of Palliative Medicine
University of Alberta, Canada

Tony O'Brien
Consultant Physician in Palliative Medicine
Marymount Hospice
St Patrick's Hospital
Cork, Ireland

J.G. O'Grady
Consultant Hepatologist
Institute of Liver Studies
King's College Hospital
London, UK

Deborah Parker
International Institute of Hospice Studies
Flinders University of South Australia

Peter Pitcher
Clinical Nurse Specialist
Hospital Palliative Care Team
Southampton General Hospital
UK

David M. Poppel
Western New England Renal & Transplant
Association
Massachusetts, USA

Gary S. Reiter
Medical Director Holyoake Hospital,
Director River Valley HIV Service,
Associate Director Hospice Life Care
Massachusetts, USA

Angie Rogers
Research Associate
Dept. of Palliative Care and Policy
Guy's, King's & St Thomas' School of Medicine
London, UK

Ildiko Schuller
Consultant Paediatrician
Queen Mary's Hospital
Sidcup, Kent, UK

Penny Snow
Rural Organiser for the Princes Royal Trust for
Carers
Bristol, UK

Charles Shee
Consultant Physician
Queen Mary's NHS Trust
Sidcup, Kent, UK

Peter W. Speck
Senior Chaplain
Southampton General Hospital
Southampton, UK

Katherine Wasson
Senior Research Ethicist
Whitefield Institute
London, UK

Abbreviations

ABCD	Americans for Better Care of the Dying
ACE	angiotensin converting enzyme
ACS	acute chest syndrome
ACT	The Association for Children with Life Threatening Terminal Conditions and their Families
AIDS	acquired immune deficiency syndrome
ALS	amyotrophic lateral sclerosis
BTS	British Thoracic Society
CEO	chief executive officer
CHD	coronary heart disease
CHF	congestive heart failure
CNS	clinical nurse specialist/central nervous system
COPD	chronic obstructive pulmonary disease
CQI	continuous quality improvement
CSF	cerebrospinal fluid
CSSCD	Co-operative Study of Sickle Cell Disease
DN	district nurse
DSCU	dementia special care units
DSM-IV	diagnostic and statistical manual of mental disorders, 4th edition
EEG	electroencephalogram
ESAS	Edmonton symptom assessment system
ESRD	End stage renal disease
FAST	functional assessment staging
GABA	gamma-amino butyric acid
GDS	global deterioration rate
GFR	glomerulariltration rate
GP	general practitioner
HAART	highly active antiretroviral therapy
HbF	foetal haemoglobin
HbS	sickle cell carrier state
HbSS	haemoglobin horiozygous for sickle cell disease
HBV	hepatitis B virus
HCV	hepatitis C virus
HD	Huntington's disease
HDCRG	Huntington's Disease Collaborative Research Group
HIMP	Health Improvement Programme
HIV	human immunodeficiency virus
HPCT	hospital palliative care team

HRS	hepatorenal syndrome
ICU	Intensive Care Unit
IHD	ischaemic heart disease
IM	intramuscular
IPPV	intermittent positive pressure ventilation
IV	intravenous
KCW	Kensington & Chelsea and Westminster Health Authority
LMN	lower motor neurone
LOC	locus of control
LTOT	long-term oxygen therapy
MMSE	'Mini-mental state examination'
MND	motor neurone disease
MND/ALS	motor neurone disease/amyotrophic lateral sclerosis
MRI	magnetic resonance imaging
MRSA	methicillin-resistant Straphylococcus aureus
MS	multiple sclerosis
NSAIDS	non-steroidal anti-inflammatory drugs
NCHSPCS	National Council for Hospice and Specialist Care Services
NG	naso-gastric tube
NHS	National Health Service
NIPPV	non-invasive positive pressure ventilation
NYHA	New York Heart Association
ONS	Office of National Statistics
OT	occupational therapist
PCA	patient controlled analgesia
PCG	primary care group
PCT	primary care trust
PD	Parkinson's disease
PEG	percutaneous endoscopic gastrostomy
PET	position emission tomography
PFE	pulmonary fat embolism
PG	percutaneous gastrostomy
PO	by mouth
PR	pulmonary rehabilitation
PT	physiotherapist
QOL	Quality of Life
qam	every morning
qhs	at bedtime
qod	every other day
RCPCH	The Royal College of Paediatrics and Child Health
RHA	Regional Health Authority
RSCD	'Regional study of care for the dying'
SBP	spontaneous bacterial peritonitis
SCD	sickle cell disease
SL	sub lingual

STAS	Support Team Assessment Schedule
SUPPORT	'Study to understand prognosis and preferences for outcomes and risks of treatment'
TENS	transcutaneous Electric Nerve Stimulation
TIPS	transjugular intrahepatic porto-systemic shunt
TLTC	traditional long-term care units
TPN	total parenteral nutrition
UMN	Upper motor neurone
VAS	visual analogue scale
WHO	World Health Organisation

Introduction

Julia M. Addington-Hall and Irene J. Higginson

This is, to our knowledge, the first book to consider specifically the palliative care needs of people who die from causes other than cancer and, in particular, to discuss how these needs might best be met. Like most people working in palliative care our initial experiences as researchers and as a clinician (Irene Higginson) were in terminal cancer. One of us (Julia Addington-Hall) became interested in palliative care for non-cancer patients when working on the 'Regional study of care for the dying', a large population based survey in the UK of deaths from all causes (Addington-Hall and McCarthy 1995). It became clear from the data that dying from cancer did not look so different from dying from congestive heart failure (CHF), chronic obstructive pulmonary disease (COPD), or stroke, and that many people dying from these conditions had un-met health and social care needs in the last year of life; Addington-Hall et al. 1995; McCarthy, Lay and Addington-Hall 1996; Addington-Hall, Fakhoury and McCarthy 1998). All clinicians will encounter patients with progressive conditions with a wide range of diagnoses. Epidemiological data demonstrates what clinicians see in day-to-day practice—that cancer forms only one quarter of all causes of death (Higginson 1997).

The complexities of addressing the needs of non-cancer patients quickly became apparent. Suggestions that hospices and palliative care services in the UK might expand to include more non-cancer patients were met with fears that existing services would be overwhelmed, that clinicians lacked the necessary expertise, that funding would not be forthcoming, and that cancer patients would suffer (Field and Addington-Hall 1999). Existing service providers feared 'empire-building' on the part of hospices and palliative care services; and many believed that they were already providing good holistic care and that patients would not benefit from the involvement of hospice services. Thinking about these issues raised fundamental questions about the nature of hospice and palliative care—is it, for example, about death and dying, or is about providing holistic care and symptom control regardless of prognosis? From both our perspectives, we found ourselves increasingly drawn to this difficult and challenging debate. The fact that we have been able to persuade so many excellent clinicians and thinkers from both within and without palliative care to contribute to this book indicates that we are not alone in seeing this issue as important. We believe that it is not only central to the development of hospice care in the twenty-first century but also to the question of how we can best meet the needs of the growing numbers of people living with chronic conditions.

In this chapter, we start with an overview of developments in medicine in the twentieth century and a brief look at the evidence that people with chronic conditions have not always been served well by these. We go on to describe the development of hospice care to meet the needs of another group ill served by modern medicine: terminally ill cancer patients. We summarise developments in hospice and palliative care, focusing particularly on the UK, and describe the patients currently served by these services. We then introduce the debate about the appropriate provision of palliative care services for non-cancer patients, and outline the contents of this book.

Twentieth-century medicine

Medicine changed dramatically in the twentieth century. Scientific and technological discoveries transformed understanding of the human body and, as a consequence, doctors for the first time had effective therapies for many illnesses. Infectious illnesses, the major killer in the early twentieth century as in previous centuries, ceased to be a formidable enemy in the developed world. Doctors who previously had had little to offer patients except care could now hope to cure. The proliferation in the number of hospitals which had started in the mid-nineteenth century alongside the development of medicine continued, and the site of medical endeavour moved from patients' homes to institutions dominated by the requirements of the new medical era. Hopes were high that the science of medicine could find a cure for all ills, and most patients were therefore willing to submit to the authority of doctors in the expectation that a cure would result. People no longer died in large numbers from infectious illnesses, usually rapidly and with little warning. Instead, they survived to succumb eventually to the new killers: cancer and chronic diseases such as CHD and chronic lung diseases. Much had been gained.

However, during the second half of the twentieth century there was increasing recognition that something had also been lost: new possibilities of cure had shifted the focus of medicine to the malfunctioning body and away from the individual. Impersonal hospital care might be an acceptable price to pay for cure—when Aneurin Bevan presented the NHS (National Health Service) bill to the UK parliament he stated he would 'rather be kept alive in the efficient if cold altruism of a large hospital than expire in a gush of warm sympathy in a small one'. But such care was less appropriate for the growing numbers of people with chronic diseases, for whom the emotional and physical costs of such care could, on occasion, outweigh the benefits. By the end of the century modern disease-focused medicine was increasingly challenged, both from within and without medicine. The increasing use of alternative therapies reflected both disillusionment in medicine's ability to cure all ills, and the attraction of practitioners interested in caring for the 'whole person' (Ernst 2000). The growth of the 'quality of life' movement within medicine marked an increasing recognition of the legitimacy of exploring the impact of disease and treatment on the individual, rather than focusing solely on the body (Clinch, Dudgeon and Schipper 1998). At the beginning of the twenty-first century, there is growing recognition that new models of care need to be developed to meet the needs of people living with chronic diseases, particularly as the population in the developed world ages.

The development of hospice care

The second half of the twentieth century saw the rapid development of a new model of care for a second group of patients who fared badly from the changing emphasis of medicine from care to cure: terminally ill patients, particularly those dying from cancer. Homes for the dying poor had been founded by religious orders in the late nineteenth century, and several survived into the middle of the twentieth century. Apart from these, the needs of the dying were largely ignored. Before the founding of the NHS in the UK in 1947 the growing numbers of voluntary hospitals (which included specialist and teaching hospitals) focused on curing patients with acute illnesses and were therefore reluctant to take patients less likely to benefit from the new advances: the chronically ill, the aged, and the dying. These patients were therefore cared for in under-resourced local authority hospitals, in Poor Law work-houses, and in the small number of homes specifically for the dying; or they remained at home. After 1947, the situation remained much the same. However, there was growing evidence of the unremitting distress experienced by many terminally ill cancer patients and the poor conditions in which patients often lived (Marie Curie Memorial Foundation 1952). This led the Marie Curie Memorial Foundation, a cancer charity, to supplement existing homes for the dying in the 1950s by opening a number of nursing homes for dying cancer patients, and to develop a basic nursing service for people at home. According to a survey conducted at the end of the decade, care in contemporary terminal care homes was characterised by good intentions but poorly developed techniques (Hughes 1960). Better care was still urgently needed.

Cicely Saunders, an Oxford graduate who trained as a nurse and medical almoner (social worker) was personally motivated to improve care for terminally ill cancer patients, and trained as a doctor specifically to be able to address their needs. Within ten years of completing her medical training she has succeeded in opening St Christopher's Hospice in Sydenham, initially a 54-bedded in-patient unit, dedicated to patient care, research, and education. This differed from existing homes for the dying poor because of its emphasis on care based on solid research, and its aim to promote palliative care through education. Her success, and the speed with which her ideas spread and were adapted to other settings, was in no small part due to Dame Cicely's (as she now is) personal skills and drive. However, her ideas and entreaties for support fell onto fertile ground. There was a growing disquiet at the terrible pain experienced by many terminally ill cancer patients, set alongside the increasing scientific evidence that such pain could be controlled; there was growing evidence from sociological and psychological studies that these patients were largely ignored within health care settings and consequently left isolated and abandoned and, in the US, by a growing movement challenging orthodox medical views and medical power. Dame Cicely showed that cancer pain could normally be controlled by the appropriate use of opiates. However, she argued that controlling pain was not the end point in itself, instead patients should be enabled to live until they died, accompanied on their journey, and with their total pain (physical, psychological, social and spiritual) addressed (Saunders 1998; Clark 1999).

The modern hospice movement is generally considered to have begun when St Christopher's Hospice opened in 1967. The movement quickly spread, with its ideas and ideals adapted to suit differing health care systems and cultural norms. By Janaury 2000, 89 countries across the world had hospice and palliative care initiatives operational or under development (Hospice Information Service 2000). These services are called by a variety of names. St Christopher's was called a hospice after the 'hospices' provided in the UK by medi-aeval monasteries to offer pilgrims shelter, and the 'hospices' in France which provided care for the dying in the nineteenth century. Many countries have adopted this label. It was not, however, appropriate for use in French-speaking countries, where the term 'hospice' implies custodial care. The term 'palliative' was therefore used instead in 1975 to describe the new hospice-type service in Montreal, Canada.

Until the early 1980s most hospices or palliative care services described the care they provided as 'terminal care'. This was, however, in the UK felt to be a barrier to health professionals referring patients sufficiently early to benefit from care, and to patients themselves accepting the care. At the same time, the value of hospice-type care earlier in the cancer trajectory was being recognised. Some services therefore chose to describe themselves as providing palliative rather than terminal care, and this has become in many countries the usual term for hospice-type services. In the UK the term 'palliative medicine' was chosen to describe hospice medicine when it was recognised as a sub-specialty of the Royal College of Physicians in 1987. However, countries such as the UK where palliative medicine is a recognised specialty remain in the minority. In the US there is an increasing division between hospice care, a network of largely community based hospice programmes which developed initially as an alternative to mainstream health care, and palliative care, which are primarily medically driven programmes within mainstream health care (Byock 1998). The terms used to describe hospice-type care therefore varies across and within countries. This is reflected in the chapters in this book. Many, however, are written from the UK perspective and refer to UK hospice services and to commonly accepted UK definitions of palliative care. These are therefore described here.

Palliative care in the UK

As outlined above, modern hospice care in the UK began with the opening of an in-patient unit to provide high quality care for terminally ill cancer patients until death. Other in-patient hospices followed, and by 2000 there were 199 hospices and palliative units for adults, with a total of 3048 beds (Hospice Information Service 2000).

It quickly became apparent, however, that many patients wanted to remain at home for as long as possible, and in 1969 St Christopher's therefore began a home care service to provide hospice-like care to patients at home, in conjunction with the primary health care team. There has been a rapid growth in the number of community palliative services—to 340 in the UK in 2000, and many more world-wide (Hospice Information Service 2000). More than two-fifths of cancer patients who died in the UK in the year ending 31 March 1995 were estimated to have had support from these nurses (Hospice Information Service 1998). The cancer charity, Macmillan Cancer Relief, has played a key role in providing initial funding for these nurses, and they have therefore become synonymous in many areas with the title of 'Macmillan nurse'. Others, however, are known as hospice home care nurses, or are named after the local hospice charity. Their working arrangements, the care they provide and their funding vary widely (Bosanquet and Salisbury 1999). They may work alone, with other nursing colleagues, or within a multidisciplinary team which includes specialists in palliative medicine. Patients may be referred by hospitals on discharge, by their GP (general practitioner), or by the district nurse. Some teams accept direct referrals from patients and families. Most offer patients and families counselling and support, as well as providing education to other health professionals. Some augment the hands-on nursing care provided by the NHS district nursing service. Most work primarily with cancer patients, some have significant HIV (human immunodeficiency virus)/AIDS (acquired immune deficiency syndrome) case loads, whilst others accept referrals for patients with any advanced disease. Many take on terminally ill patients, whilst others are involved with the care of patients from diagnosis. Some are funded by the NHS, many initially by Macmillan Cancer Relief, and others by local hospice charities.

In 1976 St Thomas' Hospital in London started the first hospital support team in the UK to provide expert advice and support to terminally ill patients and their care providers whilst in hospital. Again, the number of these services has grown rapidly, particularly since the recognition of palliative medicine as a specialty. By January 2000 there were 215 hospital palliative care teams and 118 hospital support nursing services. These services vary from a single clinical nurse specialist (CNS) plus consultants in palliative medicine, to a full multi-professional team (including, for example, consultants in palliative medicine, CNSs, counsellors or social workers, OTs, PTs, dieticians, and chaplains).

More recent developments in the UK include day care services. Day hospices now outnumber in-patient units. They vary in whether their emphasis is in providing medical and nursing care (including, for example, consultations with doctors, adjustment of medication, medical procedures (including blood tranfusions), baths, etc.) or on providing a therapeutic and creative environment to enable patients to 'live fully until death'. Some areas have also now started hospice-at-home services to provide nursing care 24 hours a day for a limited period, to enable patients to avoid hospital admission and to die at home.

Most hospices and palliative care services in the UK have been initiated by local people and funded by community fund-raising. Most in-patient hospices and day hospices are independent charities, managed by boards of trustees, with the NHS making varying contributions towards their costs (an average of 32%). A few hospices are directly managed and funded by the NHS. As outlined above, the charity Macmillan Cancer Relief has played a major role in funding community palliative care teams and hospital services; they also provided initial funding for most NHS hospices. After three years funding reverts to the NHS. The NHS therefore contributes more towards the cost of community and hospital services, but voluntary fund-raising still plays an important role. Although health districts in the UK are required by law to develop local strategies for palliative care provision, most services have developed within the voluntary sector in response to local opinion that a service is needed rather than as a planned NHS response to formally established need.

Definitions of palliative care

The NHS Executive in EL(96)85 defines the palliative care approach, palliative interventions and specialist palliative care as the principal components of the spectrum of palliative care provision. These definitions are referred to explicitly in several chapters, and underlie several others. They are therefore provided here (NHS Executive 1996; NCHSPCS 1995).

The palliative care approach aims to promote both physical and psychosocial well-being. It is a vital and integral part of all clinical practice, whatever the illness or its stage, informed by a knowledge and practice of palliative care principles and supported by specialist palliative care. The key principles underpinning palliative care which should be practised by all health professionals in primary care, hospital, and other settings comprise:

◆ focus on quality of life, including good symptom control;

◆ whole person approach taking into account the person's past life experience and current situation;

◆ care which encompasses both the person with the life-threatening disease and those individuals who matter to that person;

- respect for patient autonomy and choice (e.g. over place of care, treatment options, access to specialist palliative care);
- emphasis on open and sensitive communication, extending this to patients, informal carers, and professional colleagues.

Palliative interventions are non-curative treatments given by specialists in disciplines other than specialist palliative care aimed at controlling symptoms and improving a patient's quality of life, for example through the use of palliative radiotherapy, chemotherapy, surgical procedures and anaesthetic techniques for pain relief.

Specialist palliative care services are those services with palliative care as their core specialty. Specialist palliative care services are needed by a significant minority of people whose deaths are anticipated, and may be provided directly though specialist services, or indirectly through advice to a patient's present professional advisers/carers. These services provide physical, psychological, social, and spiritual support, and will involve practitioners with a broad mix of skills, including medical and nursing, social work, pastoral/spiritual care, physiotherapy, occupational therapy, pharmacy, and related specialties.

Palliative care for non-cancer patients

The hospice movement was initially developed in response to the perceived need of terminally ill cancer patients, and also because an effective remedy was available, but not widely used at the time, for pain, their most dreaded symptom. Although St Christopher's Hospice did (and does) provide care for some patients with progressive, fatal, neurological conditions (specifically motor neurone disease (MND)), the main focus of the early hospice movement was on terminal cancer. It was recognised that the ideas and philosophy of hospice care might benefit patients dying from other conditions:

> ... many of the symptoms to be treated and much of the general management will be relevant to other situations. . . . Terminal care should not only be part of oncology but of geriatric medicine, neurology, general practice and throughout medicine.

> (Saunders and Baines 1983)

However, the emphasis was on encouraging other medical disciplines to take up the challenge and develop services for their patients.

The emergence of AIDS/HIV in the 1980s presented a major challenge to this philosophy. There was considerable debate within the hospice movement about whether AIDS patients would be admitted to hospices. Concerns included fears about the risk of infection, anxieties that community fund-raising would be adversely affected, and a perception that hospice staff lacked the necessary expertise. The overtly Christian ethos of many hospices was in its turn off-putting to many people with AIDS, who at the time were largely from the gay community. AIDS specific hospices opened in the UK and the US, and specialist AIDS/HIV community palliative care services developed. The availability in England and Wales of ring-fenced NHS funds specifically for AIDS services was an important factor in the development of specialist services. Over time most hospices and palliative care services in the UK have expanded their admission criteria to include people with AIDS/HIV although separate services also exist (see Chapter 11). Nevertheless, almost everyone who used hospice services in the UK in 1994/5 had a diagnosis of cancer (in-patient hospices 96.7%, community palliative care services 96.3%) (Eve, Smith and Tebbit 1997).

Changes in the organisation of the NHS in the early 1990s separated the function of purchasing health care from that of providing it. District health authorities no longer directly managed services, instead their role was to determine local need for health care, to purchase it and to monitor its quality. The new focus on needs assessment was accompanied in palliative care by increasing recognition that cancer patients were not alone in needing palliative care. An expert report to the Department of Health in 1992 argued that 'all patients needing them should have access to palliative care services . . . although often referred to as equating with terminal cancer care, it is important to recognise that similar services are appropriate for and should be developed for patients dying from other diseases' (Standing Medical Advisory Committee, Standing Nursing and Midwifery Advisory Committee 1992). With its emphasis on the development of similar, but presumably separate, services it was consistent with the approach to non-cancer patients adopted by the hospice movement since its inception.

However, in 1994 a Scottish Office Management Executive letter (Scottish Office 1994) said that 'palliative care is currently provided mainly for people suffering from cancer, but it is increasingly recognised that people with a range of life threatening diseases may also benefit from it'. Similarly, in 1996, an Executive letter from the NHS Executive on palliative care stated that

> purchasers are asked to ensure that provision of care with a palliative approach is included in all contracts of services for those with cancer and other life-threatening diseases . . . although this letter is focused on services for cancer patients, it applies equally to patients with other life threatening conditions, including AIDS, neurological conditions, and cardiac and respiratory failure.

> (NHS Executive 1996)

The epidemiologically based needs assessment on palliative and terminal care provided guidance on the numbers of people within health authority populations with different diseases who may have need for palliative care (Higginson 1997). The focus was on providing care informed by the palliative care approach for non-cancer patients, rather than arguing specifically that hospices and specialist palliative care services should care for non-cancer patients. These services primarily lie outside the NHS and at best are only partially funded by it: it does not, therefore, have the authority to insist on this.

However, the emphasis on providing palliative care on the basis of need, not diagnosis, continued throughout the 1990s. It is now a key principle in guidance on the commissioning of palliative care services for adults that 'it is the right of every person with a life-threatening illness to receive appropriate palliative care wherever they are'. The government, in the recent National Service Framework for cardiac disease, stated that there should be access in all health districts to specialist palliative care services for patients with end stage heart failure (Department of Health 2000). The clear message from the government and NHS in the UK is, therefore, that palliative care should not be restricted to terminally ill cancer patients. The reality continues, however, to be that almost all patients who access hospice and specialist palliative care in the UK have cancer.

Hospice services in other countries have developed in different ways to those in the UK, in response to local circumstances and health systems. In the US the majority of patients who receive care from hospice programmes have cancer, but non-cancer patients make up a much higher proportion than in the UK. The National Hospice Organisation fact sheet for spring 1999 stated that in 1995 (according to the NHS 1995 Census), 60% of hospice patients had cancer, 6% heart-related diagnoses, 4% had AIDS, 1% renal (kidney) diagnoses, 2% Alzheimer's, and 27% 'other' diagnoses. Some of the reasons why hospice care for non-cancer patients is more common in the US than the UK are explored in Chapter 15. In both care settings, as elsewhere in the world, meeting the palliative care needs of non-cancer patients presents a number of difficult and largely unresolved challenges. These are discussed in detail elsewhere in this book, but include difficulties caused by prognostic uncertainties, funding issues, boundary disputes between professionals and between services, and a lack of relevant expertise (Addington-Hall 1998). Underlying many of these problems is the lack of scientific, empirical evidence on the needs of non-cancer patients, on the best ways of meeting these needs, and on the effectiveness and acceptability of services.

In an era of increasing emphasis on evidence based health care, the lack of evidence in this area is striking. Two of the main purposes of this book are, therefore, to bring together the available evidence and to highlight priorities for research. In the first section of the book (Chapters 1–11) authors were specifically asked to make their contribution research based, and to ensure that their conclusions were based on evidence. These chapters each address a specific disease or patient group. The authors were asked to consider which patients are likely to benefit from palliative care, the numbers of patients likely to be affected, the problems they have, and the effectiveness of interventions or services. They also suggest priorities for future research and discuss the implications of their findings for clinical management. We are grateful for the diligence with which these authors sought to be research based, even when the lack of evidence made this extremely difficult. In the second section of the book, the challenges of providing palliative care for non-cancer patients in four care settings are discussed: in nursing homes (Chapter 12), acute hospitals (Chapter 13), community and primary care (Chapter 14), and in hospices and specialist palliative care services (Chapter 15). Again, the authors were asked to ensure their work was evidence based wherever possible.

The final section of the book brings together a variety of perspectives on future issues in the development of palliative care for non-cancer patients. These include the views of a potential service user (Chapter 16), a commissioner of health services (Chapter 18), and two ethicists (Chapter 20). The needs of informal carers are considered (Chapter 19), as are cultural issues (Chapter 21). Lessons learnt from efforts in the US to improve rapidly care at the end of life in a variety of care settings are discussed in Chapter 17. The clinical implications of the material presented in the book are discussed in Chapter 22. In the final chapter of the book (Chapter 23) we reflect on the future of palliative care provision for non-cancer patients, in the light of the varied, challenging and influential views expressed in the book.

Our original aims in editing this book were to summarise current knowledge of the needs of and appropriate service provision for people dying from causes other than cancer, to debate some of the important issues identified from research and by those with expertise in this field, to highlight areas for future developments, and to help set the research agenda for the coming decade. We hope we have succeeded. If we have, this will be due primarily to the individual contributors who worked so hard at identifying the limited evidence in this area, and who have thought so carefully about the issues raised. We are enormously indebted to them.

References

Addington-Hall, J.M. (1998). *Reaching Out: Specialist Palliative Care for Adults with Non-malignant Disease*. London: National Council for Hospices and Specialist Palliative Care Services.

Addington-Hall, J.M., Fakhoury, W., and McCarthy, M. (1998). Specialist palliative care in non-malignant disease. *Palliative Medicine* 12: 417–27.

Addington-Hall, J.M., Lay, M., Altmann, D., and McCarthy, M. (1995). Symptom control, communication with health professionals, and hospital care of stroke patients in the last year of life as reported by surviving family, friends and officials. Stroke 26: 2242–8.

Addington-Hall, J.M. and McCarthy, M. (1995). The Regional study of care for the dying: methods and sample characteristics. *Palliative Medicine* 9: 27–35.

Bosanquet, N. and Salisbury, C. (1999). *Providing a Palliative Care Service: Towards an Evidence-base*. Oxford: Oxford University Press.

Byock, I. (1998). Hospice and palliative care: a parting of the ways or a path to the future? *Journal of Palliative Medicine* 1: 165–76.

Clark, D. (1999). 'Total pain', disciplinary power and the body in the work of Cicely Saunders, 1958–1967. *Social Science and Medicine* 49: 727–36.

Clinch, J., Dudgeon, D., and Schipper, H. (1998). Quality of life assessment in palliative care. In Doyle, D., Hanks, G., and MacDonald, N. (eds), *Oxford Textbook of Palliative Medicine* (2nd edn). Oxford: Oxford University Press.

Department of Health (2000). *National Service Framework For Coronary Heart Disease*. London: Department of Health.

Ernst, E. (2000). Prevalence of use of complementary/alternative medicine: a systematic review. *Bulletin of the World Health Organization*. 78: 252–7.

Eve, A., Smith, A.M., Tebbit, P. (1997). Hospice and palliative care in the UK 1994–5, including a summary of trends 1990–5. *Palliative Medicine* 11: 31–43.

Field, D. and Addington-Hall, J.M. (1999). Extending specialist palliative care to all? *Social Science and Medicine* 48: 1271–80.

Higginson, I.J. (1997). *Health Care Needs Assessment: Palliative and Terminal Care*. (Series editors: Stevens, A. and Raftery, J.) Health Care Needs Assessment, 2nd Series. Oxford: Radcliffe Medical Press.

Hospice Information Service (1998). *Directory 1998: Hospice and Palliative Care Services in the UK and Republic of Ireland*. London: Hospice Information Service at St Christopher's.

Hospice Information Service (2000). Palliative care facts and figures. http:/www.hospiceinformation.co.uk

Hughes, H.L.G. (1960). *Peace at the Last*. London: Gulbenkian Foundation.

McCarthy, M., Lay, M., and Addington-Hall, J.M. (1996). Dying from heart disease. *Journal of the Royal College of Physicians of London* 30: 325–8.

Marie Curie Memorial Foundation. (1952). *Report on a National Survey Concerning Patients Nursed at Home*. London: Marie Curie Memorial Foundation.

NHS Executive. (1996). *A Policy Framework for Commissioning Cancer Services: Palliative Care Services*. EL(96)85: NHS Executive.

National Council of Hospices and Specialist Palliative Care Services. (1995). *Specialist Palliative Care: A Statement of Definitions*. Occasional Paper 8. London: NCHSPCS.

Saunders, C. (1998). Foreword. In Doyle, D., Hanks, G., and MacDonald, N. (eds), *Oxford Textbook of Palliative Medicine* (2nd edn). Oxford: Oxford University Press.

Saunders, C. and Baines, M. (1983). *Living with Dying: The Management of Terminal Disease.* Oxford: Oxford University Press.

Scottish Office. *Contracting for specialist palliative care.* MEL(1994)104: Scottish Office.

Standing Medical Advisory Committee, Standing Nursing and Midwifery Advisory Committee (1992). *The Principles and Provision of Palliative Care.* London.

Chapter 1

Stroke

Angie Rogers

Introduction

Despite high levels of mortality (Ebrahim 1990) and morbidity the palliative care needs of people following a stroke remain under-researched. This contrasts with the substantial research base on the prevention and treatment of cerebrovascular disease, and on the rehabilitation of people following a stroke.

There have been recent signs that the palliative care needs of stroke patients are being brought to the research agenda. For example an editorial in 'Stroke Matters' (the newsletter of the Stroke Association, the major UK stroke charity) highlighted the need for more research (Jarrett 1997). The Stroke Association has funded a two-year qualitative study in this area (Rogers *et al.* 1998). The British Medical Association's recent publication on withdrawing and withholding treatment highlights the need for greater clarification of best practice in cases of severe stroke (BMA 1999).

This chapter indicates the likely number of people with stroke for whom palliative care is considered to be appropriate. It then considers the needs of two distinct groups: those whose strokes leave them heavily dependent and usually unconscious, whose prognosis is very poor and who are unlikely to leave the hospital setting ('poor prognosis stroke'); and a less severely afflicted group whose strokes reduce their previous physical, psychological and social functioning. Those in the second group are likely to remain dependent on others for most of their daily living activities and have higher mortality rates than their non-stroke counterparts, but are usually able to leave hospital. I will conclude with some suggestions for future research.

The only published study that has looked specifically at the needs of people dying from stroke is the 'Regional study of care for the dying' (RSCD) (Addington-Hall and McCarthy, 1995; Addington-Hall *et al.* 1995; Addington-Hall *et al.* 1998). This study sought the views of bereaved relatives and others on the quality of care received by people dying from all causes in their last year of life. It included information on 237 people who had died following a stroke. Because of its unique position in the literature, this chapter draws on the RSCD as well as the research literature on specific *sequelae* of stroke.

The extent of the problem

Reports of the number of people suffering a stroke and case fatality rates vary significantly because of difficulties with recording (Ebrahim 1990). However, it is estimated that a typical health authority in England of 250 000 people may expect 500 new strokes and 1000 recurrent strokes each year. At any one time there may be 1500 survivors of stroke living in the community, half of whom will have significant disability: 12% of stroke survivors will be admitted to institutional care within a year (Effective Health Care Bulletin 1992). Best estimates suggest that 20% of people suffering a stroke will die within one month, 10% throughout the following year and a further 5% in the subsequent year (Ebrahim 1990). Therefore, in a typical health authority, of the 1500 people suffering a stroke in any one year, 300 would die within one month of their stroke, 150 during the following year and a further 75 patients in the subsequent year.

Recently, the number of people who die following a stroke appears to be declining (Maheswaran et al. 1997; Ebrahim 1997; Shahar et al. 1995). Shahar et al. (1995), in their longitudinal study of deaths from acute cerebrovascular disease in the US, found improved 28-day and two-year survival between 1980 and 1990. Better treatment and rehabilitation may account for much of this change, but also the natural history of stroke may be changing. However, this study failed to show any improvement in the fatality rate for patients who were comatosed on admission to hospital (Shahar et al. 1995). A longitudinal study of deaths from stroke in the over-65s between 1967 and 1985 found decreased death rate and decline into coma at one month and increased median survival, but no significant change in the incidence of stroke over this period (Barker and Mullooly 1997). Nevertheless, much of the research suggests people who have suffered from stroke are at an increased risk of morbidity from other causes and mortality than those of the same age who have not suffered from stroke. A recent study showed that even minor strokes carry an increased risk of ten-year mortality and major stroke recurrence (Prencipe et al. 1998).

There are several predictors of early mortality following stroke, some of which have been known for over a hundred years (Ebrahim 1990). A meta-analysis of 78 research articles on the prognosis of stroke patients found that only 13 satisfied the pre-defined inclusion criteria. Age, previous stroke, urinary continence, consciousness at onset, disorientation in time and place, admission activities of daily living score, level of social support and metabolic rate of glucose outside the infarct area in hypertensive patients were all valid predictors for functional recovery after stroke (Kwakkel et al. 1996). Many of these factors, for example unconsciousness and dense hemiplegia or incontinence, are interdependent and are, by themselves, good indicators of death. Severe strokes appear to be more common in older age groups. Further, significant co-morbidity is likely to be present among older people, particularly pre-stroke incontinence and dependency.

While it is difficult to get good estimates on the numbers of people with stroke for whom palliative care may be appropriate not least because of the lack of clarity about the role of palliative care in stroke, it can be concluded that approximately a third of people having a stroke will have died within two years. Information from studies of prognostic indicators suggest people living with stroke but with poor prospects of functional recovery will have medical, health-related and social needs (Kwakkel et al. 1996).

What are the problems likely to be?

For those patients with poor prognosis stroke who are unlikely to regain consciousness, aspects of palliative care expertise can usefully make a contribution. These include communication, feeding, terminal care and bereavement support. Stroke survivors, living in the community but functionally dependent on others, are likely to be concerned with coping with on-going uncertainty and disability, incontinence, post-stroke pain and depression. Their informal carers may need respite care. However, there is overlap between the two groups: although some issues may be highlighted for one group this does not imply similar problems or issues are not important to the other group of patients.

Communication

The literature suggests that, at least in terms of functional recovery, stroke patients and their families are eager for information on their likely prognosis but that health professionals tend to avoid this subject (Hoffman 1974; Becker and Kaufman 1995). The RSCD found that that two-fifths of stroke patients were thought to have definitely or probably known that they were dying and that stroke patients and their families would have liked improved communication in all care settings (Addington-Hall *et al.* 1995). This suggests that a significant minority of stroke patients would benefit from more open discussion of their prognosis. Communication is also crucial in symptom control, both in assessing severity and in gaining compliance with treatment. In poor prognosis stroke, an open dialogue between health care workers and the patient's relatives is essential in establishing the patient's previous abilities or quality of life, which is likely to be key in any decision regarding the withdrawal or withholding of treatment (BMA 1999).

One of the consequences of stroke is aphasia, which affects a patient's ability to comprehend language and to express themselves. This is an area which seems to have been particularly under-researched. Prolonged aphasia and dysphasia (difficulty speaking, but with full comprehension) are associated with poor prognosis, and communication with patients and those close to them is likely to be time-consuming and often problematic.

Feeding

Dysphagia (the inability to swallow) is common after hemispheric stroke, and is in itself a predictor of poor outcome and mortality following stroke (Gordon *et al.* 1987). Research has found that 30% of conscious patients have an impaired swallow on the day following their stroke, 16% of survivors at one week and 2% at one month (Barer 1989).

Studies that have assessed nutritional status after stroke report malnutrition in 8–40% of stroke patients (Dennis 1998). The physical consequences of stroke may result in these patients eating slowly due to facial weakness, poor arm function and general fatigue. Poor nutrition has been linked to reduced muscle strength, resistance to infection and impaired wound healing in older people (Fiatarone and Evans 1993); among stroke patients muscle weakness, infections and pressure sores have all been found to account for a significant proportion of mortality and morbidity (Davenport *et al.* 1996).

Patients with persistent dysphagia may receive enteral tube feeding through a naso-gastric tube (NG). This can be uncomfortable and often dislodges. Alternatively they may be given a percutaneous gastrostomy (PG), a tube that is surgically inserted directly into the stomach. This is thought to be better tolerated (Wollman *et al.* 1995). There is conflicting evidence about the risks associated with and the outcomes of both NG and PG feeding (Norton *et al.* 1996). A random controlled trial of PG and NG feeding found greater mortality and decreased nutritional intake among NG-fed patients (Norton *et al.* 1996). However a review of 37 patients who had a PG tube inserted post-stroke found that only 12 patients survived for 3 months; median survival was 53 days. Taking these facts together, it is likely that patients with persistent dysphagia who require enteral feeding have a relatively short prognosis; they and their relatives would benefit from open communication on this issue.

The question of whether to feed poor prognosis stroke patients can be a crucial issue and one which families and friends are likely to have strong feelings about (BMA 1999). Poor nutritional status has been linked to the development of pressure area sores (Finucane 1995) and resultant muscular weakness may inhibit rehabilitation (Wanklyn et al. 1995). Decisions not to feed might better be based on the notion of 'why not feed' rather than 'why feed'. Again, making decisions about whether or not to feed this group of patients requires open and honest communication with families. Palliative care as a specialty has a particular interest and familiarity with difficult end-of-life decisions: the input of palliative care specialists may therefore be appropriate, particularly if there are disagreements within the medical team or between health professionals and patients or their representatives.

Incontinence

There is a high level of incontinence among stroke survivors, which has been associated with mortality, morbidity and discharge destination (Nakayamah et al. 1997; Ween et al. 1996). Meta-analysis of studies of urinary incontinence among stroke patients found that 32–79% of patients had been incontinent on admission, 25–8% on discharge and 12–19% suffered episodes of incontinence some months after discharge. Fecal incontinence was found in 31–40% of patients on admission, 18% on discharge and 7–9% six months after discharge. Incontinence may not be related to the stroke itself; it may be a functional consequence of reduced ability to express oneself and reduced mobility (Borrie et al. 1986). It is also believed that incontinence may have a role in reducing morale and thus adversely influencing the achievement of optimum recovery (Reddy and Reddy 1997).

In poor prognosis stroke urinary incontinence is managed with a catheter, which carries a risk of infection. Poor management of fecal incontinence may compromise the patient's skin and result in increased pain, discomfort and distress. Fecal incontinence is a very distressing symptom for both patients and their informal carers (Addington-Hall et al. 1995). Constipation, a common symptom following stroke of all kinds, requires regular monitoring and appropriate medical treatment.

Pain

Stroke patients may suffer pain from a variety of sources. It may be stroke specific, the result of hemiplegia or contracture, or stem from on-going chronic conditions such as arthritis. Up to 72% of stroke patients have been found to suffer from 'shoulder-hand syndrome' (Bohannon et al. 1986), in which the patient's affected upper limb becomes stiff due to reduction in movement and, as a result, their hand becomes swollen, blue, hot and clammy (Atkins and Duthie 1987). Approximately 18–32% suffer from post-stroke headaches (Ferro et al. 1995). Additionally 8% of patients suffer from 'central post-stroke pain' (Anderson et al. 1995)—a neuropathic pain syndrome, which is thought to arise from the vascular lesion and is characterised by pain in the corresponding body part (Vestergaard 1995). This pain is thought to be partially resistant to opioids (Bainton et al. 1992) and remains difficult to treat (Jensen and Lenz 1995). The expertise of specialist palliative care in pain management may be relevant here.

There is some evidence to suggest that stroke patients with aphasia receive less medication for pain than those without aphasia. This is thought to relate to aphasic patients' inability to express their need for medication that is prescribed 'to be given when required' (Kehayia *et al.* 1997). This indicates a need for better pain control in this particular group of patients, and hence the importance of analgesia being taken regularly rather than 'as required'. Patients who have been taking regular medication for pain prior to their stroke will need to be assessed and assisted in continuing these therapies.

Depression and anxiety

Post-stroke depression is described as a common problem, thought to occur in 25–30% of stroke patients (Tiller 1992). The exact nature and cause of such depression remains controversial. A follow-up study of 123 stroke survivors in south east England found that 29% were severely or moderately disabled and 36% were depressed or had borderline depression nearly five years post-stroke (Wilkinson *et al.* 1997). The RSCD found that people dying following a stroke both in hospital and in the community were reported to have needed increased psychosocial support and that those who cared in the community for depressed and anxious relatives would have liked more help and support (Addington-Hall *et al.* 1995). Gainottie *et al.* (1997) found that stroke patients' depressive symptoms were primarily a reaction to the 'devastating consequences of stroke' rather than a consequence of their strokes *per se*. Depression in stroke patients can be treated with anti-depressant medication. Post-stroke depression is a common problem, with both organic and psychological causes, and may be relieved with appropriate psychological or medical therapies.

Informal carers

Most informal care of people following a stroke is provided by spouses (Grevson *et al.* 1991). There have been various studies seeking to address the extent of the 'burden' of care on this group. The level of care needed is predicted usually by the severity of stroke and the patient's ability to undertake activities of daily living. However the 'burden' experienced by informal carers is also associated with the carer's personal characteristics rather than the level of care required (Schotte *et al.* 1998). Ill health and an overall decrease in the quality of lives of informal carers has been reported (Anderson *et al.* 1995). Stroke survivors living in the community are under-served by both the health and social services and have un-met personal and psychosocial needs, and both of these factors increase the load on informal carers (Wilkinson *et al* 1997; Addington-Hall *et al.* 1995)

In the case of poor prognosis stroke, the needs of informal carers are more likely to be associated with coping in a situation where a loved one's death is imminent. In many cases relatives will have been involved in decision-making regarding the withdrawal or withholding of treatment, which may add considerably to their distress and anxiety. Such family members may need help in coming to terms with this situation and, following the death of their loved one, may benefit from some form of bereavement support. The needs of families of these stroke patients, both at the time end-of-life decisions are made and in bereavement, have been largely neglected to date.

Care in the last days of life

People suffering a poor prognosis stroke must be well managed to ensure their comfort through the last days of life. Good supportive nursing care should include mouth care to prevent the build up of oral candida, a system of turning the patient to avoid sores developing in pressure areas, and the management of feeding, incontinence, constipation and pain. Dysphagic patients are particularly prone to chest secretions, which can be distressing for both patient and family; this difficulty can be managed with appropriate suction and medication. Guidelines relevant to these patients are available in *Changing Gear—Guidelines for Managing the Last Days of Life in Adults*. Their adoption may help to improve care (Working Party on Clinical Guidelines in Palliative Care 1997).

Future research

Natural history of stroke leading to death

As this chapter has shown there are several prognostic indicators of early mortality following stroke. However there is little systematic information on the experiences of people who have suffered a poor prognosis stroke and on those of their families, or of those who are at increased risk of death and are now living in the community. There is a need for more information on the physical and psychological consequences of severe stroke, and development of appropriate interventions for patients and their families.

Feeding

An international trial of different feeding policies for stroke patients is in progress. Results from this trial will not be available until 2003 (International Stroke Trials Collaboration. Food Trial—*http://www.dcn.ed.ac.uk/food*). Information from this trial will provide up-to-date information on the consequences of feeding stroke patients in terms of recovery. There is, however, a need for more information on the effects of both feeding and hydration among poor prognosis severe stroke patients, including the effect on the mode and 'quality' of dying. There is no objective information on the consequences of decisions to commence or withhold feeding in this group. While the practical and ethical problems in conducting a randomised control trial in this area are likely to be prohibitive, a research strategy should be developed to assess the financial, social and ethical costs of such feeding.

Symptom management

Patients suffering a stroke have a complex combination of symptoms that all require management. Effective management needs to be determined—particularly for pain, dysphasia, incontinence and depression.

Communication in decision-making

Future research should investigate not only the ways in which clinicians elicit concerns, communicate with and make decisions about the care of stroke patients but also how patients and carers are involved in these decisions. End-of-life decision-making will be of direct relevance in poor prognosis stroke but there is a need for more information on how decisions are made concerning arrangements for community based care for people following a severe stroke.

Carers and bereavement

Future research should address the needs of informal carers in poor prognosis stroke, as they may have been directly involved in both the care of the patient and in decisions about withdrawing or withholding treatment, acting as the patient's proxy. There is a need for more information on the bereavement consequences for these relatives.

Finally, whether specialist palliative care has a role in the care of stroke patients and, if so, what this should be, needs to be investigated further. As this chapter indicates, stroke patients raise difficult end-of-life decisions, have symptom control and communication needs, and, together with their families, have un-met psychosocial needs for help in adjusting to disability and death. These are areas in which specialist palliative care has expertise: the challenge is to establish how best to enable stroke experts and specialists in palliative care to work together to improve the care of these patients.

References

Addington-Hall, J.M. and McCarthy, M. (1995) The Regional Study of Care for the Dying: Methods and Sample characteristics. *Palliative Medicine* 9 (12): 27–35.

Addington-Hall, J.M., Lay, M., Altmann, D., and McCarthy, M. (1995b). Symptom control, and communication with health professionals, and hospital care of stroke patients in the last year of life as reported by surviving family, friends, and officials. *Stroke* 26 (12): 2242–8.

Addington-Hall, J.M., Lay, M., Altmann, D., and McCarthy, M. (1998). Community care for stroke patients in the last year of life: results of a national retrospective survey of surviving family, friends and officials. *Health and Social Care in the Community* 6,112–19.

Anderson, G., Vestergaard, K., Ingeman-Nielsen, M., and Jensen, T.S. (1995). Incidence of post-stroke pain. *Pain* 61,187–93.

Anderson, G.S., Linto, J., and Stuart-Wynne, E.G. (1995). A population-based assessment of the impact and burden of care giving for long term stroke survivors. *Stroke* 26: 843–9.

Atkins, R.M. and Duthie, R.B. (1987). Algodystrophy (reflex sympathetic dystrophy or Sudeck's atrophy). In Weatherall, D.J., Ledingham, J.G.G., and Warrell, D.A. (eds), *Oxford Textbook of Medicine* (2nd edn). Oxford: Oxford University Press.

Bainton, T., Fox, M., Bowsher, D., and Wells, C. (1992). A double-blind trial of naloxone in central post-stroke pain. *Pain* 48: 159–62.

Barer, D.H. (1989). The natural history and functional consequences of dysphagia after hemispheric stroke. *Journal of Neurosurgical Psychiatry* 52: 236–41.

Barker, W.H. and Mullooly, J.P. (1997). Stroke in a defined elderly population, 1967–1985—A less lethal and disabling but no less common disease. *Stroke* 28: 284–90.

Becker, G. and Kaufman, S. (1995). Managing an uncertain illness trajectory in old age: patients' and physicians' views of stroke. *Medical Anthropology Quarterly* 9: 13–18.

Borrie, M.J., Campbell, A.J., Caradoe-Davis, T.H., and Spears, G.F.S. (1986). Urinary incontinence after stroke: a prospective study. *Age and Ageing* 15: 177–81.

Bohannon, R.W., Larkin, P.A., and Smith, M.B. (1986). Shoulder pain in hemiplegia; statistical relationship to five variables. *Archives of Physical Medical Rehabilitation* 67: 514–16.

British Medical Association Discussion Document. (1999). *Withholding and Withdrawing Life-prolonging Medical Treatment: Guidance for Decision Making.* London: BMJ Books.

Davenport, R.J., Dennis, M.S., Wellwood, I., and Warlow, C.P. (1996). Complications after acute stroke. *Stroke* 27: 519–24.

Dennis, M. (1998). Nutrition after stroke. *Stroke Review* 2: 6–10.

Ebrahim, S. (1990). *Clinical Epidemiology of Stroke*. Oxford: Oxford University Press.

Ebrahim, S. (1997). Stroke mortality—secular and geographic trends: comment on papers by Maheswaran and colleagues. *Journal of Epidemiology and Community Health* **51**: 132–3.

Effective Health Care Bulletin (1992). *Stroke Rehabilitation*. Leeds: University of Leeds.

Ferro, J.M., Lelo, T.P., Oliveira, V., Salgalo, A.V., Crespo, M., Canhac, P., and Pinto, A.N. (1995). A multivariate analysis of headache associated with ischemic stroke. *Headache* **35**: 315–19.

Fiatarone, M.A. and Evans, L.J. (1993). The etiology and reversibility of muscle dysfunction in the aged. *Journal of Gerontology* **48**: 77–83.

Finucane, T.E. (1995). Malnutrition, tube feeding and pressure sores: data are incomplete. *Journal of American Geriatric Society* **43** (4): 447–51.

Gainottie, G., Azzoni, A., Razzano, C., Lanzillotta, M., Marra, C., and Gasparini, F. (1997). The post-stroke depression rating scale: A test specifically devised to investigate the affective disorders of stroke patients. *Journal of Clinical and Experimental Neuropsychology* **19**: 340–56.

Gordon, C., Laughton Hewer, R., and Wade, D.T. (1987). Dysphagia in acute stroke. *British Medical Journal* **295**: 411–14.

Greveson, G.C., Gray, C.S., Fench, J.M., and James, C.F.W. (1991). Long-term outcome for patients and carers following hospital admission for stroke. *Age and Ageing* **29**: 337–44.

Hoffman, J.E. (1974). 'Nothing can be done'- social dimensions of the treatment of stroke patients in the general hospital. *Urban Life and Culture* **3**: 50–70.

Jarrett, D. (1997). Palliative care and stroke. *Stroke Matters* **1**: 4.

Jensen, T.S. and Lenz, F.A. (1995). Central post-stroke pain: a challenge for the scientist and the clinician. *Pain* **61**: 161–4.

Kehayia, E., Korner-Bitensky, N., Singer, F., Becker, R., Lamarche, M., Georges, P., and Retik, S. (1997). Differences in pain medication use in stroke patients with aphasia and without aphasia. *Stroke* **28**: 1867–70.

Kwakkel, G., Wagenaar, R.C., Kollen, B.J., and Lankhorst, G.J. (1996). Predicting disability in stroke— A critical review of the literature. *Age and Ageing* **25**: 479–89.

Maheswaran, R., Strachan, D., Elliott, P., and Shipley, M. (1997). Trends in stroke mortality in Greater London and south east England—evidence for a cohort effect? *Journal of Epidemiology and Community Health* **51**: 121–6.

Nakayama, H., Jorgensen, H.S., Pedersen, P.M., Raaschon, H.O., and Olsen, T.S. (1997). Prevalence and risk factors of incontinence after stroke: the Copenhagen Stroke Study. *Stroke* **28**: 58–62.

Norton, B., McLean, K.A., and Holmes, G.K. (1996). Outcome in patients who require a gastrostomy after stroke. *Age and Ageing* **25** (6): 493.

Prencipe, M., Culasso, F., Rasura, M., Anzini, A., Beccia, M., Cao, M., Giubilei, F., and Fieschi, C. (1998). Long term prognosis after a minor stroke—10-year mortality and major stroke recurrence rates in a hospital-based cohort. *Stroke* **29**: 126–32.

Reddy, M.P. and Reddy, V. (1997). After a stroke: strategies to restore function and prevent complications. *Geriatrics* **52** (9): 59–62.

Rogers, A., Addington-Hall, J.M., and Pound, P. (1998) Annual Palliative Care Congress. Palliative Care Research Forum (September 1998) Abstracts. Leeds: University of Leeds.

Schotte, W.J.M., de Hain, R.J., Rijinders, P.T., Limburg M., and Van der Bos, G.A.M. (1998). Burden of care after stroke. *Stroke* **29**: 1605–11.

Shahar, E., McGovern, P.G., Sprafka, J.M., Pankpow, J.S., Doliszny, K.M., Luepker, R.V., and Blackburn, H. (1995). Improved survival of stroke patients during the 1908s—the Minnesota stroke survey. *Stroke* **26**: 1–6.

Tiller, J.W.G. (1992). Post-stroke depression. *Psychopharmacology* **106**: 5130–3.

Vestergaard, K., Nielsen, J., Andersen, G., Arendt-Nielsen, L. and Jensen, T.S. (1995). Sensory abnormalities in consecutive unselected patients with central post-stroke pain. *Pain* **61** (2): 177–86.

Wanklyn, P., Cox, N., and Belfield, P. (1995). Outcome in patients who require a gastrostomy after stroke. *Age and Ageing* **24**: 510–14.

Ween, J.A., Alexander, M.P., D'Esposita, M., and Roberts, S. (1996). Incontinence after stroke in a rehabilitation setting: outcomes, associations and predictive factors. *Neurology* **47**: 659–63.

Wilkinson, P.R., Wolfe, C.D.A., Warburton, F.G., Rudd, A.G., Howard, R.S., Ross-Russell, R.W., and Beech, R.R. (1997). A long-term follow-up of stroke patients. *Stroke* **28**: 507–12.

Wollman, B., D'Agostino, H.B., Walus-Wigle, J.R., Easter, D.W., and Beale, A. (1995). Radiologic, endoscopic and surgical gastrostomy: an institutional evaluation and a meta-analysis of the literature. *Radiology* **197**: 699–704.

Working Party on Clinical Guidelines in Palliative Care (1997). *Changing Gear—Guidelines for Managing the Last Days of Life in Adults.* London: The National Council for Hospice and Palliative Care Services.

Chapter 2

Respiratory disease

Charles Shee

Introduction

Prognosis in severe chronic obstructive pulmonary disease (COPD) is poor. This chapter is concerned predominantly with the respiratory and non-respiratory complications of COPD. The effectiveness of interventions such as oxygen therapy, drug treatment of breathlessness and 'pulmonary rehabilitation' is reviewed. It is suggested that the un-met needs of people with COPD are becoming more apparent and that emphasis needs to shift from management of acute exacerbations towards a more palliative approach to care, focusing on the health and social care interface.

Patients likely to benefit from palliative care

Chronic obstructive pulmonary disease

This chapter concentrates primarily on palliative care in chronic obstructive pulmonary disease, as this is by far the most common non-malignant chronic lung disorder. COPD is a general term which covers many previously used clinical labels such as chronic bronchitis, emphysema and chronic airflow limitation. Palliative care is concerned with the treatment of patients with disease that is active, progressive, far advanced and with a limited prognosis. Patients with COPD and severe hypoxia (lack of oxygen) fall into this category in that the majority will be dead within three years if not given long-term oxygen (Report of the Medical Research Council Oxygen Working Party 1981). Numerically asthma is one of the most important respiratory disorders affecting up to 4% of the population at some time, but the issue of palliative care only arises in the very small number of people with chronic severe asthma, within the COPD label. Similarly, only a minority of people with bronchiectasis develop end-stage lung disease.

Cystic fibrosis

Survival in cystic fibrosis has improved progressively over the last 20 years and the median survival in developed countries approaches 30 years. For those with end-stage lung disease, transplantation is the only hope, but as there is a severe shortage of donor organs 'heroic measures to prolong life are no more appropriate for the terminally ill patient with cystic fibrosis than they were ten years ago' (Smyth *et al.* 1991).

Other diseases

Some patients with severe fibrotic lung disease (e.g. due to fibrosing alveolitis or sarcoidosis) may enter a phase where active treatment is no longer successful and where palliative treatment for breathlessness and other symptoms is required. Respiratory failure can also occur with respiratory muscle disorders (e.g. muscular dystrophy or old poliomyelitis) or with severe chest wall disease (e.g. scoliosis). Various positive and negative pressure devices are available for domiciliary respiratory support which can improve quality of life and reduce mortality (Simonds 1994; Shneerson 1997). In view of the major symptomatic improvement that can occur in some of these patients following ventilatory support, it is always worth considering referral to an interested specialist.

Numbers of patients likely to benefit

COPD causes substantial morbidity. In the UK chronic respiratory disease causes 13% of adult disability and COPD is the commonest of these respiratory causes (Royal College of Physicians 1986). In a survey of all medical admissions in a UK health region, a quarter of admissions were due to respiratory diseases and over half of these were COPD (Pearson et al. 1994). The annual health service workload for COPD greatly exceeds that for asthma, and in older patients general practice consultation rates are two to four times the equivalent rates for angina (BTS 1997). Cystic fibrosis affects about 1 in 2500 children, but many will now survive into their fourth decade. Fibrosing alveolitis is rare. It is predominantly a disease of older patients, and in a recent survey there was a 45% mortality for patients over a two- to four-year period (Johnston et al. 1997). Sarcoidosis is more common than fibrosing alveolitis. Most patients will have a complete remission, and very few will die of their disease due to respiratory failure. Patients with chronic respiratory failure due to neuromuscular disease or chest wall deformity are uncommon, and tend to be under the care of specialist centres.

As a cause of mortality COPD dwarfs the other chronic respiratory conditions. It predominantly affects the older population and mortality figures for England and Wales show approximately 250–300 deaths per 100 000 persons aged 65–84 years per annum (Rijcken and Britton 1998). For comparison with the 26 000 deaths per year in England and Wales attributed to COPD, there are thought to be only about 800 deaths per year for the whole UK from fibrosing alveolitis.

Problems associated with severe respiratory disease

The main problems associated with severe respiratory disease are breathlessness (or difficulty in breathing), hypoxia, immobility and psychosocial problems (including depression). Breathlessness is a frightening symptom and, in order to avoid it, many patients practise exercise avoidance with subsequent deconditioning. Because mental factors can influence breathlessness and exercise capacity, it is not surprising that in severe lung disease there is a poor relationship between lung function, breathlessness and exercise capacity (Morgan et al. 1983).

COPD is often associated with social isolation and economic disadvantage, and depression is much more common than might be expected (Dudley et al. 1980; Heaton et al. 1983; Morgan et al. 1983). Fear and uncertainty over prognosis may contribute to the psychiatric morbidity. Unlike patients with lung cancer, patients with COPD may go from one crisis to another over some years before a fairly rapid final event. In one study patients with end-stage COPD were more likely to suffer from clinical depression and/or anxiety than terminal lung cancer patients, but did not receive specific treatment for emotional problems and, in contrast to the cancer patients, were not targeted for formal palliative care (Gore *et al.* 1997).

People with COPD can also suffer from cough, malnutrition, hypoxia and sleep disturbance (including sometimes obstructive sleep apnoea). Non-respiratory symptoms such as pain, fatigue and thirst are also common (Skilbeck *et al.* 1998). Looking after a respiratory invalid can be both distressing and a burden for family or carers. Great insight into the problems and uncertainties associated with chronic respiratory disease is revealed in the book *Chronic Respiratory Illness* (Williams 1993) which emphasises the impact on social life and family relationships.

Effectiveness of interventions

Only stopping smoking and long-term oxygen therapy have been shown to improve survival in COPD and thus most other interventions are effectively 'palliative'. Smoking cessation is advisable at all stages of the disease and, although it will not restore loss of lung function, it can prevent the accelerated decline seen in many patients. Participation in an active smoking cessation programme leads to a higher sustained quit rate, especially when nicotine replacement therapy is included (Raw *et al.* 1998).

Long-term oxygen therapy

Long-term oxygen therapy (LTOT) improves survival in advanced hypoxic COPD. In a British randomised controlled study oxygen was given via nasal cannulae at a flow rate of 2 litres/min for at least 15 hours daily. At three years, the mortality was 45% in the treated group and 67% in the controls (Report of the Medical Research Council Oxygen Working Party 1981). Quality of life was not assessed. In a major American trial, patients were randomised to continuous oxygen (in practice, for 18 hours daily) or 12 hours nocturnal treatment. At two years, the mortality was 22% in the group given 'continuous' oxygen and 41% in patients receiving nocturnal treatment (Nocturnal Oxygen Therapy Trial Group 1980). Despite mild neuropsychological improvement, patients reported little change in emotional status or life quality (Heaton *et al.* 1983).

LTOT must be given for at least 15 hours daily to achieve benefit, and is best provided by an oxygen concentrator and nasal prongs. The concentrator should be set at a flow of 2–4 litres/min depending on the blood gas assessments (Walters *et al.* 1993; BTS 1997). Patients with COPD who have a PaO_2 of less than 7.3 kPa should be considered for LTOT. There is no evidence of benefit for people with mild hypoxia (Gorecka *et al.*1997). In the UK, LTOT can also be prescribed for relief of hypoxia in patients with interstitial lung disease and other causes, but this palliative benefit has rarely been studied.

It might seem logical to use ambulatory oxygen to reduce effort-induced breathlessness and to extend walking distance, however double-blind studies suggest that only a minority of patients derive clear benefit (Walters *et al.* 1993). Portable cylinders are the only form of ambulatory oxygen therapy available in the UK and provide two hours of use at 2 litres/min. Many patients use intermittent oxygen at home for alleviation of breathlessness, but it is not always certain that it is the oxygen *per se* that helps, and there are no data to support or refute this practice.

Bronchodilators

Bronchodilators are the cornerstone of symptomatic treatment for the reversible component of airways obstruction. Inhaled agents are as efficacious as oral preparations, have fewer side effects and are therefore preferred. Short-acting beta-2 receptor agonists or inhaled anticholinergics are used as required depending upon symptomatic response. Inhaler technique should be optimised and an appropriate device selected to ensure efficient delivery. The results of clinical tests comparing metered dose inhalers and nebulisers in stable patients with COPD are inconsistent. Theophyllines are of limited value in the routine management of COPD.

Corticosteroids

It is difficult to predict the minority of patients with COPD who will respond to corticosteroids (Stokes *et al.* 1982) and so most chest physicians suggest a 'steroid trial' (e.g. oral Prednisolone 30 mg daily for two weeks). If benefit is shown (e.g. more than 20% increase over pre-treatment spirometry results), inhaled steroids are normally substituted. Two large controlled studies reporting on whether inhaled steroids slow progression of COPD are due to be published shortly. Preliminary reports suggest that the rate of decline in lung function is not altered but that the number of exacerbations is reduced and quality of life improved in those patients with the most severe lung disease. There is no evidence to support the use of prophylactic antibiotics, mucolytics or respiratory stimulants (BTS 1997).

Other drugs to reduce breathlessness

If bronchodilators fail to relieve breathlessness, are there any drugs that can reduce the sensation of breathlessness? Mitchell-Heggs *et al.* suggested in 1980 that oral diazepam was useful in treating breathlessness in 'pink and puffing' patients with COPD. However, a later study found that diazepam had no effect on breathlessness, and it reduced exercise tolerance (Woodcock *et al.* 1981). Other drugs tried for their effect against breathlessness include promethazine, dihydrocodeine, alcohol, caffeine, carbimazole, indomethacin and local anaesthetics. In general, the therapeutic benefit has been marginal and side effects considerable (Stark 1988).

Nebulised morphine has been used in palliative care with varying degrees of success in treatment of breathlessness in cancer patients. Initial reports suggested nebulised morphine might improve exercise endurance in patients with chronic lung disease (Young *et al.* 1989), but further studies, even using inhaled doses of morphine as high as 40 mg, have not borne this out (Jankelson *et al.* 1997). Oral morphine might have some effect on breathlessness (Light *et al.* 1996), but further evidence is needed. Many chest physicians are reluctant to prescribe opioids routinely for chronic stable breathlessness. This is partly due to a lack of firm evidence of efficacy, and partly due to anxiety over causing respiratory depression and drowsiness. Indeed, some authors suggest that, in many studies where reduction in breathlessness has been shown, it is likely to be due to changes in ventilatory drive and consequent decreased respiratory work rather than a modification in the perceptive process (Burdon *et al.* 1994).

Terminal breathlessness

The principles of the treatment of breathlessness in the dying are similar, whether one is dealing with end-stage lung disease or cancer. Distraction, reassurance, breathing exercises and nebulisers are sometimes useful, but hard evidence to support these actions is lacking. One paper that showed some benefit from morphine on breathlessness in terminal cancer patients actually excluded patients with airways obstruction (Bruera *et al.* 1990). There is little scientific evidence about which drug is best for terminal breathlessness; diazepam, morphine, chlorpromazine and promethazine are all used (Ahmedzai 1998). Anecdote suggests that some patients prefer to take morphine 4-hourly for breathlessness, rather than 12-hourly by sustained release preparation, as would commonly be used for pain control. Lorazepam (0.5–1.0 mg sub-lingually) can help respiratory panic attacks. As death approaches, subcutaneous midazolam or diamorphine are frequently used, where one is prepared to accept a degree of respiratory depression that would be otherwise unacceptable.

Ventilatory support

Respiratory problems can impair the quality of life for patients with neuromuscular and skeletal disorders. Ventilatory support (which is often only required at night) can, however, reduce breathlessness, relieve right heart failure, improve the quality of life, reduce daytime sleepiness and fatigue and abolish early morning headaches (Shneerson 1997). In acute respiratory failure in COPD non-invasive positive pressure ventilation (NIPPV) has been shown in randomised trials to reduce the number of patients requiring endotracheal intubation and the length of stay in hospital (BTS 1997). However, the role of domiciliary ventilatory support in COPD is unclear. Continuous positive airways pressure at night can improve daytime symptoms in patients with obstructive sleep apnoea (Douglas 1998), but whether positive pressure ventilatory support is helpful in severe COPD *in general* needs clarifying.

Surgery

In selected patients, particularly those who are young with alpha-1 antitrypsin deficiency, lung transplantation (usually single lung) may be recommended, but problems with late bronchiolitis obliterans after transplantation remain. Recent reports from the US have described lung volume reduction surgery in which various forms of surgical ablation of severely affected areas of emphysematous lung have been used. Surprising improvements in lung function can be seen, particularly in patients with severe disease and very marked air trapping (Davies and Calverley 1996). Improvement persists for at least one to two years but it seems that by three years lung function is often back to baseline (Roue *et al.* 1996). This 'palliative' major surgery should still be regarded as experimental pending further research.

Pulmonary rehabilitation

Pulmonary rehabilitation (PR) uses a multidisciplinary programme of physiotherapy, education, exercise training and psychotherapy to help the patient return to the highest possible functional capacity. Rehabilitation has now been shown to be effective in prospective randomised clinical studies and in a recent meta-analysis of the literature (Lacasse *et al.* 1996). PR probably does not improve survival. There is usually no change in spirometry values or arterial blood gases (Belman 1993). The evidence is that PR reduces symptoms and the number of hospital admissions and improves performance, exercise endurance and quality of life (Petty 1993; Lacasse *et al.* 1996). Better exercise endurance in the absence of objective cardiopulmonary improvement suggests that a reduction in breathlessness perception is important (Belman 1993). In the UK, facilities for PR are limited but protocols are currently being developed and increasing numbers of hospitals are now making programmes available. There is no evidence that respiratory muscle training has any clinically important benefit in COPD (Goldstein 1993).

Most studies of PR have looked at moderately severe disease. A recent paper has looked at the effect of PR in patients with severe advanced respiratory disease. Wedzicha *et al.* (1998) performed a randomised controlled trial of PR in moderately severe patients (Medical Research Council, MRC, breathlessness score 3/4) and severe patients (MRC 5). The severely dyspnoeic patients were treated at home. Patients with moderate breathlessness, who were regularly mobile outside the home, showed quite large improvements in exercise capacity after physical training, but in the severely disabled group, who were largely housebound owing to breathlessness, there was no improvement following individualised exercise training. Similarly, there was little improvement in 'health status' in the severely dyspnoeic treated group (Wedzicha *et al.* 1998).

Respiratory specialist nurses are increasingly being appointed, but at present there is insufficient knowledge about what kind of nursing care makes a difference to patient outcomes (Heslop 1993). These nurses are usually hospital based but also make community visits. Patients under the care of these nurses may live longer, but, despite the finding that quality of life is not necessarily improved, patients value these visits and want them to continue (Cockcroft *et al.* 1987; Littlejohns *et al.* 1991). Treatments for non-respiratory symptoms are similar to those used in cancer (Ahmedzai 1998). Malnutrition is common in COPD and, although nutritional support seems logical, controlled trials on its effect are not available. In the UK, various sources of financial help are available for patients with COPD (BTS 1997) and the British Lung Foundation has set up a postal club 'Breathe Easy' to help these patients.

Priorities for further research

Smoking cessation

As most COPD is caused by the smoking of tobacco it is largely a preventable disease. Health education may help and research continues into behavioural intervention, nicotine receptor antagonists and pharmacological methods to reduce addictive behaviour (Barnes 1998). Smoking cessation guidelines have recently been produced (Raw *et al.* 1998). The reduction of tobacco consumption is also a political issue and depends on the will of governments to tax tobacco and restrict advertising. It remains important to identify the factors that determine why only 15% of smokers actually develop COPD.

Drug therapies to slow progression of COPD

Studies are in progress to see if inhaled steroids slow progression of COPD, and results should be available soon. Several new drugs are in development that may be useful. These include leukotrione and 5-lipoxygenase inhibitors, new phosphodiesterase inhibitors, new antioxidants and neutrophil elastase and matrix metalloproteinase inhibitors (Barnes 1998).

It will be difficult to demonstrate the efficacy of such treatments as determination of the effect of any drug on the rate of decline in lung function will require large studies over at least two years.

Therapies for breathlessness

Successful drug treatment for breathlessness remains elusive. Nebulised morphine looks less promising than it did a few years ago. It is not clear if the anti-dyspnoeic and sedative actions of drugs can be separated. Some patients do seem to benefit from low dose oral morphine, and further studies are needed to elucidate this, as well as to assess the effect of other drugs such as the newer antidepressants and relatively non-sedative anxiolytics such as buspirone. If opioids, or other drugs, can be shown conclusively to reduce the sensation of breathlessness it will be necessary to determine if they are best used on a regular or 'as required' basis. The role of lung volume reduction surgery in improving breathlessness and quality of life needs to be further elucidated. Results of a large-scale European study comparing non-invasive ventilation/LTOT with LTOT are awaited, but it is probable that non-invasive ventilation will become an important additional home therapy for some COPD patients with nocturnal hypoventilation.

Models of service provision

Pulmonary rehabilitation is now an accepted modality of treatment (Lacasse *et al.* 1996). As there is increasing emphasis on the cost-effectiveness of medical interventions, future studies will try and separate out which are the essential components of this multidisciplinary intervention and will assess the *minimum* duration of these programmes, and how long the effects last. Studies are needed on how to adapt the principles of pulmonary rehabilitation in order to benefit severely dyspnoeic housebound patients. Further research is needed into the best use of respiratory specialist nurses, including their role in supervising *domiciliary* pulmonary rehabilitation. As the multiple needs of COPD patients become more apparent (Gore *et al.* 1997; Skilbeck *et al.* 1998), work is required to see whether involvement of specialist palliative care can improve symptoms and quality of life. Further development is required in designing lightweight portable oxygen cylinders and in deciding which patients will benefit from these.

Implications for clinical management

For some time there was an air of therapeutic nihilism around the management of COPD. That attitude is now changing. There is a greater awareness of the psychosocial aspects of the disease, respiratory specialist nurses are being appointed and chest physicians increasingly are convinced of the value of pulmonary rehabilitation. The profile of COPD has been further raised by publication of the British Thoracic Society (BTS) 'Guidelines for the management of COPD' (1997).

The BTS guidelines suggest that general practitioners need to consider smoking cessation policies and provide assessment in clinics, with spirometric tests, for smokers aged over 40 years. General practitioners should offer influenza vaccination to severely affected patients, and be aware of indications for specialist referral. Practice nurses might benefit from formal training to cover the substantial un-met needs of COPD patients. Possibly 'obstructive airway' clinics similar to asthma clinics might be worthwhile. Patients with moderate or severe

COPD should have a formal trial of oral steroids. Spirometry must be documented and the patient's ability to cope assessed. There should be an assessment of the inhaler technique and the patient's understanding of the recommended treatment regime. In severe COPD, the need for long-term oxygen and/or home nebuliser must be assessed.

The BTS guidelines (1997) recommend that each district general hospital should have a specified respiratory physician with responsibility for COPD, and a specialised respiratory nurse attached to each district hospital with responsibility for liaising with primary care over the care plan. Resources should be available to develop pulmonary rehabilitation, and there should be provision for terminal and respite care for patients with the most severe COPD.

The prognosis for patients with severe COPD can be worse than for patients with metastatic breast or prostate cancer. Should they be under the aegis of palliative medicine specialists? If the practice of caring for non-malignant disease were to develop, hospices would need a substantial increase in resources (Wilson *et al.* 1995). A recent paper has pointed out that current service provision in COPD is focused on acute exacerbations and that there is a need to manage the health and social care interface more effectively, with a shift from reactive *ad hoc* provision (Skilbeck *et al.* 1998). Perhaps this is where the palliative approach to care is best suited to meet the needs identified? Palliative care specialists would not take over patients' care, but rather work in partnership with general practitioners, chest physicians and respiratory nurse specialists. Specialist palliative care could provide a coherent approach to assessment, facilitate access to community services and help in management of symptoms such as pain, constipation and cachexia (muscle wasting). As training improves in the principles of palliative medicine it is to be hoped that patients suffering from chronic lung disease will no longer be dismissed with the comment 'nothing more can be done for you'.

References

Ahmedzai, S. (1998). Palliation of respiratory symptoms.). In Doyle, D., Hanks, G.W.C., MacDonald, N. (eds), *Oxford Textbook of Palliative Medicine* (2nd edn). Oxford: Oxford University Press, 583–616.

Barnes, P.J. (1998). New therapies for chronic obstructive pulmonary disease. *Thorax* **53**: 137–47.

Belman, M.J. (1993). Pulmonary rehabilitation in chronic respiratory insufficiency: 2—Exercise in patients with chronic obstructive pulmonary disease. *Thorax* **48**: 936–46.

Bruera, E., Macmillan, K., Pither, J., and Macdonald, R.N. (1990). Effects of morphine on the breathlessness of terminal cancer patients. *Journal of Pain Symptom Management* **5**: 341–44.

BTS (1997). Guidelines for the management of chronic obstructive pulmonary disease. *Thorax* **52**: Supplement 5.

Burdon, J.G.W., Pain, M.C.F., Rubinfeld, A.R., and Nana, A. (1994). Chronic lung disease and the perception of breathlessness: a clinical perspective. *European Respiratory Journal* **7**: 1342–9.

Cockcroft, A., Bagnell, P., Heslop, A., Andersson, N., Heaton, R., Batstone, J., Allen, J., Spencer, P., and Guz, A. (1987). Controlled trial of respiratory health worker visiting patients with chronic respiratory disability. *British Medical Journal* **294**: 225–8.

Davies, L. and Calverley, P.M.A. (1996). Lung volume reduction surgery in chronic obstructive pulmonary disease. *Thorax* **51**(2): 529–34.

Douglas, N.J. (1998). Systematic review of the efficacy of nasal CPAP. *Thorax* **53**: 414–15.

Dudley, D.L., Glaser, E.M., Jorgenson, B.N., and Logan, D.L. (1980). Psychosocial concomitants to rehabilitation in chronic obstructive pulmonary disease. *Chest* **77**: 413–20.

Goldstein, R.S. (1993). Pulmonary rehabilitation in chronic respiratory insufficiency: 3-ventilatory muscle training. *Thorax* **48**: 1025–33.

Gore, J.M., Brophy, C., and Greenstone, M.A. (1997). Palliative care and anxiety and depression in end-stage chronic obstructive pulmonary disease (COPD): a comparison with lung cancer. *Thorax* **52**(6): A77.

Gorecka, D., Gorzelak, K., Sliwinski, P., Tobiasz, M., and Zielinski, J. (1997). Effect of long-term oxygen on survival in patients with chronic obstructive pulmonary disease with moderate hypoxia. *Thorax* **52**: 674–9.

Heaton, R.K., Grant, I., McSweeny, A.J., Adams, K.M., and Petty, T.L. (1983). Psychologic effects of continuous and nocturnal oxygen therapy in hypoxemic chronic obstructive pulmonary disease. *Archives of Internal Medicine* **143**: 1941–7.

Heslop, A. (1993). Role of the respiratory nurse specialist. *British Journal of Hospital Medicine* **50**: 88–90.

Jankelson, D., Hosseini, K., Mather, L.E., Seale, J.P., and Young, I.H. (1997). Lack of effect of high doses of inhaled morphine on exercise endurance in chronic obstructive pulmonary disease. *European Respiratory Journal* **10**: 2270–4.

Johnston, I.D.A., Prescott, R.J., Chalmers, J.C., and Rudd, R.M. (1997). British Thoracic Society study of cryptogenic fibrosing alveolitis: current presentation and initial management. *Thorax* **52**: 38–44.

Lacasse, Y., Wong, E., Guyatt, G.H., King, D., Cook, D.J., and Goldstein, R.S. (1996). Meta-analysis of respiratory rehabilitation in chronic obstructive pulmonary disease. *Lancet* **348**: 1115–19.

Light, R.W., Stansbury, D.W., and Webster, J.S. (1996). Effect of 30 mg of morphine alone or with promethazine or prochlorperazine on the exercise capacity of patients with COPD. *Chest* **109**: 975–81.

Littlejohns, P., Baveystock, C.M., Parnell, H., and Jones, P.W. (1991). Randomised controlled trial of the effectiveness of a respiratory health worker in reducing impairment, disability and handicap due to chronic airflow limitation. *Thorax* **46**: 559–64.

Morgan, A.D., Peck, D.F., Buchanan, D.R., and McHardy, G.J.R. (1983). Effect of attitudes and beliefs on exercise tolerance in chronic bronchitis. *British Medical Journal* **286**: 171–3.

Mitchell-Heggs, P., Murphy, K., Minty, K., Guz, A., Patterson, S.C., Minty, P.S., and Rosser, R.M. (1980). Diazepam in the treatment of dyspnoea in the 'Pink Puffer' syndrome. Quarterly *Journal of Medicine* **49**: 9–20.

Nocturnal Oxygen Therapy Trial Group. (1980). Continuous or nocturnal oxygen therapy in hypoxic chronic obstructive lung disease. *Annals of Internal Medicine* **93**: 391–8.

Pearson, M.G., Littler, J., and Davies, P.D.O. (1994). An analysis of medical workload by speciality and diagnosis in Mersey: evidence of a specialist to patient mismatch. *Journal of the Royal College of Physicians of London* **28**: 230–4.

Petty, T.L. (1993). Pulmonary rehabilitation in chronic respiratory insufficiency: 1—Pulmonary rehabilitation in perspective. *Thorax* **48**: 855–62.

Raw, M., McNeill, A., and West, R. (1998). Smoking cessation guidelines and their cost effectiveness. *Thorax* **53**(5).

Report of the Medical Research Council Oxygen Working Party. (1981). Long-term domiciliary oxygen therapy in chronic hypoxic cor pulmonale complicating chronic bronchitis and emphysema. *Lancet* **1**: 681–5.

Rijcken, B. and Britton, J. (1998). Epidemiology of chronic obstructive pulmonary disease. Management of chronic obstructive pulmonary disease. *European Respiratory Monograph* **7**: 41–73.

Roue, C., Mal, H., Sleiman, C., Fournier, M., Duchatelle, J.P., Baldeyrou, P., and Pariente, R. (1996). Lung volume reduction in patients with severe diffuse emphysema. *Chest* **110**: 28–34.

Royal College of Physicians. (1986). Physical disability in 1986 and beyond. *Journal of the Royal College of Physicians of London* **3**: 160–94.

Shneerson, J. (1997). Quality of life in neuromuscular and skeletal disorders. *European Respiratory Review* 7: **42**: 71–3.

Simonds, A.K. (1994). Sleep studies of respiratory function and home respiratory support. *British Medical Journal* **309**: 35–40.

Skilbeck, J., Mott, L., Page, H., Smith, D., Hjelmeland-Ahmedzai, S., and Clark, D. (1998). Palliative care in chronic obstructive airways disease: a needs assessment. *Palliative Medicine* **12**: 245–54.

Smyth, R.L., Higenbottam, T., Scott, J., and Wallwork, J. (1991). The current state of lung transplantation for cystic fibrosis. *Thorax* **46**: 213–16.

Stark, R.D. (1988). Breathlessness: assessment and pharmacological manipulation. *European Respiratory Journal* **1**: 280–7.

Stokes, T.C., Shaylor, J.M., O'Reilly, J.F., and Harrison, B.D.W. (1982). Assessment of steroid responsiveness in patients with chronic airflow obstruction. *Lancet* **2**: 345–8.

Walters, M.I., Edwards, P.R., Waterhouse, J.C., and Howard, P. (1993). Pulmonary rehabilitation in chronic respiratory insufficiency: 4—long term domiciliary oxygen therapy in chronic obstructive pulmonary disease. *Thorax* **48**: 1170–77.

Wedzicka, J.A., Bestall, J.C., Garrod, R., Graham, R., Paul, E.A., and Jones, P.W. (1998). Randomised controlled trial of pulmonary rehabilitation in severe chronic obstructive pulmonary disease patients, stratified with the MRC breathlessness scale. *European Respiratory Journal* **12**: 363–9.

Williams, S.J. (1993). *Chronic respiratory illness*. London: Routledge.

Wilson, I.M., Bunting, J.S., Curnow, R.N., and Knock, J. (1995). The need for inpatient palliative care facilities for non-cancer patients in the Thames Valley. *Palliative Medicine* **9**: 13–18.

Woodcock, A.A., Gross, E.R., and Geddes, D.M. (1981). Drug treatment of breathlessness: contrasting effects of diazepam and promethazine in pink puffers. *British Medical Journal* **283**: 343–6

Young, I.M., Daviskas, E., and Keena, V.A. (1989). Effect of low dose nebulised morphine on exercise endurance in patients with chronic lung disease. *Thorax* **44**: 387–90.

Chapter 3

Heart disease

J. Simon R. Gibbs

Introduction

Heart disease is a common cause of death and a major public health issue. This chapter addresses the potential for palliative care in the two commonest forms of heart disease.

Which patients are likely to benefit from palliative care?

Chronic heart failure

Most cardiovascular diseases which affect the heart, such as hypertension, coronary artery disease, significant heart valve stenosis or regurgitation, and primary myocardial diseases, cause myocardial damage resulting in chronic heart failure. The clinical definition of heart failure is a syndrome associated with symptoms, signs and objective evidence of left ventricular dysfunction (The Task Force on Heart Failure of the European Society of Cardiology 1995).

Pulmonary hypertension

Severe pulmonary hypertension caused by pulmonary vascular disease has similar clinical features to heart failure but symptoms are usually more severe. Although there are a number of causes of pulmonary vascular disease, severe pulmonary hypertension itself is rare. Many of the problems of severe heart failure also apply to pulmonary hypertension and this condition is not considered further here.

Intractable angina

In some patients with coronary artery disease angina becomes refractory to optimal medical and surgical treatment. Refractory angina is defined as persistence of angina pectoris in Canadian Cardiovascular Society class III or IV (Campeau 1976) despite maximally tolerated conventional treatment. Verification of myocardial ischaemia as the cause of pain is essential and conventional coronary artery surgery and coronary angioplasty must be deemed unsuitable on the basis of a recent coronary angiogram (Schoebel et al. 1997). Most patients have triple vessel coronary artery disease and approximately 70% will have previously undergone coronary artery surgery. Heart transplantation is rarely an option. These patients should be differentiated from patients with chest pain, coronary disease, and with no evidence of myocardial ischaemia in whom the cause of chest pain is not readily identified.

Congenital heart disease

Some patients with certain types of congenital heart disease may develop heart failure and/or pulmonary hypertension at any time during their life. Many will have undergone cardiac surgery early in life. Since this population is generally younger than adults with acquired heart disease, the impact of symptoms on their lives is different. They are used to aggressive treatment which may include complex surgery, interventions in the cardiac catheterisation laboratory, and transplantation. The expectations of patients and their families may differ from patients with acquired heart disease. These issues are beyond the scope of this chapter.

How many patients are likely to be affected?

Heart failure

Heart failure is the only major cardiovascular disease with increasing prevalence, incidence, and mortality. It is mainly a disease of old age. The estimated prevalence (per 1000 population) is between 3.8 and 29.4 rising to 80.5 over the age of 65 years and up to 190 over the age of 75 (Cowie *et al.* 1997). The incidence (per 1000 population per annum) is between 2.3 and 3.3 rising to 43.5 over the age of 75 (Cowie *et al.* 1997). In the UK heart failure causes about 60 000 deaths per annum. With age adjusted mortality rates from cardiovascular disease declining and the size of the elderly population growing, the absolute number of individuals with compromised cardiac function is expected to increase dramatically over the next few decades (Madsen *et al.* 1994).

Intractable angina

There is no data on the prevalence of refractory angina (Schoebel *et al.* 1997) but it affects a minority of patients with coronary disease. The number of patients will increase as the long-term prognosis of coronary artery disease improves.

What problems do they have?

Heart failure

Heart failure is a progressive condition associated with symptomatic deterioration over a period of time which is unpredictable. With the exception of heart transplantation which is available to a minority of patients, modern treatments for heart failure slow but do not arrest progression of the disease.

Symptoms

The majority of patients have mild symptoms. The typical symptoms are breathlessness and an unpleasant sensation of fatigue. These are associated with physical restriction of activity with consequent loss of mobility, loss of well-being, anxiety, and low mood.

The cause of breathlessness and fatigue is not a direct effect of poor cardiac function: functional ability of patients with heart failure correlates poorly with objective measures of left ventricular dysfunction (Franciosa *et al.* 1981; Willens *et al.* 1987; Gorkin *et al.* 1993a). Both symptoms may be generated by the same pathophysiological process since the dominant symptom depends on the type of activity undertaken while haemodynamic changes are the same (Gibbs *et al.* 1990). Patients with heart failure ventilate excessively for a given level of exercise (Franciosa *et al.* 1984) which may be only partially explained by ventilation–perfusion mismatch (Sullivan *et al.* 1988a) since arterial oxygenation remains normal (Clark and Coats 1994). Instead the pathophysiological explanation for breathlessness and fatigue has focused on the periphery. This may involve deconditioning, wasting and metabolic changes in skeletal muscle which activate ergo- (Clark *et al.* 1996) and chemoreflexes (Chua *et al.* 1996) and influence sympathetic activation.

Quality of life in chronic heart failure is poor and may be worse than other chronic medical conditions (Stewart *et al.* 1989). Psychological factors may have more influence on quality of life than physical incapacity (Rideout and Montemuro 1986; Dracup *et al.* 1992). Psychosocial function is impaired (Wenger 1989) and often goes unrecognised (Jessup and Brozena 1988). Major depression (DSM-IV criteria) is present in a third (36.5%) and is significantly more common than in heart disease not associated with heart failure (17.0%) (Koenig 1998). It is more common in patients with severe illness, severe functional impairment and co-morbid psychiatric disorders. These patients do not make greater use of mental health resources than patients who are not depressed but they have almost double the rate of hospital admission. A cause for concern is that less than half of depressed patients receive any treatment at all for depression and they are no more likely than non-depressed patients to see a mental health specialist (Koenig 1998).

Patients are prone to episodes of acute decompensation of their heart failure causing recurrent fluid retention with symptomatic deterioration. These episodes are often unexpected and result in hospital admission which may be prolonged with an in-hospital mortality of about 8% (Rich and Freedland 1988; Rich *et al.* 1995; Krumholz *et al.* 1997). The readmission rate is 29–47% within 3 months (Rich and Freedland 1988; Vinson *et al.* 1990; Rich *et al.* 1995) and 36–44% within 6 months (Gooding and Jette 1985; Krumholz *et al.* 1997). This is the highest readmission rate for all hospitalised patient groups and has been increasing progressively for over a decade (McMurray *et al.* 1993). Symptomatic deterioration and reduced life expectancy may be caused by a lack of compliance with drug therapy. This is a common problem, especially since diuretics cause urinary incontinence and can result in constipation. Other causes of hospital readmission include dietary indiscretion with respect to salt and alcohol intake (Ghali *et al.* 1988; Vinson *et al.* 1990), failed social support and follow-up (Vinson *et al.* 1990), intercurrent infection, myocardial ischaemia, or pulmonary embolism. Survivors of hospital admission for acute exacerbation of heart failure have improved functional status and health perception on follow-up (Jaagosild *et al.* 1998).

Progressive deterioration may result in fluid retention with peripheral oedema, pleural effusions, and ascites. There is symptomatic worsening with breathlessness at rest, difficulty in breathing unless in an upright position, difficulty sleeping, anorexia, cachexia, muscle weakness, sexual dysfunction, nausea, and vomiting (Jaarsma *et al.* 1996). Pain has been reported to be an important symptom of patients dying from heart failure (McCarthy *et al.* 1996) although its nature is not yet understood. In the 'Study to understand prognosis and preferences for outcomes and risks of treatments (SUPPORT), a five centre study of seriously ill hospitalised adults in the US (Lynn *et al.* 1997b), pain was inadequately controlled in 9% of patients dying from heart failure (Desbiens *et al.* 1997).

Co-morbid disease is common in heart failure (Hakim *et al.* 1996; Lynn *et al.* 1997a) increasing the total burden of disease and hospital admissions (Krumholz *et al.* 1997) in these patients. Administration of drugs such as non-steroidal anti-inflammatory agents, tri-cyclic antidepressants, and steroids to treat co-morbid disease cause salt and water retention and may worsen heart failure.

Dying from heart failure

Poor prognosis in heart failure is predicted by poor left ventricular function, severe symptoms (Konstam *et al.* 1992), and metabolic markers (Lee and Packer 1986; Swedberg *et al.* 1990; Cohn *et al.* 1993). Assessment of prognosis by New York Heart Association (NYHA) functional class is the simplest approach (The Criteria Committee of the New York Heart Association 1998). The applicability and interpretation of more complex prognostic models (Campana *et al.* 1993; Aaronson *et al.* 1997) is uncertain and there is no accepted marker to determine which patients will die suddenly (Uretsky and Sheahan 1997).

Dying from chronic heart failure may be worse than cancer in terms of symptoms and distress (Hinton 1963; Hockley *et al.* 1988). In hospital based studies chronic heart failure has a mortality rate of 31–48% at 1 year and 76% at 3 years (Franciosa *et al.* 1983; Brophy *et al.* 1994; Bonneaux *et al.* 1994). The average annual mortality is about 10% (Konstam *et al.* 1994).

Heart failure differs fundamentally from cancer in that prognosis when close to death is more uncertain (Lynn *et al.* 1997a). This is mainly because of sudden death in symptomatically stable patients. In NYHA functional class II heart failure symptoms are mild and the annual mortality is 5–15%, of which 50–80% die suddenly (Gradman *et al.* 1989; Konstam *et al.* 1992; Benedict *et al.* 1996; Franciosa *et al.* 1983; Kjekshus 1990). In contrast in NYHA class IV annual mortality is 30–70% with only 5–30% of deaths being sudden (The CONSENSUS Trial Study Group 1987; Califf *et al.* 1997).

The main cause of sudden death is probably cardiac arrhythmias. This raises the issue of cardiopulmonary resuscitation. The wishes of patients regarding resuscitation is not always considered or discussed with them. In SUPPORT, physicians did not seem to be aware of the preferences of patients for resuscitation and attempted to project their own values on these patients (Hakim *et al.* 1996; Tsevat *et al.* 1998). Although 69% of the heart failure population in SUPPORT wanted resuscitation (Hakim *et al.* 1996), it has previously been shown that the majority of older patients do not want resuscitation when they understand the probability of survival after the procedure (Murphy *et al.* 1994). Training in cardiopulmonary resuscitation has been advocated for the carers of patients who wish to be resuscitated (Konstam *et al.* 1994) but this may have adverse psychological consequences (Dracup *et al.* 1986) and should be undertaken cautiously (Dracup *et al.* 1997).

Sudden death makes the classification of terminal illness in heart failure enigmatic if the definition of 'terminal' is only fulfilled after reaching a certain clinical state akin to cancer. It also means that the ability of physicians to recognise impending death in heart failure is often seriously inaccurate and they are unlikely to classify the majority of such patients as terminally ill (Lynn *et al.* 1996).

Angina

These patients are disabled by angina on mild exercise which may severely limit daily activities. Recurrent angina at rest results in repeated hospital admission for stabilisation of the pain.

'Regional study of care for the dying'

The only UK study to investigate symptoms in terminal heart disease was the 'Regional study of care for the dying' (Addington-Hall and McCarthy 1995). This was a population based retrospective survey of a random sample of people dying in 20 English health districts in 1990. Sudden deaths were excluded. This study did not identify the cardiac diagnosis. People who died from heart disease mainly did so in hospital and were reported to have experienced a wide range of symptoms, which were frequently distressing and often lasted for more than six months (McCarthy et al. 1996; McCarthy et al. 1997). Poor quality of life was determined by distressing symptoms (in particular low mood, anxiety, and incontinence) and the need for assistance with self care.

At least one in seven had symptom severity comparable to those of cancer patients managed in hospices or by specialist palliative care services (McCarthy et al. 1996). Although half were thought to have known, or probably known, that they were dying, open communication with health professionals was rare (McCarthy et al. 1996). The findings suggested that these patients might benefit from the expertise of palliative care in symptom control, psychological support, and open communication, with emphasis on maintaining quality of life.

Summary of research on effectiveness of interventions/ services

The primary treatment of all heart disease is appropriate evidence-based treatment to improve symptoms, prevent further deterioration, and prolong life. This includes advising and educating patients and their families about lifestyle (including diet, management of obesity, exercise, smoking, and alcohol consumption), providing rehabilitation, prescribing drug therapy, and performing surgery and interventional cardiac procedures. These aspects are well documented in the literature and are not covered here.

Heart failure

Diuretics to control fluid balance and angiotensin converting enzyme (ACE) inhibitors to improve symptoms, reduce left ventricular damage, hospital admissions and prolong life are the mainstay of therapy (The Task Force of the Working Group on Heart Failure of the European Society of Cardiology 1997). ACE inhibitors achieve this by reducing the production of angiotensin II from angiotensin I and the breakdown of bradykinins; this results in vasodilatation, reduced sodium retention, and exerts a favourable effect on myocardial and vascular remodelling. In heart failure the need to identify patients with left ventricular dysfunction and treat them with ACE inhibitors has been emphasised (Anonymous 1995; Konstam et al. 1994). In severe disease, optimisation of such therapy improves breathlessness and fatigue but may require specialist advice particularly since prescription of ACE inhibitors is often suboptimal (EUROASPIRE Study Group 1997). Randomised controlled trials have also provided evidence for the advantageous use of other drugs such as beta blockers (Australia/New Zealand Heart Failure Research Collaborative Group 1997) and digoxin (The Digitalis Investigation Group 1997).

Randomised trials to investigate the effects of antidepressants have not been performed. This is because tricyclic antidepressants and related drugs are cardiotoxic and may precipitate sudden death, although selective serotonin re-uptake inhibitors have fewer car-diotoxic effects. Acute dosing with dihydrocodeine improves breathlessness by suppressing chemosensitivity with associated reduction of exercise ventilation (Chua *et al.* 1997). This effect has not been investigated with chronic opioid administration.

Exercise training improves exercise capacity and symptoms (Sullivan *et al.* 1988b; Coats *et al.* 1990; Coats *et al.* 1992). This effect is associated with improvements in blood flow to skeletal muscle (Sullivan *et al.* 1988b) and muscle metabolism (Adamopolous *et al.* 1991). A randomised trial of exercise training is planned in Europe.

Patients with heart failure frequently express a preference to be managed at home but lack the confidence to be self-sufficient in their own care (Vinson *et al.* 1990). In one study the problem of compliance with therapy was improved by patient directed group meetings and reduced readmissions (Rosenberg 1971), but another showed that while compliance improved there was no significant effect on quality of life (Goodyer *et al.* 1995). Social sup-port may have a greater role in influencing mortality than functional status (Frasure and Prince 1985; Willund *et al.* 1992; Gorkin *et al.* 1993b).

Although the use of nurse specialists has been advocated to improve outcomes (Cintron *et al.* 1983; Frasure and Prince 1985; Dracup *et al.* 1994; Konstam *et al.* 1994), evidence of benefit from this is limited. A nurse directed intervention for hospital in-patients failed to improve communication, issues surrounding resuscitation, days spent on an intensive care unit, or control of pain (The SUPPORT Principal Investigators 1995). This finding was not peculiar to heart failure and applied to other chronic illnesses.

In the community, one randomised study has shown that nurse directed multidisciplinary care was more effective and reduced hospital admissions compared to conventional care (Rich *et al.* 1995). This multifaceted approach included education, dietary instruction, review of drug therapy, and intensive follow-up at home and was not designed to identify which elements were most important.

Such success has not been universal. A randomised trial of a structured care programme based on a nurse monitored out-patient clinic to improve symptom management failed to reduce hospital readmissions and if anything tended to increase the length of hospital stay (Ekman *et al.* 1998). Twenty-nine per cent of patients in the intervention group were unable to participate despite being judged suitable by a doctor and themselves. This poor partici-pation rate was associated with the need for assistance at home. In another randomised study of severely ill patients suffering mainly from heart failure, hospital admissions actu-ally increased during intensive care in the community by a nurse and a primary care physi-cian (Weinberger *et al.* 1996). Although patient satisfaction improved in the intensive care group, quality of life scores did not differ from the control group. Since patients with heart failure may experience worsening symptoms for a relatively long time prior to hospitalisa-tion (Friedman 1997) it has been proposed that an intensive care programme may lead to the detection of previously unrecognised medical problems (Ekman *et al.* 1998). Among a cohort of high risk patients with heart failure, home based intervention was associated with reduced frequency of unplanned readmissions plus out-of-hospital deaths within 6 months of discharge from hospital (Stewart *et al.* 1998). Home based intervention comprised a single home visit (by a nurse and pharmacist) to optimise medication management, identify early clinical deterioration, and intensify medical follow-up and caregiver vigilance as appropriate.

The disparity of the results in these studies may be caused by differences in the severity of heart failure, differences in the intervention and selection of patients by high risk of readmission, or differences in social circumstances. This limited evidence favours a home based approach to continuing care in selected patients.

Intractable angina

The pathophysiology of this condition is not well understood and therapeutic options are limited. In assessing therapy it must be appreciated that drug therapy elicits a placebo effect on symptoms of almost two-fifths (Benson and McCallie-DP 1979). Surgery may also derive considerable placebo benefit (Dimond *et al.* 1960; Effler *et al.* 1965). Over-treatment with conventional anti-anginal drugs may cause iatrogenic symptoms including dizziness, tiredness, and subjective discomfort (Tolins *et al.* 1984). A number of new therapies are being developed and these include transmyocardial revascularisation, long-term intermittent urokinase therapy, and transcutaneous and spinal electrical nerve stimulation. An analgesic approach is considered contraindicated because it may mask signs of life-threatening myocardial ischaemia (Schoebel *et al.* 1997). This is controversial, and some of these patients are managed with long-term opiates or methadone.

In addition to an analgesic effect, nerve stimulation may have an anti-ischaemic action (De Jongste *et al.* 1994) possibly by reducing myocardial oxygen demand by decreasing sympathetic activity (Norrsell *et al.* 1997) and improving myocardial perfusion to ischaemic zones (Hautvast *et al.* 1996). It does not mask pain in myocardial ischaemia (Mannheimer *et al.* 1993) or infarction (Andersen *et al.* 1994). The treatment has been reported to be effective (Eliasson *et al.* 1993; Sanderson *et al.* 1994; Bagger *et al.* 1998) but long-term treatment has a beneficial effect in only 57% of carefully selected patients (Bagger *et al.* 1998).

Priorities for further research

Heart failure

Research into, and specialist services for, the care of patients with end stage heart disease has been neglected (Higginson 1993). A suggested approach to heart failure is to determine the following.

1 The needs of patients: there is a lack of knowledge about the impact of heart failure on patients' quality of life, the adequacy of symptom control, or the communication needs of these patients. Differences between men and women as well as ethnic minorities should be explored. The need for improved provision of care for these patients with increased emphasis on quality rather than quantity of life has been recognised (Gibbs *et al.* 1998). Services for these patients cannot be developed in the absence of good information on their needs.

2 Which interventions designed to meet the needs of these patients as part of a palliative approach are appropriate, acceptable, and cost effective. It cannot be assumed that a multidisciplinary team as used in cancer will be the most appropriate and effective approach in heart disease. Interventions in heart failure include educating patients and their carers, improving communication, providing social support, providing care by telephone, management by nurse specialists, counselling, and psychological support as well as many others. In view of the lack of a clearly defined terminal phase of the illness attention needs to be paid to interventions to improve care for all patients with severe heart failure, rather than for those judged to be terminally ill.

3 Research into which models of care provide optimal medical out-patient care: this includes the role of and level of care provided by general practitioners, general physicians, geriatricians, accident and emergency physicians, palliative care physicians, and cardiologists. A prerequisite is that the doctor should have good knowledge of heart failure. A shift from generalist to specialist care would overwhelm current resources. Consideration should be given to the role of specialist heart failure clinics.

4 Where patients are best managed at different stages of the illness warrants investigation: this includes management at home, in hospital in a secondary or tertiary centre, in a hospice, a nursing home and community care.

5 How different long term models of care influence outcomes.

Intractable angina

New approaches to myocardial ischaemia will continue to evolve. The influence of new therapies needs to be evaluated in randomised trials to assess clinical efficacy and mortality. Registry data should be collected if randomisation is not ethically or practically possible. Co-morbid psychiatric illness should be assessed. The needs of these patients with particular regard to pain relief should be assessed.

Implications for clinical management

Current evidence suggests that patients dying from heart disease have poor symptom control and un-met needs. Uncertain prognosis means that while treating heart failure to improve not just symptoms but also prognosis, the possibility of dying must be acknowledged and support provided for patients and their families about the issues surrounding death (Lynn *et al.* 1997a). For the majority of patients there will be no clearly defined terminal phase of life. Planning for death early in the course of the illness might allow anticipation and reduction of futile care.

Differences in the natural history and treatment of heart disease and cancer suggest that a palliative approach to the care of cardiac patients may necessarily differ from established palliative care in cancer. The management of heart failure will require reappraisal when it becomes clear what needs these patients have, where they are best managed and which interventions are effective in improving satisfaction and quality of life. This will have important implications for the use of health care resources.

References

Aaronson, K.D., Schwartz, J.S., Chen, T.M., Wong, K.L., Goin, J.E., and Mancini, D.M. (1997). Development and prospective validation of a clinical index to predict survival in ambulatory patients referred for cardiac transplant evaluation. *Circulation* 95: 2660–7.

Adamopolous, S., Coats, A.J.S., Arnolda, L., Brunotte, F., Thompson, C., Meyer, T., Radda, G., and Rajagopolan, B. (1991). Effects of physical training on skeletal muscle metabolism in chronic heart failure: 31-P NMR spectroscopy study. *Circulation* 84 (Suppl. II): II-74.

Addington-Hall, J.M., Fakhoury, W., and McCarthy, M. (1998). Palliative care in non-cancer patients. *Palliative Medicine* 12: 417–27.

Addington-Hall, J.M. and McCarthy, M. (1995). Regional study of care for the dying: methods and sample characteristics. *Palliative Medicine* 9: 27–35.

Andersen, C., Hole, P., and Oxhoj, H. (1994). Does pain relief with spinal cord stimulation for angina conceal myocardial infarction? *British Heart Journal* **71**: 419–21.

Anonymous (1995). Guidelines for the evaluation and management of heart failure. Report of the American College of Cardiology/American Heart Association Task Force on Practice Guidelines (Committee on Evaluation and Management of Heart Failure). *Journal of the American College of Cardiology* **26**: 1376–98.

Australia/New Zealand Heart Failure Research Collaborative Group (1997). Randomised, placebo controlled study of the effects of carvedilol in patients with congestive heart failure due to ischaemic heart disease. *Lancet* **349**: 375–80.

Bagger, J.P., Jensen, B.S., and Johannsen, G. (1998). Long-term outcome of spinal cord electrical stimulation in patients with refractory chest pain. *Clinical Cardiology* **21**: 286–8.

Benedict, C.R., Shelton, B., Johnstone, D.E., Francis, G., Greenberg, B., Konstam, M., Probstfield, J.L., and Yusuf, S. (1996). Prognostic significance of plasma norepinephrine in patients with asymptomatic left ventricular dysfunction. SOLVD Investigators. *Circulation* **94**: 690–7.

Benson, H. and McCallie, DP, Jr. (1979). Angina pectoris and the placebo effect. *New England Journal of Medicine* **300**:1424–9.

Bonneaux, L., Barendregt, J.J., Meeter, K., Bonsel, G.J., and van der Maas, P.J. (1994). Estimating clinical morbidity due to ischemic heart disease and congestive heart failure: the future rise of heart failure. *Americal Journal of Public Health* **84**: 20–8.

Brophy, J.M., Deslauriers, G., and Rouleau, J.L. (1994). Long-term prognosis of patients presenting to the emergency room with decompensated congestive heart failure. *Canadian Journal of Cardiology* **10**: 543–7.

Califf, R.M., Adams, K.F., McKenna, W.J., Gheorghiade, M., Uretsky, B.F., McNulty, S.E., Darius, H., Schulman, K., Zannad, F., Handberg, T.E., Harrell, F.E., J., Wheeler, W., Soler, S.J., and Swedberg, K. (1997). A randomized controlled trial of epoprostenol therapy for severe congestive heart failure: The Flolan International Randomized Survival Trial (FIRST). *American Heart Journal* **134**: 44–54.

Campana, C., Gavazzi, A., Berzuini, C., Larizza, C., Marioni, R., D'Armini, A., Pederzolli, N., Martinelli, L., and Vigano, M. (1993). Predictors of prognosis in patients awaiting heart transplantation. *Journal of Heart and Lung Transplantation* **12**: 756–65.

Campeau, L. (1976). Grading of angina pectoris. *Circulation* **54**: 522–3.

Chua, T.P., Clark, A.L., Amadi, A., and Coats, A.J.S. (1996). Relation between chemosensitivity and the ventilatory response to chronic heart failure. *Journal of the American College of Cardiology* **27**: 650–7.

Chua, T.P., Harrington, D., Ponikowski, P., Webb-Peploe, K., Poole-Wilson, P.A., and Coats, A.J. (1997). Effects of dihydrocodeine on chemosensitivity and exercise tolerance in patients with chronic heart failure. *Journal of the American College of Cardiology* **29**: 147–52.

Cintron, G., Bigas, C., Linares, E., Aranda, J.M., and Hernandez, E. (1983). Nurse practitioner role in a chronic congestive heart failure clinic: in-hospital time, costs, and patient satisfaction. *Heart and Lung* **12**: 237–40.

Clark, A.L. and Coats, A.J.S. (1994). Usefulness of arterial blood gas estimations during exercise in patients with chronic heart failure. *British Heart Journal* **71**: 528–30.

Clark, A.L., Poole-Wilson, P., and Coats, A.J.S. (1996). Exercise limitation in chronic heart failure: central role of the periphery. *Journal of the American College of Cardiology* **28**: 1092–1102.

Coats, A.J.S., Adamopoulos, S., Meyer, T.E., Conway, J., and Sleight, P. (1990). Effects of physical training in chronic heart failure. *Lancet* **335**: 63–6.

Coats, A.J.S., Adamopoulos, S., Radealli, A., McCance, A., Meyer, T.E., Bernardi, L., Solda, P.L., Davey, P., Ormerod, O., and Forfar, C. (1992). Controlled trial of physical training in chronic heart failure: exercise performance, hemodynamics, ventilation and autonomic function. *Circulation* **85**: 2119–31.

Cohn, J.N., Johnson, G.R., Shabetai, R., Loeb, H., Tristani, F., Rector, T., Smith, R., and Fletcher, R. (1993). Ejection fraction, peak exercise oxygen consumption, cardiothoracic ratio, ventricular arrhythmias, and plasma norepinephrine as determinants of prognosis in heart failure. The V-HeFT VA Cooperative Studies Group. *Circulation* **87**: VI5–16.

CONSENSUS Trial Study Group, The (1987). Effects of enalapril on mortality in severe congestive heart failure. Results of the Cooperative North Scandinavian Enalapril Survival Study (CONSENSUS). *New England Journal of Medicine* **316**: 1429–35.

Cowie, M.R., Mosterd, A., Wood, D.A., Deckers, J.W., Poole, W.P., Sutton, G.C., and Grobbee, D.E. (1997). The epidemiology of heart failure. *European Heart Journal* **18**: 208–25.

Criteria Committee of the New York Heart Association, The (1998). *Nomenclature and criteria for diagnosis of diseases of the heart and great vessels.* 7th edn. Boston: Little Brown and Co, p. 286.

De Jongste, M.J., Haaksma, J., Hautvast, R.W., Hillege, H.L., Meyler, P.W., Staal, M.J., Sanderson, J.E., and Lie, K.I. (1994). Effects of spinal cord stimulation on myocardial ischaemia during daily life in patients with severe coronary artery disease. A prospective ambulatory electrocardiographic study. *British Heart Journal* **71**: 413–18.

Desbiens, N.A., Wu, A.W., Alzola, C., Mueller, R.N., Wenger, N.S., Connors, A.F., Jr., Lynn, J., and Phillips, R.S. (1997). Pain during hospitalization is associated with continued pain six months later in survivors of serious illness. The SUPPORT Investigators. Study to Understand Prognoses and Preferences for Outcomes and Risks of Treatments. *American Journal of Medicine* **102**: 269–76.

Digitalis Investigation Group, The (1997). The effect of digoxin on mortality and morbidity in patients with heart failure. *New England Journal of Medicine* **336**: 525–33.

Dimond, E.G., Kittie, C.F., and Crockett, J.E. (1960). Comparison of internal mammary artery ligation and sham operation for angina pectoris. *American Journal of Cardiology* **5**: 483–6.

Dracup, K., Baker, D.W., Dunbar, S.B., Daccy, R.A., Brooks, N.H., Johnson, J.C., Oken, C., and Massie, B.M. (1994). Management of heart failure. II. Counselling, education, and lifestyle modifications. *Journal of the American Medical Association* **272**: 1442–6.

Dracup, K., Guzy, P.M., Taylor, S.E., and Barry, J. (1986). Cardiopulmonary resuscitation (CPR) training. Consequences for family members of high-risk cardiac patients. *Archives of Internal Medicine* **146**: 1757–61.

Dracup, K., Moser, D.K., Taylor, S.E., and Guzy, P.M. (1997). The psychological consequences of cardiopulmonary resuscitation training for family members of patients at risk for sudden death. *American Journal of Public Health* **87**: 1434–9.

Dracup, K., Walden, J.A., Stevenson, L.W., and Brecht, M.L. (1992). Quality of life in patients with advanced heart failure. *Journal of Heart and Lung Transplantation* **11**: 273–9.

Effler, D.B., Sones, F.M., Jr., Groves, L.K., and Suarez, E. (1965). Myocardial revascularization by Vineberg's internal mammary artery implant. Evaluation of postoperative results. *Journal of Thorac and Cardiovascular Surgery* **50**: 527–33.

Ekman, I., Andersson, B., Ehnfors, M., Matejka, G., Persson, B., and Fagerberg, B. (1998). Feasibility of a nurse-monitored, out-patient-care programme for elderly patients with moderate-to-severe, chronic heart failure. *European Heart Journal* **19**: 1254–60.

Eliasson, T., Albertsson, P., Hardhammar, P., Emanuelsson, H., Augustinsson, L.E., and Mannheimer, C. (1993). Spinal cord stimulation in angina pectoris with normal coronary arteriograms. *Coronary Artery Disease* **4**: 819–27.

EUROASPIRE Study Group (1997). EUROASPIRE. A European Society of Cardiology survey of secondary prevention of coronary heart disease: principal results. European Action on Secondary Prevention through Intervention to Reduce Events. *European Heart Journal* **18**: 1569–82.

Franciosa, J.A., Leddy, C.L., Wilen, M., and Schwartz , D.E. (1984). Relation between haemodynamic and ventilatory responses in determining exercise capacity in severe congestive heart failure. *American Journal of Cardiology* **53**: 127–34.

Franciosa, J.A., Park, M., and Levine, T.B. (1981). Lack of correlation between exercise capacity and indexes of resting left ventricular performance in heart failure. *American Journal of Cardiology* **47**: 33–9.

Franciosa, J.A., Wilen, M., Ziesche, S., and Cohn, J.N. (1983). Survival in men with severe chronic left ventricular failure due to either coronary artery disease or idiopathic dilated cardiomyopathy. *American Journal of Cardiology* **51**: 831–6.

Frasure, S.N. and Prince, R. (1985). The ischemic heart disease life stress monitoring program: impact on mortality. *Journal of Psychosomatic Medicine* **47**: 431–45.

Friedman, M.M. (1997). Older adults' symptoms and their duration before hospitalization for heart failure. *Heart and Lung* **26**: 169–76.

Ghali, J.K., Kadakia, S., Cooper, R., and Ferlinz, J. (1988). Precipitating factors leading to decompensation of heart failure. Traits among urban blacks. *Archives of Internal Medicine* **148**: 2013–16.

Gibbs, J.S., Keegan, J., Wright, C., Fox, K.M., and Poole-Wilson, P.A. (1990). Pulmonary artery pressure changes during exercise and daily activities in chronic heart failure. *Journal of the American College of Cardiology* **15**: 52–61.

Gibbs, L.M.E., Addington-Hall, J., and Gibbs, J.S.R. (1998). Dying from heart failure: lessons from palliative care. *British Medical Journal* **317**: 961–2.

Gooding, J. and Jette, A.M. (1985). Hospital readmissions among the elderly. *Journal of the American Geriatric Society* **33**: 595–601.

Goodyer, L.I., Miskelly, F., and Milligan, P. (1995). Does encouraging good compliance improve patients' clinical condition in heart failure? *British Journal of Clinical Practice* **49**: 173–6.

Gorkin, L., Norvell, N.K., Rosen, R.C., Charles, E., Shumaker, S.A., McIntyre, K.M., Capone, R.J., Kostis, J., Niaura, R., Woods, P. *et al.* (1993a). Assessment of quality of life as observed from the baseline data of the Studies of Left Ventricular Dysfunction (SOLVD) trial quality-of-life substudy. *American Journal of Cardiology* **71**: 1069–73.

Gorkin, L., Schron, E.B., Brooks, M.M., Wiklund, I., Kellen, J., Verter, J., Schoenberger, J.A., Pawitan, Y., Morris, M., and Shumaker, S. (1993b). Psychosocial predictors of mortality in the Cardiac Arrhythmia Suppression Trial-1 (CAST-1). *American Journal of Cardiology* **71**: 263–7.

Gradman, A., Deedwania, P., Cody, R., Massie, B., Packer, M., Pitt, B., and Goldstein, S. (1989). Predictors of total mortality and sudden death in mild to moderate heart failure. Captopril-Digoxin Study Group. *Journal of the American College of Cardiology* **14**: 564–70.

Hakim, R.B., Teno, J.M., Harrell, F.E., Jr., Knaus, W.A., Wenger, N., Phillips, R.S., Layde, P., Califf, R., Connors, A.F., Jr., and Lynn, J. (1996). Factors associated with do-not-resuscitate orders: patients' preferences, prognoses, and physicians' judgments. SUPPORT Investigators. Study to Understand Prognoses and Preferences for Outcomes and Risks of Treatment. *Annals of Internal Medicine* **125**: 284–93.

Hautvast, R.W., Blanksma, P.K., De Jongste, M.J., Pruim, J., van der Wall, E.E., Vaalburg, W., and Lie, K.I. (1996). Effect of spinal cord stimulation on myocardial blood flow assessed by positron emission tomography in patients with refractory angina pectoris. *American Journal of Cardiology* **77**: 462–7.

Higginson, I. (1993). Palliative care: a review of past changes and future trends. *Journal of Public Health Medicine* **15**: 3–8.

Hinton, J.M. (1963). The physical and mental stress of dying. *Quarterly Journal of Medicine* **32**: 1–21.

Hockley, J.M., Dunlop, R., and Davies, R.J. (1988). Survey of distressing symptoms in dying patients and their families in hospital and the response to a symptom control team. *British Medical Journal* **296**: 1715–17.

Jaagosild, P., Dawson, N.V., Thomas, C., Wenger, N.S., Tsevat, J., Knaus, W.A., Califf, R.M., Goldman, L., Vidaillet, H., and Connors, A.F., Jr. (1998). Outcomes of acute exacerbation of severe congestive heart failure: quality of life, resource use, and survival. SUPPORT Investigators. The study to understand prognosis and preferences for outcomes and risks of treatments. *Archives of Internal Medicine* 158: 1081–9.

Jaarsma, T., Dracup, K., Walden, J., and Stevenson, L.W. (1996). Sexual function in patients with advanced heart failure. *Heart and Lung* 25: 262–70.

Jessup, M. and Brozena, S. (1988). Assessment of quality of life in patients with chronic congestive heart failure. *Quality Life Cardiovasc Care* 4: 53–7.

Kjekshus, J. (1990). Arrhythmias and mortality in congestive heart failure. *American Journal of Cardiology* 65: 421–81.

Koenig, H.G. (1998). Depression in hospitalized older patients with congestive heart failure. *General Hospital Psychiatry* 20: 29–43.

Konstam, M.A., Dracup, K., Baker, D.W., Bottorff, M.B., Brooks, N.H., Dacey, R.A., Dunbar, S.B., Jackson, A.B., Jessup, M., Johnson, J.C., Jones, R., Luchi, R.J., Massie, B.M., Pitt, B., Rose, E.A., Rubin, L.J., Wright, R.F., and Hadorn, D.C. (1994). Heart failure: evaluation and care of patients with left-ventricular systolic dysfunction. Clinical Practice Guideline No. 11. AHCPR Publication No. 94–0612 edn, Rockville, MD: Agency for Health Care Policy and Research, Public Health Service, US Department of Health and Human Services.

Konstam, M.A., Rousseau, M.F., Kronenberg, M.W., Udelson, J.E., Melin, J., Stewart, D., Dolan, N., Edens, T.R., Ahn, S., Kinan, D. *et al.* (1992). Effects of the angiotensin converting enzyme inhibitor enalapril on the long-term progression of left ventricular dysfunction in patients with heart failure. SOLVD Investigators. *Circulation* 86: 431–8.

Krumholz, H.M., Parent, E.M., Tu, N., Vaccarino, V., Wang, Y., Radford, M.J., and Hennen, J. (1997). Readmission after hospitalization for congestive heart failure among Medicare beneficiaries. *Archives of Internal Medicine* 157: 99–104.

Lee, W.H. and Packer, M. (1986). Prognostic importance of serum sodium concentration and its modification by converting-enzyme inhibition in patients with severe chronic heart failure. *Circulation* 73: 257–67.

Lynn, J., Harrell, F.E., Cohn, F., Hamel, M.B., Dawson, N., and Wu, A.W. (1996). Defining the 'Terminally Ill': insights from SUPPORT. *Duquesne Law Review* 335: 311–36.

Lynn, J., Harrell, F., Cohn, F., Wagner, D., and Connors-AF, J. (1997a). Prognoses of seriously ill hospitalized patients on the days before death: implications for patient care and public policy. *New Horizons* 5: 56–61.

Lynn, J., Teno, J.M., Phillips, R.S., Wu, A.W., Desbiens, N., Harrold, J., Claessens, M.T., Wenger, N., Kreling, B., and Connors-AF, J. (1997b). Perceptions by family members of the dying experience of older and seriously ill patients. SUPPORT Investigators. Study to understand prognoses and preferences for outcomes and risks of treatments. *Annals of Internal Medicine* 126: 97–106.

McCarthy, M., Addington-Hall, J.M., and Ley, M. (1997). Communication and choice in dying from heart disease. *Journal of the Royal Society of Medicine* 90: 128–31.

McCarthy, M., Lay, M., and Addington-Hall, J. (1996). Dying from heart disease. *Journal of the Royal College of Physicians of London* 30: 325–8.

McMurray, J., McDonagh, T., and Morrison, C.E. (1993). Trends in hospitalisation for heart failure in Scotland. *European Heart Journal* 14: 1158–62.

Madsen, B.K., Hansen, J.F., Stockholm, K.H., Brons, J., Husum, D., and Mortensen, L.S. (1994). Chronic congestive heart failure. Description and survival of 190 consecutive patients with a diagnosis of chronic congestive heart failure based on clinical signs and symptoms. *European Heart Journal* 15: 303–10.

Mannheimer, C., Eliasson, T., Andersson, B., Bergh, C.H., Augustinsson, L.E., Emanuelsson, H., and Waagstein, F. (1993). Effects of spinal cord stimulation in angina pectoris induced by pacing and possible mechanisms of action [see comments]. *British Medical Journal* **307**: 477–80.

Murphy, D.J., Burrows, D., Santilli, S., Kemp, A.W., Tenner, S., Kreling, B., and Teno, J. (1994). The influence of the probability of survival on patients' preferences regarding cardiopulmonary resuscitation. *New England Journal of Medicine* **330**: 545–9.

Norrsell, H., Eliasson, T., Mannheimer, C., Augustinsson, L.E., Bergh, C.H., Andersson, B., Waagstein, F., and Friberg, P. (1997). Effects of pacing-induced myocardial stress and spinal cord stimulation on whole body and cardiac norepinephrine spillover. *European Heart Journal* **18**: 1890–6.

Rich, M.W., Beckham, V., Wittenberg, C., Leven, C.L., Freedland, K.E., and Carney, R.M. (1995). A multidisciplinary intervention to prevent the readmission of elderly patients with congestive heart failure. *New England Journal of Medicine* **333**: 1190–5.

Rich, M.W. and Freedland, K.E. (1988) Effect of DRGs on three-month readmission rate of geriatric patients with congestive heart failure. *American Journal of Public Health* **78**: 680–2.

Rideout, E. and Montemuro, M. (1986) Hope, morale and adaptation in patients with chronic heart failure. *Journal of Advanced Nursing* **11**: 429–38.

Rosenberg, S. (1971) Patient education leads to better care for heart patients. *HSMHA Health Reports* **86**: 793–802.

Sanderson, J.E., Ibrahim, B., Waterhouse, D., and Palmer, R.B. (1994) Spinal electrical stimulation for intractable angina—long-term clinical outcome and safety. *European Heart Journal* **15**: 810–14.

Schoebel, F.C., Frazier, O.H., Jessurun, G.A., De Jongste, M., Kadipasaoglu, K.A., Jax, T.W., Heintzen, M.P., Cooley, D.A., Strauer, B.E., and Leschke, M. (1997) Refractory angina pectoris in end-stage coronary artery disease: evolving therapeutic concepts. *American Heart Journal* **134**: 587–602.

Stewart, A.L., Greenfled, S., Hays, R.D., Wells, K., Rogers, W.H., and Berry, S.D. (1989) Functional status and well-being of patients with chronic conditions. Results from the medical outcomes study. *Journal of the American Medical Association* **262**: 907–13.

Stewart, S., Pearson, S., and Horowitz, J.D. (1998) Effects of a home-based intervention among patients with congestive heart failure discharged from acute hospital care. *Archives of Internal Medicine* **158**: 1067–72.

Sullivan, M.J., Higginbotham, M.B., and Cobb, F.R. (1988a) Increased exercise ventilation in patients with chronic heart failure: intact ventilatory control despite hemodynamic and pulmonary abnormalities. *Circulation* **77**: 552–9 (Abstract).

Sullivan, M.J., Higginbotham, M.B., and Cobb, F.R. (1988b) Exercise training in patients with severe left ventricular dysfunction: hemodynamic and metabolic effects. *Circulation* **78**: 506–16.

SUPPORT Principal Investigators, The (1995). A controlled trial to improve care for seriously ill hospitalized patients. The study to understand prognoses and preferences for outcomes and risks of treatments (SUPPORT). [see comments] [published erratum appears in JAMA 1996 April 24; 275 (16): 1232]. *Journal of the American Medical Association* **274**: 1591–8.

Swedberg, K., Eneroth, P., Kjekshus, J., and Wilhelmsen, L. (1990) Hormones regulating cardiovascular function in patients with severe congestive heart failure and their relation to mortality. CONSENSUS Trial Study Group. *Circulation* **82**: 1730–6.

Task Force of the Working Group on Heart Failure of the European Society of Cardiology, The (1997). The treatment of heart failure. *European Heart Journal* **18**: 736–53.

Task Force on Heart Failure of the European Society of Cardiology, The (1995). Guidelines for the diagnosis of heart failure. *European Heart Journal* **16**: 741–51.

Tolins, M., Weir, E.K., Chesler, E., and Pierpont, G.L. (1984). 'Maximal' drug therapy is not necessarily optimal in chronic angina pectoris. *Journal of the American College of Cardiology* **3**: 1051–7.

Tsevat, J., Dawson, N.V., Wu, A.W., Lynn, J., Soukup, J.R., Cook, E.F., Vidaillet, H., and Phillips, R.S. (1998). Health values of hospitalised patients 80 years or older. HELP Investigators. Hospitalized elderly longitudinal project. *Journal of the American Medical Association* **279**: 371–5.

Uretsky, B.F. and Sheahan, R.G. (1997). Primary prevention of sudden cardiac death in heart failure: will the solution be shocking? *Journal of the American College of Cardiology* **30**: 1589–97.

Vinson, J.M., Rich, M.W., Sperry, J.C., Shah, A.S., and McNamara, T. (1990). Early readmission of elderly patients with congestive heart failure. *Journal of the American Geriatric Society* **38**: 1290–5.

Weinberger, M., Oddone, E.Z., and Henderson, W.G. (1996). Does increased access to primary care reduce hospital readmissions? Veterans affairs cooperative study group on primary care and hospital readmission. *New England Journal of Medicine* **334**: 1441–7.

Wenger, N.K. (1989). Quality of life: can it and should it be assessed in patients with heart failure? *Cardiology* **76**: 391–398.

Willens, H.J., Blevins, R.D., Wrisley, D., Antonishen, D., Reinstein, D., and Rubenfire, M. (1987). The prognostic value of functional capacity in patients with mild to moderate heart failure. *American Heart Journal* **114**: 377–82.

Willund, I., Gorkin, L., Pawitan, Y., Schron, E., Schoenberger, J., Jared, L.L., and Shumaker, S. (1992). Methods for assessing quality of life in the cardiac arrhythmia suppression trial (CAST). *Quality of Life Research* **1**: 187–201.

Chapter 4

Neurodegenerative disease

Tony O'Brien

Introduction

Specialist palliative care services have an important and evolving role to play in the care of patients with advanced and progressive neurodegenerative disease. The philosophies and skills that were developed in respect of cancer patients are readily applicable to selected groups of patients with non-malignant conditions, including those with neurodegenerative disease. The successful integration of patients with neurodegenerative disease into hospice care was first described by Saunders *et al.* (1981). Since then, research and experience has confirmed the important role of specialist palliative care services in the provision of care to such patients and their families (O'Brien *et al.* 1992).

The proportion of patients referred to specialist care programmes who have neurodegenerative rather than malignant disease varies depending on the age group under consideration. In the case of adults, the proportion of patients with neurodegenerative disease is quite small and rarely exceeds 5% of total referrals. In children and young adults, a large range of neurodegenerative disorders are described including the mucopolyssaccharidoses, Batten's disease, the leucodystrophies, and various forms of encephalopathies and encephalitis. Of over 300 children admitted to a children's hospice between 1982 and 1993, 41% had a neurodegenerative disease (Hunt and Burne 1995).

Neurodegenerative disorders are characterised by progressive deterioration in motor, sensory or cognitive status resulting in loss of function, increasing debility, and dependence. The causes of many of these conditions are as yet unidentified and, in general, there are no known cures. Much research is concerned with gaining a greater understanding of the precise aetiologies and in developing disease modifying drugs. Whilst the search for cures continues, these patients must be offered an optimal level of palliation to ensure that they have the best possible quality of life.

This chapter focuses on the palliative care of adult patients with the more common, progressive neurodegenerative conditions. It examines the principles of care that apply to patients with multiple sclerosis (MS), motor neurone disease/amyotrophic lateral sclerosis (MND/ALS), Parkinson's disease (PD), and Huntington's disease (HD). The neurodegenerative conditions of childhood, cerebrovascular disease and Alzheimer's disease are considered in Chapters 3, 5, and 9.

Specific disease states

Multiple sclerosis

Multiple sclerosis is a demyelinating disease that particularly affects the spinal cord, optic nerves, and brain stem. In Britain, the prevalence is 80–100 per 100 000 population. The disease is characterised by demyelination, inflammatory change, and gliosis. The age of onset is typically between 20–50 years with a mean of 29–30 years. Most patients have a relapsing and remitting illness, with varying degrees of recovery between episodes. Approximately one in four patients with MS pursue a relatively benign course characterised by mild exacerbations followed by complete recovery. At the other end of the spectrum, 10% of patients have a devastating illness, progressing rapidly to severe disability. Young age at onset, absence of Babinski's, motor and cerebellar signs, onset with optic neuritis, long interval between the first two flare- ups, and lack of residual deficit are all associated with a more favourable prognosis.

Diagnosis may be suspected on clinical evidence in patients presenting with optic neuritis or transverse myelitis. The advent of magnetic resonance imaging (MRI) of the brain and spinal cord has contributed significantly to the diagnosis and management of this disorder; a brain MRI is abnormal in 99% of patients with definite MS (Ormerod *et al.* 1987). MRI scanning may confirm the presence of demyelination in patients with clinically suspect disease; may detect asymptomatic lesions elsewhere in the CNS, and will facilitate monitoring of disease progression and response to drug therapy.

An acute exacerbation of MS is treated with high dose steroids. This will not, however, impact on the long-term course of the disease. Immunosuppressive treatments such as azathioprine, cyclosporine, cyclophosphamide, and plasma exchange have had disappointing results in clinical trials (Hawkins 1998). The role of the anti-inflammatory cytokine interferon beta is currently under review; it has been shown to cause a modest reduction in relapse rate and lesion load in patients with relapsing/remitting MS (IFNB Multiple sclerosis study group 1993).

Motor neurone disease/amyotrophic lateral sclerosis

Motor neurone disease/amyotrophic lateral sclerosis (MND/ALS) is a progressive and ultimately fatal neurodegenerative disorder. The disease impacts mainly on the corticospinal tracts and lower motor neurones of the brain stem and spinal cord. With the exception of rare familial forms that are typically inherited in an autosomal dominant fashion, the cause is unknown.

The incidence of MND/ALS varies between 1 and 2 per 100 000 population and the prevalence is 4–6 per 100 000. In the UK, about 1200 new cases are diagnosed each year, and at any one time there are approximately 6000 patients living with the disorder (Cardy 1993). The peak incidence occurs between ages 60 and 70 years, but it can affect patients aged from their late teens to the tenth decade. The male/female ratio is 3:2, although it approaches 1:1 in the very elderly. Diagnosis is based on the typical findings of upper and lower motor neurone signs in the absence of sensory and sphincter disturbances. Cognitive function is usually intact although about 2% of patients will develop a type of dementia. In 20–50% of patients, neuropsychological features indicative of frontal and temporal lobe dysfunction can be demonstrated (Kew *et al.* 1993)

There is often a long delay between the onset of first symptoms and subsequent diagnosis. O'Brien (1992) reported a mean interval of 13.5 months, whilst an earlier study reported intervals of 22 and 24 months for men and women respectively (Newrick and Langton-Hewer 1984). Patients usually present with a history of progressive weakness of limb or bulbar muscles, although some present with respiratory failure (de Carvalho *et al.* 1996). There is no specific diagnostic test, and it is often difficult to make the diagnosis in the condition's early stages. The El Escorial criteria, developed in 1990 by the World Federation of Neurology, require a combination of lower and upper motor neurone signs and disease progression (Table 4.1). Electrophysiological studies may support the criteria, but are not essential for diagnosis.

Table 4.1 El Escorial criteria

The diagnosis of MND/ALS requires the presence of:
1 LMN signs (may include EMG signs in clinically normal muscles)
2 UMN signs
3 Progression of the disorder
Subclassification of diagnostic criteria:
Definite MND/ALS – UMN and LMN signs in three regions
Probable MND/ALS – UMN and LMN signs in two regions, with UMN
signs rostral to LMN
Possible MND/ALS – UMN and LMN signs in one region, or UMN signs
in two or three regions
Suspected MND/ALS – LMN signs in two or three regions
Regions are defined as brain stem, brachial, thorax and trunk, and crural.
The diagnosis of MND/ALS is supported by the following features:
1 Fasciculation in one or more regions
2 Neurogenic change in EMG studies
3 Normal motor and sensory nerve conduction
4 Absence of motor conduction block
The diagnosis of MND/ALS requires the absence of the following clinical features:
1 Sensory signs
2 Sphincter disturbances
3 Visual disturbances
4 Autonomic dysfunction
5 Parkinson's disease
6 Alzheimer-type dementia
7 Certain mimic syndromes, e.g. lymphoma, acute infections, postradiation

LMN: lower motor neurone
UMN: upper motor neurone

The antiglutamate agent riluzole slows disease progression to a limited extent in selected patients but as yet, there is no known cure.

Parkinson's disease

Parkinson's disease (PD) was first described by James Parkinson in 1817. One per 100 000 of the population are affected: this increases to 1 per 200 among those aged over 65 years. The mean age at onset is 55–60 years. The characteristic pathological abnormality is a loss of pigmented neurones in the pars compacta of the substantia nigra. A deficiency of dopamine leads to a functional excess of acetylcholine. The degenerating neurones contain eosinophilic inclusion bodies called Lewy bodies. The underlying cause is unknown although genetic factors are likely to play an important role in a minority of patients. The pethidine derived toxin 1-methyl-4-phenyl-1,2,3,6-tetrahydropyridine (MPTP), when inadvertently injected by a group of heroin addicts, caused the classic symptoms and signs of PD (*Morbidity and Mortality Weekly Report* 1984). At present there is no cure for PD. Drug and surgical treatments are designed to achieve an improvement in symptoms and functional status.

The clinical features comprise: a medium amplitude tremor, especially at rest, that is most marked in the hands (resulting in pill-rolling movements); muscle rigidity, often affecting the neck and trunk, and when combined with tremor of the hands, gives rise to the so called 'cogwheel phenomenon'; bradykinesia/akinesia, characterised by a delay in initiation of movement; and an absence of spontaneous movements including blinking and postural changes, characterised by generalised flexion of the neck, trunk, and limbs. Patients with PD often appear to have little change in facial expression or appear to stare and speak in a soft, barely audible voice. The disease is associated with depression, personality changes, sleep disturbances, and dementia.

Huntington's disease

Huntington's disease is a chronic progressive neurodegenerative disorder affecting movement, cognition, and personality. It is genetically transmitted by an autosomal dominant gene and affects males and females equally. The prevalence of the clinical disorder is 5–10 per 100 000 population. The number of gene carriers is estimated at 20 per 100 000 population (Conneally 1984). The age of onset is typically between the ages of 35 and 40 years although a juvenile variant form may manifest before age 20 years.

Clinically, the disease is characterised by both abnormal involuntary and voluntary movement which deteriorate over the course of the disease. Choreoathetotic (swinging) movements involving the upper limbs and oro-buccal-facial regions are common. The oro-buccal movements may interfere with articulation, chewing, and swallowing. Mental disturbances are also common and include depression, mania, hypomania, violent and anti-social behaviour, and schizophrenia-like psychosis. The mental disturbances may pre-date the onset of the movement disorder. Cognitive impairment is usually apparent at the onset of the movement disorder and follows a progressive and unremitting course.

Two remarkable discoveries within the last 15 years have enabled a preclinical diagnosis to be made with confidence. The discovery in 1983 of a linkage between HD and a restriction fragment polymorphism on chromosome 4 provided a preclinical diagnostic marker with up to 98% accuracy (Gusella *et al.*1983; Magenis *et al.*1986; Tibben *et al.*1992). The discovery in

1993 of the Huntington's mutation, an expansion of a trinucleotide repeat at a gene IT-15 on chromosome 4 and its novel protein product 'huntingtin' was an important advance in the understanding of the pathogenesis of HD (Huntington's Disease Collaborative Research Group , HDCRG 1993). It enables the provision of preclinical (including prenatal) screening for the Huntington's disease gene without extensive genetic testing of family members.

These developments create complex ethical, social, and personal issues for at risk individuals. Hayes, as president of the Huntington's Society of America, commented in an editorial for the *New England Journal of Medicine:* 'In the abstract, it is easy to think that you would want to know. When it is time to find out, the possibility of a positive test is frightening. How many of us would really choose to be told how we would die?' Enthusiasm for preclinical diagnosis is not shared by all at risk individuals. Adam *et al.* (1989) reported that as few as 18% of at risk individuals had participated in predictive testing programmes.

Communicating the diagnosis

The diagnosis of these various disorders will usually be made, or at least confirmed by, a neurologist. Once the diagnosis is established, it is essential that all patients and their families are offered the opportunity to receive clear, factual information concerning their illness, treatment options, and prognosis to whatever extent they feel comfortable with. The patient sets the pace and depth of these discussions and health care professionals must be sensitive to the patient's right to deny. The question is not *whether* to tell or not, but how, how much, and at what pace?

As well as sharing factual information, the patient and family should be enabled to express their feelings and emotions. The manner in which the news is conveyed to patients and the degree to which they feel supported at the time will have a significant impact on their ability to cope with the illness and its future progression. This process of breaking bad news is not an one-off event. It is rather an evolutionary process during which patients and their families gradually come to a greater understanding of the nature and implications of their disease. All neurodegenerative diseases are characterised by a progressive series of losses in function, role, independence, and, ultimately, life itself. Patients must be confident that they can rely on their family and professional carers for support, care, and honesty.

Johnston *et al.* (1996) reported on a cross-sectional study that examined the experiences of 50 patients who had received a diagnosis of MND/ALS in the previous 6 months. Allowing for the limitations inherent in the study design, the researchers reached the following conclusions:

1 most patients see positive aspects to being told the diagnosis of MND/ALS, especially in providing a label for their condition;

2 patients prefer the diagnosis be communicated in direct, empathetic style, with someone else present;

3 being able to ask questions was associated with overall satisfaction, perhaps because it enabled patients for whom the diagnosis was worse than expected to reach a better understanding of what they had been told;

4 doctors did not give too optimistic an account of the disease and some patients found that they were unnecessarily pessimistic;

5 information on what to do, especially about obtaining further information, may be important at the time of diagnosis;

6 there was no evidence that poor communications were associated with later mood disturbances.

This final conclusion seems at variance with conventional wisdom and merits further evaluation. The researchers postulated that the results from this study on MND/ALS patients may be extrapolated to other patient groups with progressive, degenerative and incurable diseases.

Symptom control

Neurodegenerative diseases have the capacity to evoke the most negative and despondent attitudes in the minds of many health care professionals. This attitude may readily transmit to patients and their families. The fact that we cannot significantly alter disease progression is sometimes interpreted to mean that there is nothing more to be done (Norris 1992). This is both inaccurate and regrettable. It is precisely because we cannot reverse or even retard the disease process that we must do everything possible to alleviate symptoms and offer appropriate psychosocial and spiritual support.

Many of the neurodegenerative disorders are relatively rare conditions. For example, a typical general practitioner may expect to see no more than one or two new cases of MND/ALS in his/her professional life. Consequently, members of the primary health care team may not feel entirely competent in managing these disorders. However, the essential point to note is that whilst the individual disorders are rare, the symptoms that occur in association with these disorders are extraordinarily common. Symptoms such as pain, breathlessness, constipation, and insomnia are commonly encountered and their routine management should fall within the scope of all competent practitioners. Of course, more complex issues of nutritional support using an enteral feeding system, or evaluation of respiratory function with a view to possible ventilatory support, will require specialist input.

A series of 124 MND patients admitted to a hospice were compared to cancer patients admitted to the same hospice (O'Brien *et al.* 1992). Pain was less prevalent in the MND patients (57% versus 69%) whilst insomnia (48% versus 29%) and constipation (65% versus 48%) were more prevalent; breathlessness was equally common in the two groups (47% versus 50%). At referral, only 15 patients (12%) were receiving an opioid even though 71 patients (57%) had uncontrolled pain. During their hospice course, 109 patients received an opioid on at least one occasion. The mean dose used was morphine 30 mg orally every 24 hours and the mean duration of treatment was 58 (18.5) days. This study demonstrated the safety and efficacy of morphine in the management of pain, breathlessness, and insomnia in a hospice population of patients with advanced MND/ALS. Established principles of symptom control must be applied to all patients with neurodegenerative disorders.

Pain

Pain occurs in around half of patients with MS (Moulin 1989) and up to three-quarters of patients with MND/ALS (O'Brien *et al.* 1992). In MS, Moulin described three pain syndromes: dysaesthetic extremity pain, back pain, and painful leg spasms.

Musculoskeletal pain is commonly associated with spasticity, gait disturbances, and poor sitting posture. Pseudoradicular pain secondary to plaque formation on a sensory nerve is also described and often presents as paroxysmal facial pains indistinguishable from tic douloureux. In MND/ALS, pains are described as aching, cramping, burning, shock-like, and simply 'indescribable'. The stiffness associated with prolonged immobility is often troublesome and the fact of knowing that one cannot move is in itself a source of considerable distress. In PD, pain most commonly affects the lower limbs: the mechanism for this type of pain is not known.

Management involves the early introduction of physiotherapy and occupational therapy. Advice on correct posture, passive exercises and the use of appropriate aids are vitally important. Pains associated with immobility and stiffness will often respond to anti-inflammatory agents—frequently in combination with low dose opioids. Pains with a more obvious neuropathic basis will require specific therapy with a tricyclic antidepressant and/or anticonvulsant. TENS (transcutaneous electric nerve stimulation) therapy may also be of benefit in these situations. Spasticity in MS may require specific treatment with baclofen, diazepam, or dantroloene. The last is used with caution because of hepatotoxicity. More recently, tizanidine has become available as an oral treatment for spasticity associated with MS and spinal cord injury. Initial data suggests that this new agent reduces spasticity whilst maintaining muscle strength.

Dysphagia/nutritional problems

A high proportion of patients with neurodegenerative disease will develop dysphagia. Associated symptoms and concerns relate to salivary dribbling, fear of choking attacks, weight loss, progressive malnourishment, and aspiration pneumonia. Family members may feel obliged to ensure that their loved ones maintain a high calorie intake in order to sustain life. At a practical level, a single meal may take between two to three hours to complete, and ultimately meal times become a source of regular confrontation and intense frustration for all concerned.

Detailed and regular assessments should be undertaken by an inter-professional team including a speech and language therapist, an occupational therapist, a nutritionist, and a physiotherapist, in addition to the patient's own medical and nursing team. Advice on correct positioning of the neck, swallowing techniques, the use of adapted cutlery and utensils, mobile arm supports, and dietary modifications may help to maintain an independent eating pattern for longer. In some centres, more detailed evaluation of the swallowing reflex is undertaken using video fluoroscopy. This technique provides detailed information on the oral preparatory, oral, and pharyngeal phases of swallowing.

The management goals of dysphagic patients include the maintenance of independent eating and drinking for as long as possible. If a patient cannot maintain an adequate intake despite oral supplementation, they should actively consider the use of assisted enteral feeding. Specifically, assisted enteral feeding is indicated if patients are feeling hungry or thirsty, if they are losing weight (>10% of usual body weight), if meals are taking an excessive amount of time to complete, or if patients are experiencing regular 'choking' episodes.

Nasogastric tubes are generally unsatisfactory for long-term enteral nutrition. The preferred option involves the use of a gastrostomy tube which may be sited endoscopically (PEG (percutaneous endoscopic gastrostomy) tube), radiologically, or surgically. Alternatively, a jejunal tube may be employed. The patient may continue to take small amounts orally if desired. The timing of the introduction of assisted enteral feeding systems is critical. Obviously, too early an introduction deprives the patient of a very important function prematurely. However, if we delay excessively, patients will already have a serious nutritional deficit and no longer be in an in optimum condition for any procedure.

Patients who are using assisted enteral feeding systems must have access to support and advice on a 24-hour basis. They may elect to be fed continuously for a defined period e.g. overnight using a pumped system. Alternatively, they may opt to use intermittent bolus feeds of 200–300 ml every few hours using a syringe. Tube blockage is a common problem and regular flushing of the tube with water after a feed is essential. If the blockage persists, flush with warm water; alternatively, try flushing with soda water, dilute pineapple juice, or carbonated drink.

Salivary dribbling

Patients with a bulbar palsy will frequently find it difficult to swallow their own saliva. Consequently, saliva is seen to drool from the mouth which causes local soreness and excoriation. This is a source of considerable distress and embarrassment. Drug therapy is aimed at reducing the volume of saliva produced. The dose of the anticholinergic agent employed must be carefully titrated so as to avoid an excessively dry mouth or the production of very viscid secretions which are extremely difficult to expectorate. Hyoscine hydrobromide may be tried either in a patch or sublingual preparation. Alternatively, a low dose tricyclic antidepressant such as amitriptyline may be of benefit. Radiotherapy may be necessary in refractory cases but, again, achieving a balance between reducing secretions and leaving patients with an uncomfortably dry mouth is difficult.

Breathlessness/respiratory problems

Respiratory complications are a common source of morbidity and mortality in neurodegenerative diseases. A combination of immobility, aspiration, poor cough reflex, progressive weakness of the intercostal and diaphragmatic muscles, and malnutrition all, predispose these patients to infection. The clinical signs of infection may be minimal and it is important to maintain a high index of suspicion. Appropriate antibiotic therapy and physiotherapy will be required for selected patients.

In MND/ALS, death usually occurs as a result of acute or acute on chronic ventilatory failure. Many patients are very fearful of the mode and manner of their death, and will speak of their fear of 'choking'. This is an unfortunate term that is both inappropriate and inaccurate when applied to the cause of death in MND/ALS (O'Brien et al. 1992). Rarely, MND/ALS may present as acute respiratory failure in ambulatory patients without significant swallowing difficulties.

Breathlessness at rest, in the absence of reversible causes such as cardiac failure or infection, usually signifies a poor prognosis. Symptoms may be relieved by careful attention to positioning and by explanation and reassurance. Pharmacological treatments are directed towards relieving anxiety and reducing subjective distress associated with the work of breathing. In this regard, regular low dose oral morphine often in combination with a benzodiazepine will offer good symptomatic benefit. If patients are unable to tolerate oral medication, a continuous subcutaneous infusion may be initiated. Some breathless patients derive symptomatic benefit from oxygen therapy, or from the use of a strategically placed fan.

The issue of offering ventilatory support is more complex. Practice varies world-wide and seem to be more influenced by culture, custom, and tradition, rather than science. In the US, about 10% of MND/ALS patients receive home ventilatory support in the form of intermittent positive pressure ventilation (IPPV) at an average annual cost of $150 000 (Lloyd and

Leigh 1998). Traditionally, ventilation was achieved via a tracheostomy. More recently, the advent of nasal IPPV has provided an alternative (Cazzolli and Oppenheimer 1996).

It is sometimes assumed that the use of mechanical ventilation will inevitably result in a deterioration in overall quality of life. However, McDonald et al. (1996) compared the physical and psychological status of 18 MND/ALS patients on ventilatory support for between 1 and 120 months with that of 126 patients who did not receive ventilatory support. The two groups did not differ in levels of depression, hopelessness, quality of life, or psychological well-being. In another study focusing on patients receiving IPPV, 90% of patients said they were glad they had chosen the option and would do so again. However, family carers were less enthusiastic, with only 50% saying they would choose it for themselves (Moss et al. 1993).

The role of ventilatory support raises complex practical, ethical and social issues for patients, families and professional carers. These issues must be fully evaluated and explored before any mode of treatment is agreed or dismissed.

Dysarthria/anarthria/communication difficulties

In palliative care, considerable importance is attached to the principles of good communication between individual patients and their carers. In the case of neurodegenerative disease, patients may be unable to articulate clearly and, in some instances, their speech is totally unintelligible. Because communication is a two-way interaction, both parties are in fact 'paralysed'. The inability to communicate is a source of intense frustration.

Early assessment by a speech and language therapist and also by an occupational therapist is mandatory. It may be possible to teach patients techniques to enable them derive maximum benefit from grossly impaired articulation. Depending on the extent of their limb involvement and their cognitive status, it may be possible to introduce various aids to communication including picture charts and typewriters, some of which may have a voice synthesiser.

Even in the absence of any intelligible speech and a total inability to use any aids or devices, patients can often communicate at least their physical needs by means of facial gestures, grimacing, or some other muscle movement. Family carers and nurses who spend long periods of time with such patients are frequently quite expert at interpreting even the most subtle messages. If, despite your very best efforts, you are not able to understand what a patient is trying to say, it is always better to acknowledge that you cannot understand rather than to pretend that you do. In these circumstances, allow the patient to rest for a time and try again.

Bladder dysfunction

Approximately 50–80% of MS patients will develop evidence of bladder dysfunction (Augspurger 1985). Symptoms may include urgency, hesitancy, frequency, retention and incontinence. Detrusor hyperactivity is a common end-stage urodynamic pattern. Urinary frequency and urgency can be suppressed by oxybutinin. If bladder emptying is troublesome, it may be necessary to try intermittent bladder self-catherisation.

Sphincter function is usually preserved in MND/ALS. Continence may, however, be compromised by impaired mobility. An occupational therapy assessment of the patient in their usual environment is essential. Urinary tract infections are likely to occur in immobile debilitated patients, particularly if their fluid intake is less than adequate.

Depression/anxiety

Disturbances of mood are commonly associated with progressive neurodegenerative disease. Hogg *et al.* (1994) reported that in patients with MND/ALS, a correlation exists between increasing physical dependency and depression, and also between speech impairment and anxiety. In the case of MS, a number of studies reported an association between disease activity and depression. The unpredictable course of MS was cited as a potent stressor (Brooks and Matson 1982). Tedman *et al.* (1997) found no difference in the incidence and severity of depression in 40 MND/ALS patients as compared to 92 MS patients. In the MND/ALS group, there was a significant association between pain severity scores and depression, but no association between depression and functional status. In the MS group, there was a weak association increasing physical disability and depression.

Health care professionals must be aware of the possibility of depressive illness in patients with neurodegenerative disease, and if diagnosed, appropriate therapy usually with antidepressants should be instituted.

Teamwork

It is evident that the care of patients with progressive neurodegenerative disease requires input from a range of professional disciplines, in community, hospital, and hospice settings. The overall objective is to ensure that patients achieve and maintain an optimal level of symptom control and functional status at all stages of their illness. Care will inevitably involve a great deal of explanation, reassurance, and support. Voluntary bodies have an important practical and supportive role to play in this regard.

Each member of the inter-professional team must be competent in their own skills and must also have an awareness of teamwork. They must be willing to share their own expertise freely, and must have an awareness of the important role of other team members. This will require a willingness to involve other health care professionals in the caring process at the appropriate time. Clear, rapid, and comprehensive systems of communication must be established and maintained. Poor communication, often associated with professional rivalries and jealousies, is utterly destructive and very detrimental to the caring process. The concept of a co-ordinating 'key worker' has many merits.

Summary

In caring for patients with advanced neurodegenerative disease, we must focus on what is still possible and on what can still be achieved. Work to develop a greater understanding of the pathophysiology of these conditions continues, with the objective of identifying cures. In the meantime patients and families need continuing care and support. In particular, they must never again be told that there is nothing more to be done. There is always more to be done. Patients and their families expect and deserve nothing less.

References

Adam, S., Wiggins, S., Bloch, M., *et al.* Five year study of prenatal testing for Huntington's disease, demand, attitudes, and psychological assessment. *Journal of Medical Genetics*, **30**: 549–56.

Augspurger, R.R. (1985). Bladder dysfunction in multiple sclerosis. In Maloney, F.P., Burke, J.S., and

Ringel, S.P. (eds), *Interdisciplinary rehabilitation of multiple sclerosis and neuromuscular disorders.* J.B. Lippincott Co., Philadelphia, pp. 48–61.

Bensimon, G., Lacomblez, L., Meininger V., and the ALS/Riluzole study group. (1994). A controlled trial of riluzole in amytrophic lateral sclerosis. *New England Journal of Medicine* **330**: 585–91.

Brooks, N.A. and Matson, R.R. (1982) Social–psychological adjustments to multiple sclerosis: a longitudinal study. *Social Scientis and Medicine* **16**: 2129–38.

Cardy, P. (1993). Research and the associations: an era for partnership. *Palliative Medicine* **7** (Suppl. 2): 3–9.

Cazzolli, P.A. and Oppenheimer, E.A. (1996) Home mechanical ventilation for amyotrophic lateral sclerosis: nasal compared to tracheostomy-intermittent positive pressure ventilation. *Journal of the Neurological Sciences* **193** (Suppl.): 123–8.

Conneally, P.M. (1984). Huntington's disease: genetics and epidemiology. *American Journal of Human Genetics* **36**: 506–26.

de Carvalho, M., Matias, T., Coelho, F., Evangelista, T., Pinto, A., and Sales Luis, M.L. (1996). Motor neurone disease presenting with respiratory failure. *Journal of the Neurological Sciences* **139**: 117–22.

Gusella, J.F., Wexler, N.S., Conneally, P.M., Naylor, S.L., Anderson, M.A., and Tanzi, R.E. *et al.* (1983). A polymorphic DNA marker genetically linked to Huntington's disease. *Nature* **306**: 234–8.

Hawkins, C.P. (1998). Spinal features of multiple sclerosis. In Engler, G.L., Cole, J., Merton, W.L. (eds), *Spinal Cord Disease—Diagnosis and Treatment.* New York: Marcel Dekker, pp. 399–412.

Hogg, K.E., Goldstein, L.H., and Leigh, P.N. (1994). The psychological impact of motor neurone disease. *Psychological Medicine* **24**: 625–32.

Hunt, A. and Burne, R. (1995). Medical and nursing problems of children with neurodegenerative disease. *Palliative Medicine* **9**: 19–26.

Huntington's Disease Collaborative Research Group (1993). A novel gene containing a trinucleotide repeat that is expanded and unstable on Huntington's disease chromosomes. *Cell* **72**: 971–83.

IFNB Multiple sclerosis study group. (1993). Interferon beta-1b is effective in relapsing–remitting multiple sclerosis. 1. Clinical results of a multicentre, randomized, double-blind, placebo-controlled trial. *Neurology* **43**: 655–61.

Johnston, M., Earll, L., Mitchell, E., Morrison, V., and Wright, S. (1996). Communicating the diagnosis of motor neurone disease. *Palliative Medicine* **10**: 23–34.

Kew, J.J.M., Leigh, P.N., and Playford, E.D. (1993). Cortical function in amyotrophic lateral sclerosis: a positron emission tomographic study. *Brain* **116**: 655–80.

Lloyd, C.M. and Leigh, P.N. (1998). Motor neurone disease. In Engler, G.L., Cole, J., Merton, W.L. (eds), *Spinal Cord Disease—Diagnosis and Treatment.* New York: Marcel Dekker, p. 433.

McDonald, E.R., Hillel, A., Weidenfeld, S.A. (1996). Evaluation of the Psychological Status of Ventilatory – supported patients with ALS/MND. *Palliative Medicines* **10**: 35–41.

Magenis, R.E., Gusella, J., Weliky, K., Olson, S., Haight, G., Toth-Fejel, S. *et al.* (1986). Huntington disease-linked restriction fragment length polymorphism localized within band p16.1 of chromosome 4 by insitu hybridization. *American Journal of Human Genetics* **39**: 383–91.

Morbidity and Mortality Weekly Report (1984). **33**(24): 351–2.

Moss, A.H., Casey, P., Stocking, C.B., Roos, R.P., Brooks, B.R., and Siegler, M. (1993). Home ventilation for amyotrophic lateral sclerosis patients: outcomes, costs, patient, family and physician attitudes. *Neurology* **43**: 438–43.

Moulin, D.E. (1989). Pain in multiple sclerosis. *Neurologic Clinics* **7**: 321–31.

Newrick, P.G. and Langton-Hewer, R. (1984). Motor neurone disease: can we do better? A study of 42 patients. *British Medical Journal* **289**: 539–42.

Norris, F.H. (1992). Motor neurone disease—treating the untreated. *British Medical Journal* **304**: 459–60.

O'Brien, T., Kelly, M., and Saunders, C. (1992). Motor neurone disease: a hospice perspective. *British Medical Journal* **304**: 471–3.

Oppenheimer, E.A. (1993). Decision-making in the respiratory care of amyotrophic lateral sclerosis: should home mechanical ventilation be used? *Palliative Medicine* **7** (Suppl. 2): 49–64.

Ormerod, I.E.C., Miller, D.H., McDonald, W.I., *et al.* (1987). The role of NMR imaging in the assessment of multiple sclerosis and isolated neurological lesions. *Brain* **110**: 1579–1616.

Saunders, C., Walsh, T.D., and Smith, M. (1981). Hospice care in motor neurone disease. In Saunders, C., Summers, D.H., and Teller, N. (eds), *Hospice: the living idea*. London: Edward Arnold, pp. 126–47.

Swash, M. and Leigh, P.N. (1990) Workshop report—criteria for diagnosis of familial amyotrophic lateral sclerosis. *Neuromuscular Disorders* **2**(1): 7–9.

Tedman, B.M., Young, C.A., and Williams, I.R. (1997). Assessment of depression in patients with motor neurone disease and other neurologically disabling illness. *Journal of Neurological Science* **152**(1): S75–9.

Tibben, A., Vegter van der Vlis, M., Skraastad, M.I., Frets, P.G., van der Kamp, J.J., Niermeijer, M.F. *et al.* (1992). DNA testing for Huntington's disease in the Netherlands: a retrospective study of psychosocial effects. *American Journal of Human Genetics* **44**: 94–9.

Chapter 5

Children and young adults

Ann Goldman and Ildiko Schuller

Introduction

Fortunately most children grow into adulthood without experiencing serious illness. However, good support and palliative care are essential for those who are born with or develop a life-threatening disease. Focusing on the needs of children with life-threatening illness as a group and the development of paediatric palliative care as a specialty is relatively new compared with adult palliative care, but it has been developing rapidly over the last ten years. We hope this chapter will highlight some of the particular problems of care for children, the differences from adult care and the evolving models of services.

Which children need palliative care

Palliative care for children and young adults embraces a whole range of life-threatening diseases, which differ considerably from those causing anticipated deaths in adults (Table 5.1). They cover a wide variety of pathological problems, may develop at any time from birth into early adulthood and the time course of the illness may vary from a few days to many years. The recent report from ACT (The Association for Children with Life Threatening or Terminal Conditions and their Families) and the RCPCH (The Royal College of Paediatrics and Child Health) has identified four broad categories (ACT and RCPCH 1997), which can be helpful when considering the children's and families' needs (Table 5.2).

Depending on the diagnosis the introduction of palliative care for some children is not always clear cut, and various models for the relationship between palliative care and curative therapy have been suggested (Figure 5.1) (ACT and RCPCH 1997). For some children palliation may be instituted after some time when it is finally realised that the child has a terminal illness, while in others it may be commenced from the time of diagnosis. In some cases the emphasis of care shifts gradually to palliative care. In other situations, for example HIV/AIDS or cystic fibrosis, the situation is less obvious and highly technical invasive treatments may be used, entirely appropriately, alongside palliative therapy, with each becoming dominant at different stages of the disease. For some children, such as those suffering from organ failure or cystic fibrosis (Robinson *et al.* 1997), intensive therapy may be continued throughout in the hope of obtaining an organ transplant or a final cure, and some studies have revealed that the life-limiting nature of the disease can remain unacknowledged, both by professionals and families (Thornes 1998; While *et al.* 1996).

Table 5.1 Life-threatening diseases in children

Diseases	Examples
Malignant diseases	leukemia, neuroblastoma
Metabolic disorders	Mucopolysaccharidoses, disorders of lipid metabolism
Disorders of blood and of blood forming organs	Aplastic anaemia, Fanconi syndrome
Diseases of the immune system	Wiscott Aldrich syndrome, severe combined immunodeficiency syndrome
Diseases of the nervous system	Batten disease, spinal muscular atrophy, Duchenne muscular dystrophy, severe cerebral palsy
Diseases of the cardiovascular system	Congenital anomalies of the heart, cardiac myopathy
Diseases of the respiratory system	Cystic fibrosis
Diseases of the digestive system	Chronic liver failure, short bowel syndrome
Diseases of the genito-urinary system	Chronic renal failure
Congenital anomalies and chromosomal disorders	Edward syndrome (trisomy 18), Patau syndrome (trisomy 13)
Disorders of the skin and subcutaneous tissues	Epidermolysis bullosa
Musculo-skeletal disorders	Systemic lupus erythematosus

Source: OPCS Data 1995, DHS Publication 13.

Table 5.2 Groups of life-threatening diseases

Life-threatening conditions for which curative treatment may be feasible but can fail. Palliative care may be needed during times of prognostic uncertainty or when treatment fails, for example, cancer and irreversible organ failure.

Conditions where there may be long periods of intensive treatment aimed at prolonging life and enabling participation in normal childhood activities, but where premature death is anticipated, for example, cystic fibrosis, muscular dystrophy and acquired immunodeficiency syndrome.

Progressive conditions where treatment is almost exclusively palliative and may extend for years, for example, Batten disease and the mucopolysaccharidoses.

Conditions with severe non-progressive neurological disability such as severe cerebral palsy, which may lead to weakness and susceptibility to health complications.

The intensity of the need for palliative care and support may vary throughout the course of the disease. As well as at the anticipated times of diagnosis (Colville and Bax 1996; Jeffery and Jeffery 1993) and in the terminal stages, it is also important at critical points in the illness, such as when a child with cystic fibrosis is hospitalised with an infection (Bluebond-Langner 1996), when a child with Duchenne muscular dystrophy is no longer able to walk (Gagliardi 1991), or when a child with a neurodegenerative condition loses the ability to communicate.

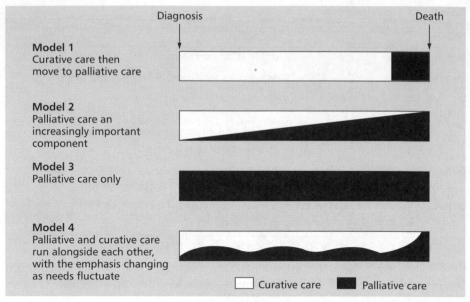

Fig 5.1 Curative and palliative care relationship.

How many children are likely to be affected

The number of children dying from life-threatening diseases is small in comparison with deaths in the adult population. Mortality and morbidity have been difficult to quantify accurately, particularly as these children have not been thought of as a cohesive group until recently. The most up-to-date information, including data from voluntary societies, suggests the figure for the annual mortality rate for children aged between 1 and 17 years with life-limiting conditions is 1 per 10 000, while the morbidity rate is approximately 10 per 10 000. A useful way to look at this is to extrapolate the figures for a district of 250 000 people with a child population of approximately 50 000. In one year 5 children are likely to die from a life-limiting condition: of these 2 would be from cancer, 1 from heart disease and 2 from other life-limiting conditions. About 50 children would be suffering from a life-limiting condition at any one time and about half of these would be needing palliative care (ACT and RCPCH 1997; While *et al.* 1996).

What problems do they have

The problems faced by children, young adults and their families are dependent on many variables (Table 5.3), and each situation will be unique. All these aspects need to be considered in planning an individual child's care. Acknowledgement of a child's current developmental level and their continuing development is essential and needs to be reflected in the management of their care. Children's changing physiological development will influence aspects such as pharmacokinetics, drug therapy and ease of nursing care, whilst their cognitive and emotional levels will affect their understanding of illness and death, their ability to communicate and their need for independence.

Table 5.3 Some factors affecting the needs of dying children and their families

Age	The time course of the disease
Cognitive awareness	Family structure
Diagnosis	Family ethos and communication pattern
The disease trajectory	Social circumstances

As with adults, palliative care in children focuses on enhancement of the quality of life for the child, but also stresses the needs of the whole family. With such a wide range of life-threatening diseases in childhood and young adult life the spectrum of problems is manifold. They fall largely into the headings of medical and nursing management of symptoms, psychosocial support for the child and family, attention to practical needs, including respite care, and educational and spiritual support.

Assessment of symptoms

Assessment of symptoms can pose particular problems in children. A range of well-validated tools, appropriate for children of different cognitive levels, has been developed for evaluating severity of acute pain (Hain 1997) but a broader view is needed for chronic pain. Psychological factors for the child and family, cultural and spiritual issues will also contribute to the picture (RCPCH 1997). Tools for assessing other symptoms barely exist, although those used for nausea and vomiting as a result of chemotherapy could potentially be adapted (Hockenberry-Eaton and Brenner 1990). Formal assessment tools are not helpful for pre-verbal children or those with severe neurological disability. In most situations a combination of approaches is needed, integrating contributions from the child with parents' and staff's observations.

Some common problems

The spectrum of symptoms encountered reflects the different diagnoses and their pathophysiology. For children with progressive cancer, pain is a very significant problem. Others may include gastrointestinal symptoms, dyspnoea, anaemia, bleeding and seizures. In contrast, for those with non-malignant illnesses, pain appears to be a less prominent symptom, although this may in part reflect assumptions on the part of staff and lack of appropriate evaluation. In those with neurological disability pain appears to be particularly associated with muscle spasm, joint pain and oesophagitis (Hunt 1990; Hunt and Burne 1995).

For these children progressive physical disability is a frequent problem causing difficulty in movement, ataxia (inability to co-ordinate), dystonia (abnormal muscle tone) and weakness. Adaptations to the home such as ramps, stair lifts, bath aids and wheelchair access may be required. Communication and speech impairment with or without intellectual impairment is common (Hunt 1990; Hunt and Burne 1995). Feeding and nutrition problems, such as difficulty in swallowing, choking, decisions relating to tube feeding and gastrostomies and difficulty in administration of medicines are frequently encountered.

Respiratory problems, frequent chest infections due to impaired mobility, muscular weakness and physical deformity occur in many children. Those with cystic fibrosis need daily physiotherapy, the administration of nebulised medication and antibiotics. Excess secretions can occur, requiring medication and suction (at home) for difficulty in swallowing and excessive drooling or choking. This is a long-term problem with neurological impairment and neurodegenerative disease, and also may occur in the terminal phase with other children.

Seizures, which may be difficult to control, are an increasing problem with many neuro-degenerative conditions, particularly Batten disease (Hunt 1990; Hunt and Burne 1995). Behaviour problems may occur as part of the disease, for example in the mucopolysaccha-ridoses (in particular San Fillipo syndrome) (Colville and Bax 1996; Bax and Colville 1996). For many children terminal agitation and restlessness may need treatment. Sleep disorders occur in particular for those children with mucopolysaccharidoses (Bax and Colville 1996) and those with hypoxia.

Particular disease related problems may occur. Cystic fibrosis in the later stages may be associated with pneumothoraces that may be treated by intercostal drainage or occasionally thoracic surgery and sometimes pleurodesis (fusion of the pleural membranes). In the later stages of liver failure portal hypertension may develop with oesophageal varices which may need sclerotherapy. Chronic heart disease and failure may be treated specifically, at least in the short term. Respiratory failure in muscular dystrophy necessitates decisions in relation to ventilatory support. Children may be waiting for organ transplants, and therefore addressing symptom management which acknowledges the life-threatening nature of their disease may be a problem for them, their family and staff.

In most cases close attention to details of routine daily care is needed to avoid causing dis-comfort to children with chronic life-threatening diseases. Skin care is important; children with immobility are particularly vulnerable and require frequent turning and special mat-tresses. Constipation requiring oral medication or enemas is a common problem secondary to feeding problems, immobility and medication. Urinary incontinence is a particularly common problem with severely intellectually impaired and disabled children.

Symptom management

Providing effective treatment for children is always dependent on working alongside and co-operatively with the child's primary carers—almost always the parents. They will know their child best and be undertaking the majority of care, so any management plans must be nego-tiated and developed with them and, where possible, the child. Many of the pharmacologi-cal approaches to symptom management are similar to those used in adults; often, however, the drugs used have not been formally recommended for use in children although a body of clinical experience has developed in the absence of trials or pharmacokinetic data (Goldman 1998; WHO 1998). Children often find taking large amounts of drugs difficult and complex regimens may not be possible. They should be offered choices of preparations. Oral drugs are usually possible though alternative routes such as subcutaneous or rectal administration may be needed in the final stages.

Psychosocial problems

While relatively few families face the task of caring for a child with a life-limiting and incur-able disorder, the literature is conclusive in suggesting that the experience takes a heavy toll on families (While *et al.* 1996; Gagliardi 1991; Davies 1996; Mastroyannopoulou *et al.* 1997; Thompson *et al.* 1992). The impact of a chronically sick and increasingly dependent child is dramatic and has social, financial, mental and physical health repercussions on the whole family (While *et al.* 1996). Therefore support for the family is fundamental as parents and siblings are especially vulnerable, often bearing an increasing responsibility for nursing and personal care; it should begin from the time of diagnosis, continue through the illness and extend into care through death and bereavement (Stein *et al.* 1989; Woolley *et al.* 1991)

The sick children themselves also need support, information and the opportunity to understand what is happening to them, and to be able to express their feelings in a way appropriate to their developmental level. However, for many, what they value most is to be able to continue as normal a life as possible for as long as they can, with minimal intrusion from the illness and professionals.

As the illness progresses, many children may find their lives increasingly difficult and the provision of suitable stimulation, recreation and education becomes hard. In While's study (1996) 50% of children were found to require wheelchairs and a significant number were found to need special equipment and furniture. Facing up to progressive disabilities coupled with their developing understanding of death and its irreversibility, and their increasing isolation and loneliness, all contribute to feelings of distress and difficulty in coping. For young adults these problems are particularly acute when they finish full-time education, are unemployed, and see their peers with similar diagnoses die.

For the families too, the burden of care results in profound psychosocial difficulties. Parents frequently become isolated and depressed. Without respite care they may find themselves exhausted both physically and mentally, suffering from anxiety, stress, depression and malaise (Mastroyannopoulou *et al.* 1997). Living in a rural area, impoverished circumstances and unemployment can make the situation even worse (While *et al.* 1996).

Siblings may suffer from lack of attention and frustration. They may be expected to take on inappropriate amounts of care in the home. Difficulties are increased in families where the child with a life-threatening illness has behavioural problems. It may be hard for family members to go out and embarrassing for them to invite friends to the home.

Many of the individual conditions are familial, so there may be more than one child affected in a family and genetic counselling will be important. Often parents are distraught and guilt-ridden at the diagnosis of a hereditary condition in their child and the implications of a genetic disorder rebound throughout the whole family. Also, since so many of the conditions are extremely rare, parents may feel themselves very isolated and this can compound their distress.

Practical problems

Daily practical tasks and time-consuming treatment can occupy many hours. The physical toll on parents may be enormous and present a considerable financial burden on a family. More than half of children with life-limiting disorders suffer from disability which often increases with age (While *et al.* 1996; Gagliardi 1991; Hunt and Burne 1995; Davies 1996). In While's study (1996), more than half of the children experienced difficulties in personal care with more than two-thirds requiring help with feeding and one-third requiring help during the night. Incontinence provides additional practical problems.

Families often experience and complain of bureaucracy and delays in obtaining funds and support for essential special equipment or adaptations within the home (While *et al.* 1996). Help in the home and respite care can potentially make a huge difference but the difficulty of finding and arranging them can itself cause stress. Transportation problems to and from hospital and clinic appointments are particularly pertinent for those children with neurological diseases, musculoskeletal diseases and Duchenne muscular dystrophy.

Spiritual support

Although spiritual support is regularly acknowledged as an important aspect of care it is one which many professionals feel uneasy with. It is easy to confuse with formal religious needs and easy to neglect.

Services

The development and provision of palliative care services for children have been the subject of two recent reports (ACT and RCPCH 1997; Thornes 1998). These have identified that there is a well developed model of palliative care for children with cancer, but that the needs of children with other life-threatening illnesses are less well addressed (ACT and RCPCH 1997; Goldman 1998; Woolley *et al.* 1991). Several models of care for these children have been set up and there is some consensus on what is needed for the future. However there is still a considerable way to go before the recommended services are established and available nationally.

Providing care for these children and families is complex and multidisciplinary, involving social services and education as well as health services, and may include input from a number of different trusts. Inevitably this causes problems with co-ordination and allocation of funding, which can put additional stress on the families. Some of the strong recommendations for the future (ACT and RCPCH 1997) include:

- a co-ordinator in each district to monitor the cases and ensure services are being offered to the families
- a flexible children's palliative care service in each district
- a key worker allocated to and co-ordinating services for each individual family
- extension of the children's community nursing service
- facilities for respite care, both at home and in children's hospices
- improved provision of professions allied to medicine in the community and to education
- a network of tertiary paediatric palliative care consultants

Psychological support is also necessary, though many of the stresses faced by families are of a practical and financial nature. If more practical help were available for families many stresses would diminish. Voluntary organisations and self help groups are available for many childhood disorders and can offer both practical and emotional support (The CAF Directory 1997). Details about them, written information on a child's condition and regular up-to-date information about the illness and management should be offered. The knowledge can help enhance the family's sense of control.

Many children die of incurable illnesses within the first four years of life, with numbers increasing again in the late teenage years and early adulthood. Those individuals in their late teenage years have often been supported by paediatricians during their lifetimes but facilities diminish for this age group; physicians who normally deal with adults have less experience with these childhood disorders. Full-time education is no longer feasible and isolation and psychological problems increase for the teenager. Often, just as the nursing burden is increasing, finding suitable care becomes even harder for the family. Services for adolescents and young adults are badly needed.

Effectiveness of interventions

In contrast to the growing literature on assessment of needs, the research and literature evaluating the interventions available is much more sparse. Many of the therapeutic and management approaches used routinely are judged as effective by clinicians, but have not been formally assessed, and depend on individual experience and anecdote.

There are various reasons contributing to this lack of research. There is only a small number of children with any one disease and most of them are cared for by different clinicians in different parts of the country. It is therefore difficult, in practical terms, to develop clinical experience and research protocols. At present many drugs used widely in general paediatrics have still not been formally assessed or licensed. There is reluctance to impose the perceived burden of a clinical trial on children and families, for whom the focus of care is quality of life. The lack of financial incentive to the pharmaceutical companies to work with such small patient populations may also contribute.

The assessment and management of pain, both pharmacological and non-pharmacological, are the areas in which there has been most formal research applicable to these children, even though it has often been based primarily on children with cancer (McGrath 1998). Many other symptoms, such as convulsions, feeding problems and disability are relatively common in children, and treatments for those with life-threatening diseases use the body of knowledge and research available in general paediatrics, which, although relevant, does not focus on their specific problems.

In relation to psychological interventions there is a significant body of descriptive literature on aspects of support, communication, coping skills and care throughout the course of the disease. This contrasts with the few formal audits and quantitative assessments of interventions. Recently qualitative approaches are becoming more widely used and valued (Bluebond-Langner 1996; Black 1996). An important observation has been made that, if practical and financial issues are addressed, the psychological needs of families diminish; this is therefore one of the most effective ways of enabling families to care for their children at home (Thornes 1998).

A recent helpful evaluation has been published: 'The pilot project programme for children with life-threatening illnesses'. It was initiated by the government in 1992 and undertaken by many different practitioners in a variety of aspects of care throughout the United Kingdom (Thornes 1998). This report found that one of the most successful factors in setting up a district-wide service for children with life-threatening diseases has been the establishment of a district co-ordinator to ensure collaboration across the many disciplines involved in the care of these children. Even though both parents and professionals favour the concept of key workers, it is evident that they are still not being nominated and used effectively. Other interesting points to emerge include the importance of children's community nursing services and information about the relationship between location and funding on the work of nurse specialists.

Priorities for further research

The priorities for further research are manifold and provide scope for investigating problems related to each disease and to each age group. Studies are necessary into the physiology and therapeutic interventions for the whole range of symptoms, both into aspects which will overlap with information needed in adult palliative care and also those specific to children. There is still a need to develop more approaches in assessment, particularly for chronic pain, other symptoms and for children who are severely intellectually impaired and have communication difficulties. There is too little information available to formally evaluate quality of life for children and their families, particularly outside oncology (Eiser and Jenney 1996). Gathering more information would help in developing studies to assess interventions in palliative care and to establish the effectiveness of the services provided. An increase in research in these areas would complement current information on the children's and families' needs.

Implications for clinical management

The most important improvement needed is the development of a more comprehensive provision of services for all children with life-threatening diseases. Particular attention needs to be given to adolescents and young adults. The individual aspects of this are outlined by the report of the joint working party and the pilot project report, which recommends a flexible co-ordinated service, led by a senior professional for each district. This should include a key worker for each family, community children's nursing teams and improved access to occupational therapy, physiotherapy, social work and respite care. A tertiary network of children's palliative care specialists should also be developed as a source of advice, training and research (ACT and RCPCH 1997).

Summary

Paediatric palliative care is a relatively new specialty. The needs for the families and children have been comparatively well defined but there is considerable scope for research in order to improve symptom management and to evaluate the current approaches to care. Recommendations to those developing services have been laid out and hopefully will be heeded.

References

Association for Children with Life Threatening or Terminal Conditions and their Families and the Royal College of Paediatrics and Child Health (1997). *Report of a Joint Working Party. A guide to the development of children's palliative care services.* Published jointly by ACT Bristol and RCPCH London.

Bax, M.C.O. and Colville, G.A. (1996). Behaviour in mucopolysaccharide disorders. *Archives of Disease in Childhood* 73(1): 77–81.

Black, N. (1996). Why we need observational studies to evaluate the effectiveness of health care. *British Medical Journal* 312: 1215–18.

Bluebond-Langner, M. (1996). *In the Shadow of Illness, Parents and Siblings of the Chronically Ill Child.* Princeton, NJ: Princeton University Press.

The CaF Directory of Specific Conditions and Rare Syndromes in Children with their Family Support Networks (1997), March, H., Partridge, L., Youngs, L., Casswell, D. (eds). London: Contact a Family.

Colville, G.A. and Bax, M.A. (1996). Early presentation in the mucopolysaccharide disorders. *Child: Care, Health and Development* 22(1): 31–6.

Davies, H. (1996). Living with dying: families coping with a child who has a neurodegenerative genetic disorder. *Axone* 18(2): 38–44.

Eiser, C. and Jenney, M.E.M. (1996). Measuring symptomatic benefit and quality of life in paediatric oncology. *British Journal of Cancer* **73**(11): 1313–16.

Gagliardi, B.A.(1991). The impact of Duchenne muscular dystrophy on families. *Orthopaedic Nursing* **10**(5): 41–9.

Goldman, A. (ed.) (1998). *Care of the Dying Child.* Oxford: Oxford University Press.

Hain, R.D. (1997). Pain scales in children: a review. *Palliative Medicine* **11**(5): 341–50.

Hockenberry-Eaton, M. and Brenner, A. (1990). Patterns of nausea and vomiting in children: nursing assessment and intervention. *Oncology Nursing Forum* **17**(4): 575–84.

Hunt, A.M. (1990). A survey of signs, symptoms and symptom control in 30 terminally ill children. *Developmental Medicine and Child Neurology* **32**(4): 341–6.

Hunt, A.M. and Burne, R. (1995). Medical and nursing problems of children with neurodegenerative disease. *Palliative Medicine* **9**(1): 19–26.

Jeffery, R. and Jeffery, A. (1993). Metachromatic leukodystrophy: two sides of a coin. *British Medical Journal* **307**: 1631–2.

McGrath, P.A. (1998). Pain control. In Doyle, D., Hanks, G.W.C., MacDonald, N. (eds), *The Oxford Textbook of Palliative Medicine* (2nd edn). Oxford: Oxford Medical Publications, pp. 1013–31.

Mastroyannopoulou, K., Stallard, P., Lewis, M., and Lenton S. (1997). The impact of childhood non-malignant life-threatening illness on parents: gender differences and predictors of parental adjustment. *Journal of Child Psychology and Psychiatry and Allied Disciplines* **38**(7): 823–9.

Robinson, W.M., Ravilly, S., Berde, C., and Wohl, M.E. (1997) End-of-life care in cystic fibrosis. *Pediatrics* **100**(2): 205–9.

Royal College of Paediatrics and Child Health (1997). *Prevention and Control of Pain in Children. A Manual for Health Care Professionals.* London: BMJ Publishing Group.

Stein, A., Forrest, G.C., Woolley, H., and Baum, J.D. (1989). Life-threatening illness and hospice care. *Archives of Disease in Childhood* **64**(5): 697–702.

Thompson, R.J., Zeman, J.L., Fanurik, D., and Sirotkin-Roses, M. (1992). The role of parent stress and coping and family functioning in parent and child adjustment to Duchenne muscular dystrophy. *Journal of Clinical Pschology* **48**(1): 11–19.

Thornes, R. (1998). *Evaluation of the Pilot Project Programme for Children with Life Threatening Illness.* Wetherby: NHS Executive, Department of Health, Health Services Directorate.

While, A., Citrone, C., and Cornish, J. (1996). Executive summary: A study of the needs and provisions for families caring for children with limiting incurable disorders. Commissioned by the Department of Health, Department of Nursing Studies, King's College London, London.

Woolley, H., Stein, A., Forrest, G.C., and Baum, J.D. (1991). Cornerstone care for families of children with life-threatening illness. *Developmental Medicine and Child Neurology* **33**(3): 216–24.

World Health Organisation (1998). *Cancer Pain Relief and Palliative Care in Children.* Geneva: WHO Publications.

Chapter 6

The management of chronic pain in palliative non-cancer patients

Eduardo Bruera and Catherine M. Neumann

Introduction

Most palliative care programmes have been developed primarily in order to address the physical and psychosocial needs of terminal cancer patients (MacDonald 1998; Woodruff 1996). A number of studies have highlighted the under-treatment of patients with cancer pain and the lack of adequate education of health care professionals on the assessment and management of patients with pain due to cancer (Foley 1998; Cleel *et al.* 1994; US DHHS 1994; Von Roenn *et al.* 1993; WHO 1990; Health and Welfare Canada 1984). A number of excellent reviews and guidelines have been produced in order to improve the assessment and management of cancer pain (WHO 1997; Levy 1996; WHO 1996; WHO 1990; Health and Welfare Canada 1984).

As a result of the intense educational effort by pain experts and scientific organisations, during the last 10 years there have been major improvements in the patterns of treatment of cancer pain around the world (US DHS 1994; WHO 1990; Health and Welfare Canada 1984). On the other hand, there has been limited research on the assessment and management of palliative care patients with non-cancer pain. There is evidence that pain control in these patients is also frequently inappropriate (Breitbart *et al.* 1996; Elander and Midence 1996; Farrell *et al.* 1996; O'Brien *et al.* 1992).

The purpose of this chapter is to suggest some guidelines for the assessment and management of non-cancer pain and to review the characteristics and patterns of care of some of the more common pain syndromes in palliative care patients with diseases other than cancer. Some possible future research areas will also be discussed. Chronic non-malignant pain will be addressed only within the context of terminal illness. The assessment and management of patients with conditions such as low back pain, chronic headache, or fibromyalgia are usually considered out of the scope of palliative care and, therefore, will not be addressed in this chapter.

Assessment

Inappropriate assessment is one of the main reasons for the inadequate management of cancer pain (Cleel *et al.* 1994; Von Roenn *et al.* 1993). There is evidence that pain is also frequently poorly assessed in palliative non-cancer patients (Breitbart *et al.* 1996; Farrell *et al.* 1996; Archibald *et al.* 1994; Marzinski 1991).

The production of pain

Figure 6.1 summarises the different components of the pain experience. The production of pain is the process by which nociception (stimulation of afferent nerves that carry the pain message to the central nervous system) occurs (e.g, a bone fracture, a local tumor, or the entrapment of a nerve). The production of pain can be significantly different from one individual to another and in different areas within the same individual. Perception is the process by which nociception reaches the brain cortex. This can also vary significantly from one individual to another (endorphins or descending inhibitor pathways can significantly confound the intensity of pain perceived). Unfortunately, these two stages cannot be measured. Finally, the expression of pain is the only measurable part of the experience and is a target of therapy. However, this stage can also be very variable from one individual to another due to beliefs about the meaning of the pain, intra-psychic factors such as depression or somatisation, and even cultural factors.

In summary, while it is very important to measure the intensity of certain symptoms such as pain or nausea, it is important to recognise that this intensity of expression does not have the same unidimensional value of blood glucose in the control of diabetes, or blood pressure in the case of control of arterial hypertension. Interpreting the intensity of the expression of pain as being only the expression of nociception would deny that in addition to variability in nociception, there is a great variability in both perception and expression of pain. Rather, pain expression should be interpreted as a multidimensional construct. In a given patient, a score of 8 out of 10 in the intensity of pain could be the result of nociception plus a wide variety of other factors—for example, somatisation (patients who express part of their emotional distress as physical symptoms), emotional concerns, other symptoms, or mild delirium. The multidimensional assessment should help in the recognition of the contribution of these different dimensions to the patient's expression, and thereby assist in the planning of care. The concept of 'total pain', that has physical, emotional, social, and spiritual concerns, as used in cancer palliative care, is helpful here. A purely unidimensional interpretation of the intensity of pain would result in assuming that complete success could be achieved with use of higher and higher doses of opioids. This simplistic approach could result in massive doses of opioids, opioid-related toxicity, and excessive reliance on pharmacological, as compared to non-pharmacological, approaches to symptom control.

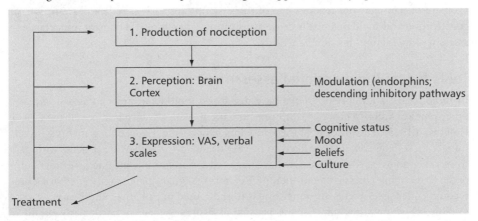

Fig 6.1 A schematic of pain experience.

Multidimensional pain assessment

Figure 6.1 identifies some of the dimensions that need to be assessed in these patients. In the case of cancer pain, a number of these factors have been identified and staging systems are available for the regular multidimensional assessment of patients (Bruera *et al.* 1995b). Unfortunately, similar staging systems do not exist for palliative non-malignant pain, and those tools available for cancer pain have not been validated in non-cancer populations.

A positive history for alcoholism or drug abuse indicates a higher risk for 'coping chemically' (using the medication as a way of coping with emotional stress). This is a major prognostic factor for the development of opioid dose escalation and opioid-related neurotoxicity (Bruera *et al.* 1995b). However, when cancer patients undergo regular screening for alcoholism and are provided with multidimensional and multidisciplinary support, both pain intensity and overall opioid dose is not significantly different compared to those of patients with no history of alcoholism (Bruera *et al.* 1995a). This assessment is particularly important for patients with AIDS pain, in whom substance abuse may be an HIV transmission risk.

Somatisation, either as a primary coping strategy or as a result of affective disorders such as anxiety or depression, is also an independent poor prognostic factor for the outcome of patients with cancer pain (Bruera *et al.*1995b). The appropriate assessment and management of affective disorders with both pharmacological and non-pharmacological techniques, and appropriate counselling of patients with a history of somatisation can result in improved symptom control and satisfaction with the level of care.

Cognitive failure is a frequent complication in patients with non-cancer terminal disease. The presence of cognitive failure makes the assessment of intensity and other dimensions of pain very difficult. In addition, cognitive failure may be aggravated by a number of pharmacological interventions for the management of pain. Therefore, the regular assessment of cognitive function using tools such as the 'Mini-mental state examination' (MMSE) should be done (Folstein *et al.* 1975). In non-communicative patients with severe neurological diseases or dementia, behavioural scales or third party assessments have been proposed (Baker *et al.* 1996). Unfortunately, validation of these tools following traditionally accepted criteria is impossible because of the characteristics of the patient population.

Palliative care patients present with a number of symptoms in addition to pain. The management of pain may not relieve some of those symptoms such as sedation, confusion, or constipation and could potentially cause aggravation. Therefore, it is of great importance to assess multiple symptoms simultaneously.

Tools for multidimensional assessment

In recent years, a number of groups have developed tool kits in order to assess pain and other physical and psychosocial symptoms in patients with advanced cancer (Bruera 1996; Higginson 1993). The majority of these tool kits have been developed for patients with terminal cancer. However, they are likely to be very useful for palliative care patients with pain from other sources. A recent review has suggested a number of outcome assessments for patients receiving chronic opioid therapy for non-malignant pain (Jamison 1996). These recommended assessments are quite similar to those used in palliative cancer care.

Table 6.1 summarises some of the bedside assessments that are particularly useful in palliative care. The 'Edmonton symptom assessment system' (ESAS) (Bruera *et al.* 1991)

Table 6.1 Useful assessments in palliative care

◆ Current stage of disease (palliative status)

◆ Symptom intensity i.e. STAS (Higginson 1993); ESAS (Bruera *et al.* 1991)

◆ Cognitive function i.e. MMSE (Folstein 1975)

◆ History of alcohol/substance abuse i.e. CAGE (Bruera *et al.* 1995)

◆ Functional status i.e. EFAT (Kaasa *et al.* 1997)

◆ History of psychiatric/psychological distress

◆ Social/family issues

◆ Spiritual assessment

consists of 9 different visual analogue scales that assess 9 different symptoms. In patients who are unable to complete the visual analogue scales, the intensity of the symptom can be reported verbally as a number or registered by circling on a numbered scale. The results, in terms of symptom intensity, can then be recorded in graphic display on the patient's chart. This allows for follow-up on a daily basis on an admitted patient, and also for comparison of changes in symptoms between an out-patient's visits. For the purpose of auditing, or for programmes delivering care to a large number of cognitive impaired or demented patients, tools that focus on the assessment by a caregiver, such as the Support Team Assessment Schedule (STAS), may be more appropriate (Higginson 1993).

Management

The goals of analgesic interventions in palliative care patients with non-cancer pain are not significantly different from those traditionally accepted for the management of patients with cancer pain (WHO 1997; WHO 1996; US DHHS 1994). Ideally, a decrease in the intensity of pain expression by the patient should be accomplished with no or minimal effects on cognitive or affective mental functions, no or minimal side effects, and the overall results should be an improvement in physical and psychosocial function. Therefore, regular monitoring of the intensity of multiple symptoms, cognitive function, psychosocial variables, and physical function, ideally using reliable tools that can be documented in the patient's chart are an important part of achieving therapeutic success.

Pharmacological interventions

Non-opioid analgesics

A number of authors have reviewed analgesic strategies for the management of malignant (WHO 1997; Levy 1996; WHO 1996; US DHHS 1994) and non-malignant (Rawlins 1998; Merskey 1997; Andersen and Leikersfeldt 1996; Portenoy 1996) pain. Most authors coincide in recommending non-opioid analgesics (e.g. Non Steroidal Anti-Inflammatory Drugs (NSAIDs) as a first step for patients with mild to moderate pain. However, most studies conducted in patients with AIDS (Breitbart *et al.* 1996; Kimball and McCormick 1996), neurological diseases (Oliver 1996; O'Brien *et al.* 1992), and sickle cell disease (Jacobsen *et al.* 1997; Elander and Midence 1996) found that the majority of patients required opioid analgesics before death.

The main limitation of NSAIDs is their relatively flat dose–response curve and the presence of gastrointestinal, renal, and bleeding side effects. These effects are related to the inhibition of cyclo-oxygenase I (Rawlins 1998). A new generation of cyclo-oxygenase II NSAIDs will soon be available for clinical use (Lane 1997). These agents will have lower frequency of toxicity and may be effective for use alone, or in combination with opioid analgesics.

Opioids

These drugs have been used in the management of pain in palliative care patients with a number of non-malignant conditions. Most groups have used these drugs following the general recommendations usually made for the treatment of cancer pain (Jacobsen et al. 1997; Breitbart et al. 1996; Elander and Midence 1996; Kimball and McCormick 1996; Oliver 1996; O'Brien et al. 1992). However, there are no specific guidelines for the use of opioids in palliative care patients with non-malignant pain.

A number of authors have reviewed the use of opioids in non-malignant chronic pain (McQuay 1997; Stacey 1996; Turk 1996; Hagen et al. 1995). While most palliative cancer and non-cancer patients will need opioids for weeks to months, many chronic non-malignant pain patients will require analgesic therapy including opioids for years. This has raised a number of concerns regarding adverse pharmacological outcomes in these patients:

1 *Major organ toxicity:* a number of longitudinal studies in methadone maintenance patients and cancer patients have failed to demonstrate consistent evidence of major organ damage (Portenoy 1996).

2 *Persistent side effects:* perhaps the side effects which cause most concern are those related to opioid-induced neurotoxicity (Ripamonti and Bruera 1997). While cognitive failure and sedation are common findings during the initial phases of opioid titration, they are less frequent in patients maintained on a regular opioid dose unless patients are receiving other centrally acting drugs, or they develop intercurrences such as renal failure, dehydration, infections, or need for significant dose increases. Unfortunately, there is limited research on the long-term cognitive effects of opioid administration.

3 *Risk of opioid addiction and abuse:* the potential for iatrogenic addiction is a major issue in the long-term use of opioids for chronic non-malignant pain. Most of the evidence available suggests that in absence of a history of substance abuse or severe psychiatric or psychological problems, patients do not develop addiction to chronic opioid therapy (Portenoy 1996).

There is emerging consensus that a selected population of patients with chronic non-malignant pain should receive trials of opioid analgesics. However, consensus is not universal (Shofferman 1993). Table 6.2 summarises some of the guidelines established by the Alberta College of Physicians and Surgeons for the use of opioids for non-malignant pain (Hagen et al. 1995). Unfortunately, there is a very small number of controlled trials on the role of opioids for non-malignant pain. Moulin et al. (1996) randomised 46 patients with chronic regional pain of soft tissue or muscular skeletal origin to morphine 60 mg twice a day versus benztropine (active placebo) 1 mg also twice daily in a double-blind, crossover study of 6 weeks. The morphine group showed a reduction in pain intensity relative to placebo. There was no significant psychological or functional improvement, the authors observed no significant changes in cognitive function or memory and there were no cases of psychological dependence or addiction. The authors conclude that further randomised

Table 6.2 Summary of guidelines for the opioid management of chronic non-malignant pain (Alberta College of Physicians and Surgeons) (Hagen *et al.* 1995)

- The underlying cause of the pain should be carefully investigated
- History of substance abuse is a relatively strong contraindication
- Previous adequate but unsuccessful trial of non-opioid analgesics
- One physician only should provide opioids to any patient
- The opioid treatment should be considered a treatment trial. Effective therapy can be defined as meaningful partial analgesics with no adverse effects capable of compromising comfort or function
- Frequent monitoring of analgesia, side effects, and behaviour consistent with substance abuse is required

controlled trials are required to define the role of oral morphine in the management of chronic non-cancer pain. Arkinstall *et al.* (1995) conducted a randomised, double-blind, placebo-controlled study of slow release codeine every 12 hours in 46 patients with chronic non-malignant pain. Thirty patients completed the study. Pain intensity measured with both visual analogue scales and categorical scores were significantly better in patients who received codeine. In addition, patients' and investigators' blinded treatment preference was significantly in favor of codeine relative to placebo. The authors conclude that treatment with codeine resulted in reduced pain and pain-related disability.

In summary, a number of uncontrolled trials (Portenoy 1996) and controlled trials (Moulin *et al.* 1996; Arkinstall *et al.* 1995) support the use of opioid trials in selected patient populations with chronic non-malignant pain. However, at the present time it is unclear which patients are most likely to benefit from this intervention; some of the potential long-term cognitive effects, and the most effective type and dose of opioid, are also unknown.

It has been noticed with concern that in some countries, for example Denmark, the patterns of prescription of opioids have changed dramatically during the last 10 years. More than 90% of the opioid prescriptions are for pain of non-malignant origin (Clausen 1997). These results stress the urgency in conducting clinical trials and establishing universally accepted guidelines for the utilisation of opioids in chronic non-malignant pain. They also suggest that opioid consumption is not always a reliable indicator of the patterns of cancer pain relief.

Adjuvant drugs

Palliative non-cancer patients have a high frequency of neuropathic pain syndromes. As a result, their pain is likely to be less responsive to opioid analgesics. Therefore, many of these patients may benefit from trials of adjuvant drugs. Table 6.3 summarises some of the most common groups of adjuvant drugs.

The overall effectiveness of adjuvant drugs for neuropathic pain is highly variable, ranging from less than 20% for some neuropathic cancer pain syndromes to more than 75% for neuropathic pain associated with post-herpetic neuralgia (Hanks *et al.* 1998; Hewitt and Portenoy 1998). Unfortunately, there are very few randomised controlled trials comparing different adjuvant analgesics for specific pain syndromes. Therefore, at the present time it is frequently necessary to use sequential trials of two, three, or even more, different adjuvant

Table 6.3 Adjuvant analgesic drugs (most commonly used agents)

- Tricyclic antidepressants (Amitryptiline)
- Specific seratonin re-uptake inhibition (Paroxetine-Fluoxetine)
- Oral local anesthetics (Mexiletine-Flecainide)
- Anticonvulsants (Carbamazepine, Phenytoin, Clonazepam)
- Gabapentin
- Corticosteroids (Dexamethasone, Prednisone)
- Baclofen
- N-methyl-D-asparate antagonists (Dextromethorphan, Ketamine)
- Clonidine

analgesics in order to determine which one is the most effective and least toxic for a given patient. Most authors recommend gabapentin, tricyclic antidepressants, and mexiletine as their main choices for initial treatment (Hanks *et al.* 1998; Hewitt and Portenoy 1998).

Non-pharmacological interventions

Non-pharmacological interventions should always be considered an integral part of the management of pain in palliative care. Table 6.4 summarises the most frequently recommended techniques. Some of these approaches should be universal, such as appropriate counselling of patient and family. Other approaches, including transcutaneous nerve stimulation or physiotherapy can be attempted in most patients because of their relatively limited side effects and cost. Finally, in patients for whom pharmacological and less invasive non-pharmacological approaches are not effective, a number of invasive techniques can be attempted. While traditionally these techniques have been used for pain of non-neuropathic origin (Swarm and Cousins 1998), a number of authors recognise that many of these invasive procedures can also be helpful to patients with intractable neuropathic pain syndromes (Cramond 1998).

Pain in palliative non-cancer patients

In the following paragraphs we will summarise some of the characteristics and patterns of treatment of pain syndromes in non-cancer palliative care populations.

Table 6.4 Non-pharmacological techniques

- Patient and family counselling
- Transcutaneous nerve stimulation (TENS)
- Physiotherapy—orthotics
- Relaxation
- Massage
- Anesthetic techniques (blocks—spinal infusions)
- Neurosurgical techniques

AIDS

Pain is a frequent complication in patients with AIDS (Hewlitt *et al.* 1997; Kelleher *et al.* 1997; Breitbart *et al.* 1996; Glare and Cooney 1996; Kimball and McCormick 1996; Schofferman 1988). The frequency of pain ranges from approximately 25% of patients in the 'asymptomatic' phases to more than 80% of patients in the terminal stage (Hewlitt *et al.* 1997; Kelleher *et al.* 1997; Breitbart *et al.* 1996; Glare and Cooney 1996; Kimball and McCormick 1996; Schofferman 1988).

Table 6.5 characterises pain syndromes in patients with advanced AIDS. As in the case of cancer pain, AIDS pain may be a direct consequence of the AIDS infection, it may be related to some of the treatments, or unrelated to both the infection and its treatment. This is considered in more detail in Chapter 11.

The mechanism of pain is somatic and/or visceral in the majority of patients. However, in a series of 151 ambulatory patients with AIDS pain, 69 (46%) had at least one neuropathic pain syndrome (Hewitt *et al.* 1997). The frequency of neuropathic pain in these patients appears to be higher than that in cancer patients. Neuropathic pain is a complex pain syndrome that is frequently associated with decreased opioid responsiveness (Bruera *et al.* 1995b; Sykes *et al.* 1997). A study conducted in 59 male and 59 female AIDS patients revealed that headache and muscoskeletal pain were more frequently experienced by women, whereas neuropathic pain was experienced more frequently by men (Kelleher *et al.* 1997).

There is evidence that AIDS pain is frequently under-treated (Breitbart *et al.* 1996). Breitbart *et al.* found that 226/366 ambulatory AIDS patients surveyed (62%) reported 'persistent or frequent' pain over the two week period surveyed. Nearly 85% of patients were classified as receiving inadequate analgesic therapy, as measured by the Pain Management Index. Adjuvant analgesic drugs were prescribed in only 10% of the patients. Women, less educated patients, and patients who reported injection drug use as their HIV transmission risk factor, were most likely to have received inadequate analgesic therapy (Breitbart *et al.* 1996; Breitbart *et al.* 1997).

Treatment considerations

There are very few studies addressing the role of different analgesics for AIDS pain. Most authors propose opioids as the main therapeutic intervention for AIDS pain (Kelleher *et al.* 1997; Glare and Cooney 1996; Kimball and McCormick 1996; Schofferman 1988). The presence of incidental pain may require careful opioid titration and may be associated with

Table 6.5 Characterisation of pain syndromes in AIDS patients

◆ Frequency of pain ranges from 30% to 90% and is higher in advanced stages

◆ Most patients have more than one painful location and/or mechanism

◆ Neuropathic mechanism in approximately 50% of patients

◆ Somatic mechanism the most common (71% of patients)

◆ Directly due to AIDS in 30–50% of patients

◆ Related to AIDS treatment in <10% of patients

◆ Unclear origin in 30–40% of patients

Table 6.6 Specific challenges to adequate pain management in AIDS patients

- Frequent neuropathic mechanism
- Frequent incidental nature
- Co-morbidity of cognitive failure/dementia
- High prevalence of substance abuse
- High prevalence of psychosocial distress
- Concurrent multiple drug therapy
- Lack of studies on effective pain treatments

increased opioid neurotoxicity (Schofferman 1988). Since almost half the patients have neuropathic pain syndromes, it may frequently be necessary to add adjuvant drugs. However, these drugs are generally associated with central side effects that may be particularly toxic to AIDS patients because of the high frequency of cognitive dysfunction and dementia (Kelleher *et al.* 1997; Glare and Cooney 1996; Kimball and McCormick 1996; Schofferman 1988).

The high frequency of affective disorders and psychological distress with resulting somatisation, and 'chemical coping' associated with a history of drug dependency may have implications for the assessment and management of pain with opioid analgesics. The frequency, intensity, and functional interference did not seem to differ between patients with a history of illegal injection drug use and those without such history (Breitbart *et al.* 1997). However those patients with a history of injection drug use are more likely to receive inadequate analgesic medications, and are more likely to report lower levels of pain relief and greater degree of psychological distress (Breitbart *et al.* 1997).

Finally, the combination of antiviral therapy, multiple prophylactic antibiotic regimes, and other drugs increases the possibility of interactions between these agents and opioids, NSAIDS, or adjuvant drugs. Table 6.6 summarises some of the specific challenges related to adequate pain management in AIDS patients.

Neurological diseases

Two most common neurological disorders encountered in palliative care are multiple sclerosis and amyotrophic lateral sclerosis .

Multiple sclerosis

Pain is a common feature of well established multiple sclerosis (Houtchens *et al.* 1997; Archibald *et al.* 1994; Knudsen and Jensen 1991; Moulin 1989; Moulin *et al.* 1988). An acute or chronic pain syndrome was found in 88/159 (55%) and 45/85 (53%) patients with multiple sclerosis respectively (Archibald *et al.* 1994; Moulin *et al.* 1988). In both studies, the frequency of pain was higher in patients with longer disease duration and neurological symptom severity. The most common chronic pain syndromes relate to dysaesthesia (impaired touch sensation) and muscle spasms (Archibald *et al.* 1994; Knudsen and Jensen 1991; Moulin *et al.* 1988). Unfortunately, there is evidence that these patients are also frequently under treated (Archibald *et al.* 1994; Knudsen and Jensen 1991). This is considered further in Chapter 4.

In most cases these patients received a combination of NSAIDS, opioids, and adjuvant drugs similar to those used in the management of cancer pain (Archibald *et al.* 1997; Knudsen and Jensen 1991). Because of the high frequency of neuropathic pain in these patients, adjuvant drugs have a major role. The findings of an open study in 25 patients (Houtchens *et al.* 1997) and a double-blind, placebo-controlled, non-cancer study in 15 patients (Mueller *et al.* 1997) suggest that gabapentin is a safe and effective adjuvant. In cases of intractable pain, intrathecal octreotide was found useful in 1 multiple sclerosis patient (Paice *et al.* 1996). Because of the role of urinary tract infections in increasing the frequency and severity of painful tonic spasms of the limbs, antibiotic therapy of obvious or subclinical infections can be an effective adjuvant analgesic procedure (Andersson and Goodkin 1996).

A recent survey suggests that patients with multiple sclerosis frequently use marijuana or derivates for the management of pain associated with muscle spasms (Consroe *et al.* 1997). Most of the responders who used marijuana in the survey reported significant subjective improvement (Consroe *et al.* 1997). However, there have been no controlled trials on the role of these agents.

Amyotrophic lateral sclerosis

Amyotrophic lateral sclerosis (ALS) (motor neurone disease) is classically a disease of motor neurones and has clinical manifestations involving mostly the motor system (see Chapter 4). During the 1980s pain associated to ALS was described as a rarity (Drake 1983). However, during the 1990s palliative care groups found pain in 38/52 (73%) (Oliver 1996) and 71/124 (57%) (O'Brien *et al.* 1992) patients with ALS. But these two reports suggest that most patients were not given opioids until quite late in the course of their illnesses. In most cases, opioid therapy was started by the hospice groups (Oliver 1996; O'Brien *et al.* 1992). The types of pain syndromes have not been well characterised. However, patients appeared to improve with opioid analgesics: 36/49 patients with ALS who were treated with opioids achieved good pain control (O'Brien 1992).

Dementia

Dementia is a frequent and increasing problem that mostly effects older people (see Chapter 9). Because of progressive cognitive failure, patients develop a progressive inability to communicate. This raises serious concerns about the potential for under-recognition of pain. A number of authors have addressed issues regarding the assessment and management of pain in patients with dementia (Fisher-Morris and Gellatly 1997; Scherder and Bouma 1997; Farrell *et al.* 1996; Porter *et al.* 1996; Robinson *et al.* 1995).

Communicative patients with dementia are probably less able than non-impaired patients to recall, interpret, and articulate their experience (Farrell *et al.* 1996, see chapter 5). One of the main potential confounders for the measurement of pain in people with dementia is memory impairment, since pain experienced at one moment can be forgotten the next (Fisher-Morris and Gellatly 1997; Porter *et al.* 1996). A comprehensive study conducted in 51 controls and 44 patients with dementia concluded that dementia is capable of influencing not only the reporting but also the experience of pain (Porter *et al.* 1996). Two papers have reported cases of communicative patients with dementia who appeared to have diminished or absent self reporting of pain; behaviours displayed by the patients suggested that decreased pain perception rather than expression was the main reason for this (Fisher-Morris and Gellatly 1997; Robinson *et al.* 1995). This is considered in detail in Chapter 9.

Analgesic use has been found to be decreased in patients with dementia (Scherder and Bouma 1997). While this might be related to decreased perception or expression of pain, one of the main independent negative correlates for opioid dose in cancer patients is age (Viganó *et al.* 1998). Patients with increasing age required significantly lower opioid dose in order to achieve a similar level of analgesia as compared to younger patients (Viganó *et al.* 1998). The influence of age on opioid use could be explained by pharmacokinetic research (decreased clearance), or by possible effects of age on perception or expression of pain. More research is needed in order to better characterise these findings.

Agitated behaviours for reasons other than pain may be misinterpreted as pain and treated with opioid analgesics. This phenomenon has been previously observed in patients with agitated delirium related to cancer (Bruera *et al.* 1992). Decreased or absent self reporting of pain may make the diagnosis of acute complications such as fractures, dental problems, urinary retention, or other acute intercurrent events difficult. Decreased oral intake and self reporting of bowel habits may result in dehydration with accumulation of active opioid metabolites and severe constipation due to opioid therapy. Finally, the presence of cognitive failure significantly increases the likelihood of neurotoxicity to the use of both opioids and most of the adjuvant analgesic drugs. Table 6.7 summarises some of the specific challenges associated with the assessment and management of pain in patients with terminal dementia.

Sickle cell disease

Sickle cell disease is an inherited blood disorder that affects approximately 50 000 people in the US. It is considered in detail in Chapter 10. However, one of the main challenges associated with sickle cell disease is the presence of numerous episodes of severe acute pain requiring aggressive oral or parenteral management followed by periods during which minimal or no analgesic therapy is required (Ballas 1997; Jacobsen *et al.* 1997; Martin and Moore 1997; Westerman *et al.* 1997; Elander and Midence 1996; Steinberg 1996). Patients are usually under treated during the episodes of acute pain (Ballas 1997; Jacobsen *et al.* 1997; Martin and Moore 1997; Westerman *et al.* 1997; Elander and Midence 1996; Steinberg 1996). The risk of poor pain management is greatest for patients in adverse social circumstances, who are more severely affected by painful episodes, who are poorly adjusted, and who have less effective personal strategies for coping with pain (Elander and Midence 1996).

Table 6.7 Challenges in assessing and managing pain in patients with dementia

◆ Unreliable self reporting of pain or opioid side effects (inability to express pain)

◆ Misinterpretation of patient behaviour (over- or under-diagnosis of pain)

◆ Lack of validated assessment tools

◆ Increased risk of neurotoxicity of opioids and adjuvant drugs

◆ Poor understanding of the effects of dementia on pain perception

While most patients are initially treated with NSAIDS, there is consensus, both in Europe and North America, that severe episodes of sickle cell pain require opioid analgesia (Elander and Midence 1996). Meperidine is the most frequently used opioid in the UK and the US (Ballas 1997; Elander and Midence 1996). However, due to its shorter half-life and higher frequency of neurotoxicity, meperidine should be avoided in these patients. Regular opioids are effective in the management of this crisis, both when given as intermittent injections or continuous infusions. Selected patients can be effectively managed with oral slow release morphine (Jacobsen et al. 1997). Because of the nature of these acute episodes of pain, techniques used for post-operative pain such as patient-controlled analgesia have been tried in these patients with significant success (Martin and Moore 1997; Elander and Midence 1996).

In summary, there is evidence that opioid agonists given as intermittent injections, continuous infusions, patient-controlled analgesia, or oral slow release opioids in selected cases can all result in good pain control.

Improvement in the assessment and management of patients with sickle cell disease have resulted in significant life prolongation in these patients (Adams-Graves et al. 1997; Steinberg 1996). The management of chronic pain syndromes, developed as a result of tissue damage in the sickle crisis, requires further work—see Chapter 10.

Future research

◆ The frequency, pathophysiology, clinical course, and response to pharmacological and non-pharmacological analgesic interventions of pain syndromes in most non-malignant palliative care patients are poorly known. Simple longitudinal studies addressing issues such as intensity, location, mechanism, and psychosocial correlates of pain intensity will greatly assist in future research and planning of care.

◆ Reliable assessment tools are needed for patients with severe dementia or severe neurological deterioration.

◆ Randomised controlled trials are required in order to better define the role of opioids in the management of pain in these patients. Specifically, the best type and dose of opioids have not been clarified. Studies in non-cancer palliative care populations are important because of the frequent presence of centrally acting drugs, borderline cognition, decreased psychomotor response, and neuropathic pains resulting in decreased opioid responsiveness in this population. Results from opioid trials in cancer patients cannot be automatically generalised to non-cancer palliative care patients.

◆ The role of adjuvant drugs in addition or as an alternative to opioids in some cases needs to be defined in randomised controlled trials. Again it is very difficult to apply results from both cancer pain studies and studies conducted in chronic non-malignant pain to palliative non-cancer pain.

◆ Finally, there is great need for guidelines on the management of pain in palliative non-cancer patients. These guidelines may have to emphasise different assessment methods that will take into consideration the cognitive and psychomotor limitations of these patients, and perhaps an earlier and more significant role for adjuvant drugs as compared to opioids. Ideally, these guidelines should be evidence based. The process of generating the guidelines will assist palliative care groups with programme planning and care delivery and will also identify the specific areas where future research should be conducted.

Conclusions

Pain is a frequent and devastating complication in palliative care patients with diseases other than cancer. Unfortunately, current knowledge about the frequency, pathophysiology, and clinical course of these pain syndromes is limited as compared to pain syndromes in cancer patients. There is evidence that pain in palliative non-cancer patients is frequently under-diagnosed and under-treated. The assessment of pain intensity can be very difficult because of cognitive or psychomotor problems resulting from AIDS, dementia, or terminal neurological diseases. There is evidence that most patients require and benefit from regular opioid analgesics for the treatment of pain. However, the best type and dose of opioids has not been established.

The higher incidence of neuropathic pain in palliative patients with non-cancer pain requires treatment other than opioids, often necessitating trials of adjuvant drugs. The role of both opioids and adjuvant drugs has not been well characterised in this patient population, and more clinical research is badly needed.

References

Adams-Graves, P., Kedar, A., Koshy, M., Steinberg, M., Veith, R., *et al.* (1997). RheothRx (Poloxamer 188) injection for the acute painful episode of sickle cell disease: a pilot study. *Blood* **90**: 2041–6.

Andersen, S. and Leikersfeldt, G. (1996). Management of chronic non-malignant pain. *British Journal of Clinical Practice* **50**: 324–30.

Andersson, P. and Goodkin, D. E. (1996). Current pharmacological treatment of multiple sclerosis symptoms. *Western Journal of Medicine* **165**: 313–17.

Archibald, C. J., McGrath, P. G., Ritvo, P. G., Fisk, J. D., Bhan, V., *et al.* (1994). Pain prevalence, severity and impact in a clinic sample of multiple sclerosis patients. *Pain* **58**: 89–93.

Arkinstall, W., Sandler, A., Goughnour, B., Babul, N., Harsanyi, Z., and Darke, A.C. (1995). Efficacy of controlled-release codeine in chronic non-malignant pain: a randomized, placebo-controlled clinical trial. *Pain* **62**(2): 169–78.

Baker, A., Bowring, L., Brignell, A., and Kafford, D. (1996). Chronic pain management in cognitively impaired patients: a preliminary research project. *Perspectives* **20**(2): 4–8.

Ballas, S. K. (1997). Management of sickle pain. *Current Opinion in Hematology* **4**(2): 104–11.

Breitbart, W., Rosenfeld, B., Passik, S., Kaim, M., Funesti-Esch, J., and Stein, K. (1997). A comparison of pain report and adequacy of analgesic therapy in ambulatory AIDS patients with and without a history of substance abuse. *Pain* **72**: 235–43.

Breitbart, W., Rosenfeld, B.D., Passik, S.D., McDonald, M.V., Thaler, H., and Portenoy, R.K. (1996). The undertreatment of pain in ambulatory AIDS patients. *Pain* **65**: 243–249.

Bruera, E. (1996). Patient assessment in palliative care. *Cancer Treatment Reviews* **22**: 3–12.

Bruera, E., Fainsinger, R., Miller, M.J., and Kuehn, N. (1992). The assessment of pain intensity in patients with cognitive failure: a preliminary report. *Journal of Pain and Symptom Management* **7**(5): 267–70.

Bruera, E., Kuehn, N., Miller, M.J., Selmser, P., and Macmillan, K. (1991). The Edmonton symptom assessment system (ESAS): a simple method for the assessment of palliative care patients. *Journal of Palliative Care* **7**(2): 6–9.

Bruera, E., Moyano, J., Seifert, L., Fainsinger, R.L., Hanson, J., and Suarez-Almazoer, M. (1995a). The frequency of alcoholism among patients with pain due to terminal cancer. *Journal of Pain and Symptom Management* **10**(8): 599–603.

Bruera, E., Schoeller, T., Wenk, R., MacEachern, T., Marcelino, S., *et al.* (1995b). A prospective multi-center assessment of the Edmonton staging system for cancer pain. *Journal of Pain and Symptom Management* **10**(5): 348–355.

Clausen, T.G. (1997). International opioid consumption. *Acta Anaesthesiologica Scandinavica* **41**:162–5.

Cleeland, C.S., Gonin, R., Hatfield, A.K., Edmonson, J.H., *et al.* (1994). Pain and its treatment in outpatients with metastatic cancer. *New England Journal of Medicine* **330**: 592–6.

Consroe, P., Musty, R., Rein, J., Tillery, W., and Pertwee, R. (1997). The perceived effects of smoked cannabis on patients with multiple sclerosis. *European Neurology* **38**: 44–8.

Cramond, T. (1998). Invasive techniques for neuropathic pain in cancer. In Bruera, E. and Portenoy, R.K. (eds), *Topics in Palliative Care*, vol. 2. New York: Oxford University Press, pp. 63–90.

Drake, M.E. (1983). Chronic pain syndrome in amyotrophic lateral sclerosis. *Archives of Neurology* **40**: 453–4.

Elander, J. and Midence, K. (1996). A review of evidence about factors affecting quality of pain management in sickle cell disease. *The Clinical Journal of Pain* **12**: 180–93.

Farrell, M. J., Katz, B., and Helme, R. D. (1996). The impact of dementia on the pain experience. *Pain* **67**: 7–15.

Fisher-Morris, M. and Gellatly, A. (1997). The experience and expression of pain in Alzheimer patients. *Age and Ageing* **26**: 497–500.

Foley, K.M. (1998). Pain assessment and cancer pain syndromes. In Doyle, D., Hanks, G.W.C., and MacDonald, N. (eds), *Oxford Textbook of Palliative Medicine*. Oxford: Oxford University Press, pp. 310–31.

Folstein, M.F., Folstein, S., and McHugh, P.R. (1975). 'Mini-mental state': a paractival method for grading the cognitive state of patients for the clinician. *Journal of Psychological Research* **12**: 189–98.

Glare, P.A. and Cooney, N.J. (1996). HIV and palliative care. *Medical Journal of Australia* **164**: 612–15.

Hagen, N., Flynne, P., Hays, H., and MacDonald, N. (1995). Guidelines for managing chronic non-malignant pain. *Canadian Family Physician* **41**: 49–53.

Hanks, G., Portenoy, R.K., MacDonald, N., and Forbes, K. (1998). Difficult pain problems. In Doyle, D., Hanks, G.W.C., and MacDonald, N. (eds), *Oxford Textbook of Palliative Medicine*. Oxford: Oxford University Press, pp. 454–77.

Health and Welfare Canada (1984). Cancer pain: a monograph on the management of cancer pain. Canada, Ottawa: Health and Welfare Canada:, Minister of Supply and Services, H42–2/5.

Hewitt, D.J., McDonald, M., Portenoy, R.K., Rosenfeld, B., Passik, S., and Breitbart, W. (1997). Pain syndromes and etiologies in ambulatory AIDS patients. *Pain* **70**: 117–23.

Hewitt, D.J. and Portenoy, R.K. (1998). Adjuvant drugs for neuropathic cancer pain. In Bruera, E. and Portenoy, R.K. (eds), *Topics in Palliative Care*, vol. 2. New York: Oxford University Press, pp. 41–62.

Higginson, I. (1993). Audit methods: validation and In-patient use. In Higginson, I. (ed.), *Clinical Audit in Palliative Care*. Oxford and New York: Radcliffe Medical Press, pp. 48–54.

Houtchens, M.K., Richert, J.R., Sami, A., and Rose, J.W. (1997). Open label gabapentin treatment for pain in multiple sclerosis. *Multiple Sclerosis* **3**(4): 250–3.

Jacobsen, S.J., Kopecky, E.A., Joshi, P., and Babul, N. (1997). Randomised trial of oral morphine for painful episodes of sickle cell disease in children. *The Lancet* **350**: 1358–61.

Kaasa, T., Loomis, J., Gillis, K., Bruera, E., and Hanson, J. (1997). The Edmonton functional assessment tool: preliminary development and evaluation for use in palliative care. *Journal of Pain and Symptom Management* **13**: 10–19.

Kelleher, P., Cox, C., and McKeogh, M. (1997). HIV infection: the spectrum of symptoms and disease in male and female patients attending a London hospice. *Palliative Medicine* **11**: 152–8.

Kimball, L.R. and McCormick W.C. (1996). The pharmacologic management of pain and discomfort in persons with AIDS near the end of life: use of opioid analgesia in the hospice setting. *Journal of Pain and Symptom Management* **11**: 88–94.

Knudsen, S.E. and Jensen, K. (1991). Acute and chronic pain syndromes in multiple sclerosis. *Acta Neurologica Scandinavica* **84**: 197–200.

Lane, N.E. (1997). Pain management in osteoarthritis: the role of COX-2 inhibitors. *Journal of Rheumatology* **24**(49): 20–4.

Levy, M.H. (1996). Pharmacological treatment of cancer pain. *New England Journal of Medicine* **335**: 1124–32.

MacDonald, N. (1998). The interface between oncology and palliative medicine. In Doyle, D., Hanks, G.W.C., and MacDonald, N. (eds), *Oxford Textbook of Palliative Medicine*. Oxford University Press, pp. 11–17.

Martin, J.J. and Moore, G.P. (1997). Pearls, pitfalls, and updates for pain management. *Emergency Medicine Clinics of North America* **15**(2): 399–415.

Marzinski, L.R. (1991). The tragedy of dementia: clinically assessing pain in the confused, non-verbal elderly. *J Gerontological Nursing* **17**(6): 25–8.

McQuay, H.J. (1997). Opioid use in chronic pain. *Acta Anaesthesiologica Scandinavica* **41**: 175–83.

Merskey, H. (1997). Pharmacological approaches other than opioids in chronic non-cancer pain management. *Acta Anaesthesiologica Scandinavica* **41**: 187–90.

Moulin, D.E. (1989). Pain in multiple sclerosis. *Neurologic Clinics* **7**: 321–31.

Moulin, D.E., Foley, K.M., and Ebers, G.C. (1988) Pain syndromes in multiple sclerosis. *Neurology* **38**: 1830–4.

Moulin, D.E., Lessi, A., Amireh, R., Sharpe, W.K.J., Boyd, D., and Merskey, H. (1996). Randomised trial of oral morphine for chronic non-cancer pain. *Lancet* **347**: 143–7.

Mueller, M.E., Gruenthal, M., Olson, W.L., and Olson, W.H. (1997). Gabapentin for relief of upper motor neuron symptoms in multiple sclerosis. *Archives of Physical Medicine and Rehabilitation* **78**(5): 521–4.

O'Brien, T., Kelly, M., and Saunders, C. (1992). Motor neurone disease: a hospice perspective. *British Medical Journal* **304**: 471–3.

Oliver, D. (1996). The quality of care and symptom control—the effects on the terminal phase of ALS/MND. *Journal of the Neurological Sciences* **139**(Suppl.): 134–6.

Paice, J.A., Penn, R.D., and Kroin, J.S. (1996). Intrathecal octreotide for relief of intractable non-malignant pain: 5-year experience with two cases. *Neurosurgery* **18**: 203–7.

Portenoy, R. (1996). Opioid therapy for chronic non-malignant pain. *Pain Research and Management* **1**: 17–28.

Porter, F.L., Malhotra K.M., Wolf, C.M., Morris, J.C., Miller, J.P., and Smith, M.C. (1996). Dementia and response to pain in the elderly. *Pain* **68**: 413–421.

Rawlins, M.D. (1998). Non-opioid analgesics. In Doyle, D., Hanks, G.W.C., and MacDonald, N. (eds), *Oxford Textbook of Palliative Medicine*. Oxford: Oxford University Press, pp. 355–61.

Ripamonti, C. and Bruera, E. (1997). CNS adverse effects of opioids in cancer patients. Guidelines for treatment. *CNS Drugs* **8**: 21–37.

Robinson, D., Bucci, J., and Fenn, H. (1995). Pain assessment in the Alzheimer's patient. *Journal of the American Gerontological Society* **43**: 318–19.

Scherder, E.A. and Bouma, A. (1997). Is decreased use of anallgesics in Alzheimer disease due to a change in the affective component of pain. *Alzheimer Disease and Associated Disorders* **11**(3): 171–4.

Schofferman, J. (1988). Pain: diagnosis and management in the palliative care of AIDS. *Journal of Palliative Care* 4(4): 46–9.

Schofferman, J. (1993). Long-term use of opioid analgesics for the treatment of chronic pain of nonmalignant origin. *Journal of Pain and Symptom Management* 8: 279–88.

Stacey, B.R. (1996). Effective management of chronic pain. *Postgraduate Medicine* 100(3): 281–96.

Steinberg, M.H. (1996). Review: sickle cell disease: present and future treatment. *American Journal of Medical Science* 312(4): 166–74.

Swarm, R.A. and Cousins, M.J. (1998). Anaesthetic techniques for pain control. In Doyle, D., Hanks, G.W.C., and MacDonald, N. (eds), *Oxford Textbook of Palliative Medicine*. Oxford University Press, pp. 390–414.

Turk, D.C., (1996). Clinicians' attitudes about prolonged use of opioids and the issue of patient heterogeneity. *Journal of Pain and Symptom Management* 11: 218–30.

US Department of Health and Human Services. (1994). *Management of Cancer Pain. Clinical Practice Guideline*. Rockville, MD: AHCPR Publications.

Viganó, A, Bruera, E., and Suarez-Almazor, M.E. (1998). Age, pain intensity, and opioid dose in patients with advanced cancer. *Cancer* 83(6): 1244–50

Von Roenn, J.H., Cleeland, C.S., Gonin, R., Hatfield, A.K., and Pandya, K.J. (1993). Physicians attitudes and practice in cancer pain management. A survey from the Eastern Cooperative Oncology Group. *Annals of Internal Medicine* 119(2): 121–6.

Westerman, M.P., Bailey, K., Freels, S., Schlegel, R., and Williamson, P. (1997). Assessment of painful episode frequency in sickle cell disease. *American Journal of Hematology* 54(3): 183–8.

Woodruff, R. (1996). *Palliative Medicine* (2nd edn). Melbourne: Asperula.

World Health Organisation (1996). *Cancer Pain Relief* (2nd edn). Geneva: World Health Organisation.

World Health Organisation, Collaborating Centre for Palliative Cancer Care (1997). *Looking Forward to Cancer Pain Relief for All*. Oxford: CBC.

World Health Organisation Expert Committee.(1990). *Cancer Pain Relief and Palliative Care*. Geneva: World Health Organisation.

Chapter 7

Palliative care in liver disease

M.A. Heneghan and J.G. O'Grady

Introduction

Chronic end-stage liver disease evolves over a period of years and has a terminal phase that is appropriate to consider in the context of palliative care. The profile of terminal chronic liver disease has been modified greatly in countries with active liver transplant programmes and many patients do not develop the range of complications considered here. However, in the UK at least four people die from chronic liver disease for every one transplanted. In addition, those parts of the world with the highest incidence of liver disease have limited access to transplantation.

End-stage liver disease is a major cause of morbidity and mortality world-wide. This results in the development of a number of symptoms and signs. A few patients may develop hepatocellular carcinoma. All patients will have ascites, jaundice, or encephalopathy as elements of their disease, with the majority of patients having all three by the last days of life. Even in terminal stages, good symptomatic management is essential.

In this chapter, we outline the epidemiology of end-stage liver disease with particular emphasis on those conditions with greatest prevalence world-wide. We also focus on the occurrence of symptoms, the syndromes associated with them, and outline treatment strategies applicable to patient care. These strategies are as relevant in the setting of hospice and domicilary care as they are in secondary and tertiary referral centres particularly given the increasingly dynamic and multidisciplinary approach to palliative care.

Epidemiology

Chronic viral hepatitis and alcohol accounts for the vast majority of chronic liver disease. Cirrhosis in the remainder is caused by a range of relatively uncommon diseases: for example, autoimmune hepatitis, primary biliary cirrhosis, primary sclerosing cholangitis, drug-induced liver disease, metal-associated liver disease, and other inherited disorders.

The median mortality rate for cirrhosis in 38 selected countries of the Americas, Europe, Africa, and Asia was 10 per 100 000 inhabitants (range 3–40) between 1985 and 1990 (La-Vecchia *et al.* 1994). Considering that the median survival of patients is approximately six years following diagnosis, and that 40% of cirrhotic patients will die before their disease is recognised, the median expected prevalence of the disease is 100 per 100 000 inhabitants (range 25–400) (Pagliaro *et al.* 1994; Dufour *et al.* 1993). In

England approximately 2000 deaths per year under the age of 65 result from cirrhosis. In Italy, 18 000 people died from cirrhosis in 1988, suggesting a prevalence of about 110 000 patients with cirrhosis in that country. In the US, approximately 3 million people are estimated to have cirrhosis, and it is the eleventh leading cause of death (Dufour et al. 1993; Capocaccia and Farchi 1988).

On a world-wide basis, more than 250 million people are estimated to suffer from chronic hepatitis B virus (HBV) infection, the vast majority of these living in China and the Far East. Although most have an acute self-limiting infection, individuals with persistent infection run the major health risks. Half of chronic carriers can be expected to die prematurely, either as a result of chronic inflammation or secondary to the development of hepatocellular carcinoma (Beasley et al. 1981; Brown et al. 1984). Chronic HBV infection is relatively uncommon in Western Europe and North America compared with less developed Eastern European and third world states. In the UK, HBV is not a common cause of chronic hepatitis (Reed et al. 1973). In contrast, HBV is responsible for 25–60% of cases of chronic hepatitis and/or cirrhosis in Greece, Africa and Iraq (Hadziyannis et al. 1970; Anthony et al. 1972). Incidences of chronic HBV infection of 10–15% are seen in the Middle East, but the highest rates are found in South East Asia: in Taiwan, 70 to 90% of the population have markers which suggest exposure to HBV at some time in their life (Beasley et al. 1981).

In 1989, the cloning and sequencing of the hepatitis C virus (HCV) was a major breakthrough for virologists and hepatologists dealing with chronic liver disease. Subsequent to the discovery of HCV and the development of antibody tests for the detection of this agent, it is clear that most cases of chronic non-A, non-B hepatitis are due to this agent as are many cases of so-called cryptogenic chronic hepatitis (Martin 1990). Up to 2% of total populations in North America and in Western Europe are infected. Chronic HCV infection appears to occur all over the world. Chronicity following inoculation occurs in 80–90% of infected individuals with up to 20% of these developing cirrhosis over 20 to 30 years. It is estimated that morbidity and mortality rates from this condition alone are likely to triple over the coming decade.

The prevalence in liver disease in almost all European countries follows trends in alcohol consumption. The per capita alcohol consumption correlates so well with cirrhosis mortality that liver cirrhosis mortality has been used as a measure of the prevalence of alcoholism. Most heavy drinkers and alcoholics will develop hepatomegaly and fatty infiltration of the liver; one-fifth to one-third develop a more severe liver injury. This includes alcoholic hepatitis or cirrhosis (Leevy 1968; Lelbach 1976). Increases in the mortality due to liver cirrhosis have been documented in the UK and Europe (Saunders et al. 1981; Schubert et al. 1982). In many patients, cirrhosis of the liver remains undetected during life. Accordingly morbidity from all types of alcoholic liver diseases is much higher than mortality, but no valid data about exact numbers are available.

Principal syndromes and symptoms: their pathogenesis and management

Ascites and oedema in cirrhosis

Patients with cirrhosis frequently accumulate large amounts of fluid in the peritoneal cavities (ascites), pleural cavities, and subcutaneous tissue (oedema) as a consequence of an abnormal regulation of extracellular fluid volume (Arroyo *et al.* 1991). This is associated with alterations in renal function, predominantly salt retention, which may or may not occur in combination with water retention and vasoconstriction of the renal circulation.

The dominant factor in ascites formation in cirrhosis is probably sodium (salt) retention. This causes expansion of the extracellular fluid volume and results eventually in ascites and/or oedema. Increased reabsorption of sodium occurs in the renal tubules. Although a number of other factors are involved in enhanced sodium reabsorption, hyperaldosteronism and enhanced renal sympathetic nerve activity are the most important (Arroyo *et al.* 1996).

Cirrhosis causes marked structural abnormalities within the liver resulting in marked disturbance of both hepatic and splanchnic blood circulation. The deposition of fibrous tissue and the formation of nodules result in increased resistance to blood flow. In addition to marked effects in the venous blood flow, leading to portal hypertension, effects are also seen within arteries, which dilate. All of these changes predispose to the formation of ascites by increasing the filtration of fluid (Benoit and Grainger 1988; Sieber and Groszmann 1992).

Symptoms

The principal symptom of patients with ascites and oedema is discomfort due to abdominal and leg swelling. Respiratory function and physical activity may be impaired. Nausea and reduced appetite are frequent complaints and reflux symptoms or heartburn may also occur. In severe cases 10–15 litres of fluid may accumulate. Hernial orifices may become weakened, scrotal oedema and venous engorgement of the abdominal wall may occur. Right-sided pleural effusions tend to occur while peripheral oedema may be present as a result of low protein concentrations in the circulation.

The objective of treatment in patients with ascites and in cirrhotic patients with oedema is to reduce the patient's discomfort. In addition, the decrease in the amount of fluid present within the peritoneal cavity reduces the risk of complications.

Treatment

Fluid restriction

The most appropriate treatment of patients with ascites depends on the cause of fluid retention and the stage of illness. The serum–ascites albumin gradient, derived from a diagnostic paracentesis can be helpful therapeutically (*see* table 7.1 on page 89). Patients with low serum–ascites albumin gradient usually do not have portal hypertension and often fail to respond to salt restriction and diuretics. In contrast, patients with high serum–ascites albumin gradient have portal hypertension and usually respond to these measures. One of the most important steps in treating this form of ascites is to treat the underlying liver disease. Abstention from alcohol is critical in these cases as abstinence from alcohol has been shown to normalise portal pressure in some patients (Pokross and Reynolds 1986).

Abstention from alcohol, however, will not be pertinent during the last days of life and alcohol will provide certain relief to the dying patient. Patients may crave for merely the taste or smell of their favourite beverage. For the family, the mere approval to administer previously prohibited substances such as alcohol by the attending physician, may be helpful in their coming to terms with impending death.

Sodium restriction

Sodium restriction is critical in the management of ascites as the amount of fluid retained in the body depends on the balance between sodium ingested in the diet and sodium excreted in the urine. The reduction of sodium content in the diet to 40–60 mcg per day (1–1.5 g of salt), without any other therapeutic intervention causes a negative sodium balance and loss of ascites and oedema in patients with mild sodium retention. In patients with moderate to marked sodium retention, such salt restriction is not sufficient in itself to achieve a negative sodium balance but may slow the accumulation of fluid. These patients might respond to a more severe restriction of sodium (less than 20 mcg per day). However, such intense sodium restriction is difficult to accomplish and may impair nutritional status. Clearly, as with the issue of alcohol, salt restriction will not be pertinent in the profoundly encephalopathic patient, unresponsive to treatment in the pre-terminal days.

Diuretic therapy

The pharmacological treatment of ascites has been based for many years in the administration of diuretics. These drugs increase urinary sodium excretion by reducing reabsorption of sodium. Diuretic therapy in patients with cirrhosis is based predominantly on the administration of spironolactone, either alone or in combination with a loop diuretic, usually frusemide. Bumetanide may be substituted for frusemide in patients who have intestinal oedema. Amiloride, a potassium-sparing diuretic is an alternative to spironolactone.

Approximately 10–20% of patients with ascites may not respond to diuretic therapy or will suffer diuretic-induced complications preventing the use of these agents.

Therapeutic paracentesis

Although it has been recognised since the time of the ancient Greeks that paracentesis is an effective means in controlling ascites, it is only recently that controlled trials have demonstrated the safety of this approach. Therapeutic paracentesis has increasingly been used in the management of patients with large ascites, due to the results of several randomised studies comparing paracentesis, either total removal of all ascitic fluid, in a single tap or repeated taps of 4–6 litres per day, in association with plasma volume expansion and diuretics for those with severe ascites (Arroyo *et al.* 1994; Guazzi *et al.* 1975; Peltekian *et al.* 1997; Ginès *et al.* 1987; Runyon 1997). These studies show that paracentesis is more rapid, effective, and is associated with lower number of complications than conventional diuretic therapy. Because it does not alter pre-existing renal functional abnormalities and cirrhosis, patients should therefore be given diuretics following paracentesis to avoid reformation of ascites.

Even in patients without urinary sodium excretion, ascites can be controlled by paracentesis performed on a two-weekly basis (Runyon 1998; Runyon 1988). The sodium concentration of ascitic fluid is approximately equivalent to that of plasma, which is 130 mmol per litre in these patients. A 6-litre paracentesis therefore removes 780 mmol of sodium. Patients who consume 88 mmol of sodium per day, excrete 10 mmol per day in non-urinary losses, but fail to excrete sodium in the urine, retain a net balance of +78 mmol per day. Therefore a 6-litre paracentesis removes 10 days of retained sodium. Patients with some urinary sodium excretion should need paracentesis even less frequently.

A controversy relating to therapeutic paracentesis is that of colloid replacement. One study randomised patients to receive albumin (10 g per litre of fluid removed) versus no albumin following therapeutic paracentesis. The group that received no albumin developed statistically significantly more changes in electrolytes, plasma renin, and serum creatinine. Despite this there was no more clinical morbidity or mortality in one group compared to the other (Ginès et al. 1988). However, another study documented that a subset of patients who develop a rise in plasma renin have a decreased life expectancy.

Refractory ascites

Refractory ascites is defined as fluid overload that is unresponsive to a sodium-restricted diet and high dose diuretic therapy, in the absence of prostaglandin inhibitors such as non-steroidal anti-inflammatory drugs (Runyon 1988). Less than 10% of patients with cirrhotic ascites will be refractory to standard medical therapy. In patients in whom the diagnosis of refractory ascites is made, other strategies must be employed including serial therapeutic paracentesis, peritoneovenous shunt, or transjugular intra-hepatic porto-systemic shunt (TIPSS).

Shunts

Shunts, such as the LeVeen or Denver shunts, were popular in the 1970s as a physiological treatment of ascites. Their use, however, has decreased partly because of complications such as shunt occlusion, caval thrombosis, and peritoneal fibrosis, and partly because of the apparent safety of large volume paracentesis. Shunt placement reduced hospital stay, the number of hospitalisations, and reduced doses in patients with ascites (Bories et al. 1986; Stanley et al. 1989). Long-term potency however is poor and no survival advantage occurs when compared to conventional medical therapy in controlled trials (Stanley et al. 1989; Ginès et al. 1991). These side effects have led to almost near abandonment of these procedures. Peritoneovenous shunting should probably now be reserved for diuretic resistant patients who are not transplant candidates and who are not candidates for serial therapeutic paracentesis as a result of multiple abdominal surgical scars, or distance from a physician willing and capable of performing paracentesis.

TIPS

A number of studies recently published examine the utilisation of transjugular intra-hepatic porto-systemic shunts (TIPS) in patients with refractory ascites (reviewed in Ginès et al. 1997). As with surgical shunts, reduction in portal pressure obtained with TIPS is associated with favourable physiological effects on renal function. In addition, TIPS does not have the operative mortality and morbidity associated with surgical shunting. However, the shunt may block, and impairment of liver function occurs as a result of shunting of blood between the portal and systemic circulation causing hepatic encephalopathy. A recent study in a small number of patients with refractory ascites showed increased mortality in patients with poor liver function treated with TIPS, compared with patients treated with paracentesis plus albumin (Lebrec et al. 1996). However, larger controlled studies will be needed to define whether TIPS has a role in the management of these patients. At present, the TIPS shunt has been designated as 'unproven' for the treatment of refractory ascites by a National Institute of Health Consensus Conference (Shiffman *et al.* 1995).

Spontaneous bacterial peritonitis

Even in patients receiving palliative care, onset of symptoms compatible with spontaneous bacterial peritonitis (SBP) (sudden onset of fever in association with worsening or new-onset encephalopathy, with/without abdominal pain) and an increased polymorpho-nuclear leukocyte count of more than 250 mm^{-3}, antibiotic therapy should be started. Delaying treatment until ascitic fluid culture grows bacteria may result in the death of the patient or overwhelming sepsis.

The diagnosis is made when there is a positive bacterial culture from ascitic fluid and an increased absolute polymorphonuclear leukocyte count greater than 250 cells mm^{-3}, without an evident intra-abdominal and surgically treatable source of infection. A paracentesis must be performed and ascitic fluid analysed before confident diagnosis of ascitic fluid infection can be made.

In patients with alcoholic hepatitis and end-stage disease, a fever, white cell count elevation, and abdominal pain can occur without bacterial peritonitis. However, in these patients an elevated neutrophil count in the ascitic fluid represents spontaneous bacterial peritonitis.

Broad-spectrum antibiotic therapy is warranted in patients with suspected ascitic fluid infection until the results of susceptibility testing are available. Cefotaxime or similar third generation cephalosporins appear to be the treatment of choice for suspected SBP as they cover 95% of the flora, including the three most common isolates which are *Escherichia coli*, *Klebsiella pneumoniae* and *Streptococcus pneumoniae* (Runyon 1998). A follow up ascitic fluid analysis is not necessary in patients with SBP.

The majority of patients who develop this complication will have advanced cirrhosis with typical symptoms. Sucessful treatment with antibiotics results in a dramatic clinical response with cessation of abdominal pain, normalisation of temperature, and resolution of encephalopathy. Oral ofloxacin has been reported as being as effective as intravenous cefotaxime in the treatment of SBP in patients who are not vomiting or in shock (Navasa *et al.* 1996). Alternatively oral ciprofloxacin can be utilised.

Summary

The two year survival of patients with cirrhosis and ascites is approximately 50%. In addition, once patients become refractory to routine medical therapy, 50% will die within 6 months, and only 25% of patients with a refractory ascites will be alive at 12 months (Bories *et al.* 1986). In the past, patients with ascites frequently occupied hospital beds for long periods of time. Although it would be desirable to have no clinically detectable fluid present within the abdominal cavity, this should not be a prerequisite for discharge from hospital. Patients who are stable, with ascites as their main problem can be discharged after it has been determined that they are responding to their medical regimen. However, patients should probably be observed either at home or in a clinic setting within a week of discharge from hospital. Figure 7.1 shows an algorithm for management of ascites in patients with cirrhosis applicable in both home and hospital settings.

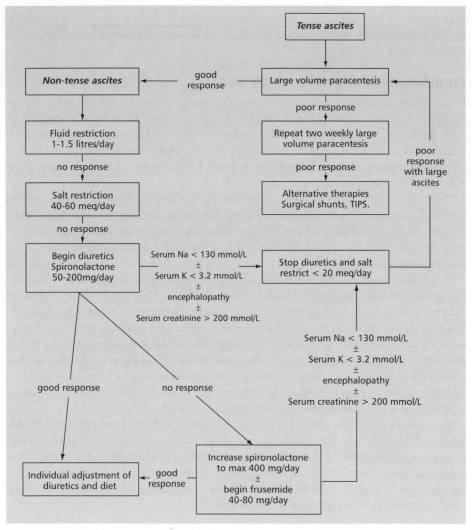

Fig. 7.1 Algorithm for the management of ascites in patients with cirrhosis.

Hepatorenal syndrome

Hepatorenal syndrome (HRS) is a common and serious complication of cirrhosis characterised by impaired renal function and disturbance of the arterial circulation in conjunction with the activity of the vaso-active systems (Runyon 1988). Although the kidney is structurally normal there is a marked increase in vascular resistance in the setting of a reduction in systemic vascular resistance. The mechanism of vasoconstriction is not fully understood, but probably involves increased vasoconstrictor and reduced vasodilator reactors.

Hepatorenal syndrome occurs in approximately 10% of hospitalised patients with cirrho-

Table 7.1 Recommendations of the American Association for the Study of Liver Diseases in relation to appropriate management of patients with ascites related to cirrhosis

1 Abstinence from alcohol.

2 A sodium restricted diet together with oral spironolactone and frusemide.

3 Fluid restriction if the serum sodium is less than 120 mmol per litre.

4 Bed rest is not recommended.

5 A single 4 to 6 litre abdominal paracentesis performed in patients with tense ascites. This should be followed by a sodium restricted diet and diuretics administered orally.

6 Urinary sodium excretion determination in patients where compliance is suspect or diuretic resistance is suspected.

7 Diuretic sensitive patients should be treated with salt restricted diet and oral diuretics rather than serial paracentesis.

sis. Two types of hepatorenal syndrome exist. Type I is characterised by rapid progressive deterioration of renal function with the doubling of the initial serum creatinine or a 50% reduction in the initial 24 hour creatinine clearance to a level lower than 20 ml per minute in less than two weeks. Renal failure in patients like this is often associated with progressive oliguria, marked sodium retention, and hyponatraemia. These patients will have signs of advanced liver failure. In 50% of patients, type I HRS develops spontaneously without any identifiable cause. In others it may relate to the development of bacterial infection, especially SBP, or to paracentesis without plasma expansion. Type II hepatorenal syndrome is characterised by moderate and stable reduction of GFR glomerular filtration rate that does not meet the criteria proposed for type I. These patients will have relatively preserved hepatic function but the main consequence of this type of hepatorenal syndrome is diuretic resistant ascites. HRS is diagnosed based on the exclusion of other causes of renal failure that can occur in patients with cirrhosis. This includes pre-renal failure, acute tubular necrosis, administration of nephrotoxic agents especially non-steroidal anti-inflammatory agents, or aminoglycosides.

Treatment options for patients with HRS are limited and the prognosis for patients with HRS is poor. Median survival time of these patients is less than two weeks, a survival time shorter than that of patients with acute renal failure from other causes (Kleinknecht 1992). The combination of several factors including renal failure and liver failure probably accounts for this poor outcome. For type II HRS the median survival time is usually several months. This is longer than those with type I HRS but shorter than patients with ascites without renal failure. The development of HRS at home will be inevitably fatal, and its recognition will usually herald a rapid deterioration in the patient's clinical condition.

Hepatic encephalopathy

It was recognised by Hippocrates in the fifth century BC that 'those who [are] mad from bile are vociferous, malignant and will not be quiet'. Although this association of altered mentation in patients with disordered liver function was described over 2500 years ago, the precise mechanisms associated with this development remain unknown.

Hepatic encephalopathy occurs when blood from the portal circulation carrying nitrogenous degradation products of dietary and gut bacterial origin reaches the brain, either because of liver cell failure or in patients with chronic liver disease and portal hypertension, because of collateral venous circulation bypassing the liver and emptying directly into the systemic blood. Most patients have a combination of both hepatocellular failure and portosystemic shunting contributing to the neuropsychiatric disturbance.

The development of neuropsychiatric disturbance in patients with chronic liver disease results in depression of the central nervous system with varying degrees of severity. However, it is a potentially reversible metabolic abnormality. In the majority of patients with chronic liver disease encephalopathy is subclinical. Reaction times in activities of daily living such as driving and operating machinery may be affected and will be detected in EEG abnormalities or as impairment of psychometric performance (Conn et al. 1977; Conn 1977). Encephalopathy becomes overt in approximately 30% of patients with chronic liver disease resulting in abnormalities in mood, personality, behaviour, and altered consciousness. In some patients, reversal of day/night sleep patterns will occur.

In normal circumstances, the biochemical and metabolic milieu of the brain remains relatively undisturbed mainly as a result of the blood brain barrier. Several studies confirm increased blood brain barrier transport of neutral amino acids and a reduction in the transport of basic amino acids and ketone bodies into the brain in advanced liver disease. The underlying mechanism responsible for this change is not understood although increased levels of ammonia and methanthiols have been implicated (Grippon et al. 1986). Recently, PET scanning has demonstrated an increased rate at which ammonia is taken up into the brain in patients with chronic hepatic encephalopathy (Lockwood et al. 1992). Regional variation in cerebral blood flow has also been found in these patients, with glucose metabolism reduced in the cortex and increased in the cerebellum, thalamus, and the caudate nucleus. These changes in blood flow and glucose may be related to global depression of CNS (central nervous system) function rather than being the primary cause.

In patients with encephalopathy, blood ammonia levels are frequently but not always increased. In the past, ammonia has been considered the most important factor in the genesis of encephalopathy. In patients with cirrhosis, loss of hepatocellular cellular function and shunting of blood contributes to increased ammonia concentrations in the blood stream. EEG activity in humans with hepatic encephalopathy is not characteristic of that produced by hyperammonaemia in animals. It is possible however that persistent hyperammonaemia facilitates the synergistic effects on the central nervous system of other neuro toxins and also primes the neurones to acute increases in ammonia (Raabe and Onstad 1985).

Other compounds which have been implicated in the development of encephalopathy include extremely volatile and toxic sulphur-containing compounds which are the products of gut bacterial metabolism. Methanthiol has been shown to exert adverse effects upon the blood brain barrier and may be synergistic with ammonia. Phenols also come into this category (Martensson et al. 1985). Other potential candidates which may result in the development of encephalopathy include medium chain fatty acids such as butyrate, valerate and octanoate.

Neurotransmitters such as glutamate have also been identified as being potentially important in the development of encephalopathy. Regulation of these cells is impaired in patients with hepatic encephalopathy. Increased cerebral glutamine has been found in the brain and CSF (cerebrospinal fluid) of patients with hepatic encephalopathy (Taylor-Robinson et al. 1994).

Gamma-amino butyric acid (GABA) is the major inhibitory neurotransmitter in the CNS. In health, a fine balance exists between glutamate and GABA activity. This is mediated through GABA receptors. Benzodiazepines modulate the activity of these receptors, binding at a different but closely linked site from GABA. Derangements in GABA have been suggested as being causally related to the development of encephalopathy. Increased levels of endogenous benzodiazepines have been reported in patients with hepatic encephalopathy. Benzodiazepine antagonists have therefore been used as treatment in some patients.

Other theories in the evolution of hepatic encephalopathy include production of ammonia by the bacterium *Helicobacter pylori* while manganese accumulation has been noted on MRI examination of the basal ganglia.

Treatment of encephalopathy

Treatment of encephalopathy is aimed primarily at reducing the absorption of potentially neurotoxic material from the gastrointestinal tract and is achieved by dietary alterations and the use of agents which may alter the nature and metabolism of intestinal flora. Newer agents have not yet been confirmed as beneficial in clinical trials.

Treatment aimed at reducing the intestinal absorption of neurotoxins

Patients with chronic liver disease will need protein restriction in the face of increased energy requirements. Approximately 40–60 g of protein daily appears optimum. Clinical trials have shown that vegetable protein is better tolerated than meat protein, which may relate to a greater fibre content. Dietary fibre in the colon is subject to fermentation from bacteria, and acidification of colonic lumenal contents occurs in the setting of high fibre: a fall in pH may reduce the formation of toxic fatty acids and ammonia from amino acids in the gut lumen. Poor patient compliance however frequently limits the use of such diets.

The use of non-absorbable disaccharides such as lactulose and lactitol have been an accepted part of the management of encephalopathy for over three decades. Intestinal absorption of neurotoxic compounds is reduced by altering ammonia absorption and metabolism of gut flora. These agents also reduce bowel transit time and alters both bowel acidity and flora. Lactulose may stimulate the incorporation of ammonia into bacterial protein thus reducing the amount available for absorption (Vince *et al.* 1978). It may also inhibit the generation of ammonia in the gut mucosa by interfering with the uptake of glutamate and its metabolism. A range of side effects, including flatulence, abdominal cramps, and pain may result from treatment with the non-absorbable disaccharides and may require treatment discontinuation in some patients.

Lactitol (beta glactosido-sorbitol) was first used to treat hepatic encephalopathy in 1982 and has been found to be as effective as lactulose. Meta-analysis of all randomised control trials comparing the two agents suggests that lactitol may produce fewer gastrointestinal side effects (Blanc *et al.* 1992). Any evidence or suspicion of intestinal obstruction precludes the use of either of these agents.

Antibiotics: Until recently the use of oral antibiotics was widespread in the treatment of chronic hepatic encephalopathy. Early studies suggested that oral neomycin was at least as effective as lactulose in the treatment of chronic hepatic encephalopathy. However, a controlled study showed no clinical benefit from neomycin compared with placebo. In addition, up to 3% of an orally administered dose of neomycin is absorbed systemically and therefore the toxic effects of aminoglycosides such as nephrotoxicity and ototoxicity can result. The long term use of oral aminoglycosides in chronic hepatic encephalopathy is therefore not advised. Anecdotal evidence suggests that the combination of an antibiotic with an unabsorbable disaccharide may be of some use in patients unresponsive to lactulose alone. However, a controlled trial in 80 patients found that a lactulose–neomycin combination was no better than placebo (Blanc *et al.* 1990). The use of oral antibiotics in the management of patients with encephalopathy should not be considered routine, although metronidazole may be of benefit in some patients.

Treatment based on elimination of nitrogenous waste

Sodium benzoate has been used to treat congenital urea cycle enzymopathies. Excretion of urinary nitrogen is increased from the defective urea cycle to hippurate synthesis. In a large prospective controlled trial in India, sodium benzoate (5 mg twice daily) was as effective as lactulose in improvement of mentation and EEG findings (Sushma *et al.* 1992). A further advantage of sodium benzoate is that it can be administered intravenously if necessary in addition to being a cheaper alternative to lactulose.

Other interest has focused on the use of 1-ornithine-1-aspartate, which promotes hepatocyte glutamine synthesis. Blood ammonia levels have been reduced in patients with cirrhosis and although its clinical efficacy needs to be fully established, oral ornithine has been found to be at least as effective as lactulose in terms of improvement in clinical grade of encephalopathy.

Besides the use of pharmacological agents, the control of precipitating factors such as constipation, gastrointestinal haemorrhage, electrolyte imbalance, and infection are the critical factors in the management of hepatic encephalopathy. In addition, given the potential role of neurotransmitter agents in the pathophysiology it is also prudent to stop all sedatives, tranquillisers, hypnotics, and opiate agents.

Jaundice and pruritus

Effective treatment for pruritus (itching) complicating cholestatic liver disease remains a difficult and highly significant problem. Pruritus can markedly impair the quality of life and may lead to sleep deprivation or even suicidal ideation. The efficacy of conventional and some heroic therapies that have been tried are usually partial and often insufficient to provide patients with adequate relief. Some of the current treatments have tried to address this by looking at the scientific basis behind pruritus.

The onset of jaundice in patients with malignant disease usually heralds a rapid deterioration in the clinical course. However, in patients with cirrhosis without hepatocellular cancer, an aggressive approach to evaluating this sign is merited. In some patients, symptomatic treatment of pruritus may be the only achievable goal, whereas in others, a more

Table 7.2 Classification and causes of jaundice

Pre-hepatic	Intra-hepatic	Extra-hepatic
Gilbert's disease	*Hepatitis*	*Malignant*
Haemolytic processes	Viral	Pancreatic carcinoma
Haematoma	Alcoholic	Ampullary tumours
	Autoimmune	Cholangiocarcinoma
	Cholestatic liver disease	Lymphadenopathy
	Primary biliary cirrhosis	External biliary compression
	Primary sclerosing cholangitis	*Benign*
	Ischaemia	Gallstone disease
	Hepatic artery thrombosis	Choledochal cysts
	Left ventricular failure	Chronic pancreatitis
	Venous outflow block	Biliary stricture
	Congestive cardiac failure	
	Veno-occlusive disease	
	Budd Chiari syndrome	
	Infiltrative conditions	
	Malignancy	
	Lymphoma	
	Gauchers	
	Other	
	Drugs	
	TPN (total parenteral nutrition)	
	Sepsis	

aggressive approach will almost certainly improve quality and duration of life. The more aggressive approach will involve multidisciplinary care between biliary endoscopists, radiologists, and physicians in order to best define the appropriate strategy. In patients with non-malignant liver disease, the presence of jaundice may be part of the natural history of the condition, such as primary biliary cirrhosis or primary sclerosing cholangitis. It is therefore critical to define the primary cause of jaundice, identify treatable disease, and, where these ideals are not met, palliate the disturbing symptoms for both patients and their relatives.

Jaundice is classified as relating to pre-hepatic, intra-hepatic and post-hepatic causes (Table 7.2) and most patients who present to palliative care services should at an early stage have their cause of jaundice identified.

Pruritus is a sensation that stimulates an urge to scratch. Extra-hepatic biliary obstruction is a frequent presenting complaint. The commonest proposed theory is that bile salts contribute to pruritus by their deposition on nerve endings in the skin (Varadi 1974). This is supported by the fact that pruritus can be induced by the administration of bile salts on the skin (Ghent *et al.* 1977). Indirect evidence exists in that bile salts are usually elevated in patients with pruritus, and lowering of serum bile salts by cholestyramine is associated with the relief of pruritus (Carey andWilliams 1961; Sharp *et al.* 1967). Moreover, external biliary drainage relieves pruritus in patients with biliary tract obstruction. It is not clear, however, which bile salts are the most pruritogenic as the relative proportions of bile acids in disease states differ considerably (Varadi 1974). Pruritus can occur in patients with relatively low concentrations of serum bile salts (Osborne *et al.* 1959), while relief of pruritus can occur in patients with rising levels of bile salts (Hanid and Levi 1980).

It has recently been postulated that pruritus is related to a direct effect on the hepatocyte rather than its effect on nerve endings in the skin (Ghent 1987). Bile salt accumulation could occur and cause release of a pruritus-inducing substance from the hepatocyte. It is known that bile salts have a detergent effect, which can alter membrane dynamics. The nature and site of action of this pruritus has not been identified.

Evidence has emerged that the pruritus of cholestasis is associated with increased neuro-transmission—neuromodulation which is mediated by endogenous opioids in the central nervous system (Bergasa and Jones 1995). Three lines of evidence support this hypothesis. First, administration of morphine or other opioid agonistic drugs induces pruritus particularly if the drug is administered centrally rather than peripherally (Thomas *et al.* 1992). Second, the syndrome of cholestasis is associated with phenomena consistent with increased opioidergic tone (Thornton and Losowsky 1988). Finally, the pruritus of cholestasis can be ameliorated by parenteral administration of the opioid antagonist naloxone (Bergasa *et al.* 1992). However, most opioid antagonists are given parenterally whereas the best way to give these agents to patients with jaundice is orally. Two studies using oral nalmefene have found it to be efficacious (Thorntorn and Losowsky 1988; Bergasa *et al.* 1998). This agent appears to be useful in the long term. It has been found to have low toxicity, good bio-availability following oral dosage, greater potency than naloxone in antagonising opioid agonists at their receptors, and has a half-life of 8.6 hours. This potency appears critical as it seems increasingly likely that endogenous opioids contribute to the itch of cholestasis, and that greater antagonism of opioid receptors appears to be required to reverse the effects of endogenous opioids than exogenous ones. Oral nalmefine has given new impetus to the search for effective remedies in cholestasis and randomised double-blind controlled trials will probably be performed with this agent. Other agents which appear to be responsible for the pruritus of cholestasis include histamine, calorcrines, prostaglandins, substance P, and ceratonone.

Treatment of jaundice and pruritis

Several strategies have been applied to the treatment of jaundice and can be categorised as general, local, and specific therapies. Where a focal stricture exists, for example in patients with biliary obstruction secondary to pancreatic cancer, cholangiocarcinoma, and malignant disease, surgical bypass or non-operative stenting via percutaneous cholangiography or endoscopic stent placement will achieve drainage of bile. In patients with cholestatic jaundice without evidence of stricturing in the biliary tree, it will be more difficult to gain good control of pruritus.

General measures: Cool temperatures and an air-conditioned environment reduce the sensation of itch (pruritis). Reduced perspiration as a result of cooling may also reduce the itch threshold. Local measures in the treatment of itch includes moistening agents such as oatmeal and oil baths or astringents such as calamine lotion cream. Calamine preparations typically contain a combination of calamine, zinc oxide, glycerol, and sodium citrate in a liquid or paraffin preparation. Topical corticosteroids may also have an effect. These should be discouraged, however, especially if long-term administration is anticipated. Numerous topical antihistamines are available in the treatment of pruritus but they will have the best effect in situations where an allergic rash is present. These agents include mepyramine, diphenhydramine, and antazoline, and may be suitable for some patients.

Systemic agents: Antihistamines are relatively ineffective and the rationale for their use is in part their sedative effect. Those most commonly used are chlorpheniramine or promethazine. Newer, less sedating antihistamines, including astmizole or loratadine, are of unproven value. Antihistamines can cause headache, psychomotor impairment, and antimuscarinic effects such as urinary retention, dry mouth, and blurred vision. Other antihistamines, such as the H2 receptor antagonist cimetidine, have been found to be useful in patients with pruritus, but other H2 receptor blockers such as ranitidine or nizatidine do not share the drug metabolism inhibitory properties of cimetidine. Phenothiazines such as trimepraxine and prochlorperazine have also been recommended as anti-pruritic therapies and seem to manifest their effects by acting centrally rather than peripherally. Routine and widespread use of the neuroleptic drugs is not recommended given their propensity to a large number of side effects.

Other agents which have been useful in treating pruritus include cholestyramine resin, which mediates its effect by its capacity to bind bile salts, preventing their reabsorption and so eliminating them in the faeces. Cholestyramine should be administered one hour before and after meals so that the arrival of the drug in the duodenum coincides with gall bladder emptying. The maintenance dose is usually 12 g per day. At higher doses, cholestyramine may impair the absorption of vitamins A, D, E, and K by reducing intestinal lumenal concentrations of bile acids. Therefore patients needing long-term treatment may need vitamin supplements. Care should also be taken that other drugs are taken at different times to that of cholestyramine.

Ursodeoxycholic acid has been found to be useful in patients with itch secondary to primary biliary cirrhosis. This may be due to a choleretic effect or by reduction of bile acids. Although its use has been associated with biochemical improvement in bilirubin in patients with both drug-induced cholestasis and primary biliary cirrhosis, it is unproven as an anti-pruritic agent. Paradoxically, ursodeoxycholic acid may cause or aggravate itch.

Rifampicin (300–500 mg per day) has been used in the treatment of pruritus and chronic cholestasis secondary to primary biliary cirrhosis and other cholestatic disorders (Ghent and Carruthers 1988; Gregorio et al. 1993). It usually mediates its effect within seven days. The mechanism of rifampicin is unknown but may relate to the ability of the drug to inhibit bile acid uptake into hepatocytes thus preventing release of other putative pruritus-inducing agents. Alternatively, its mechanism of action relates to enzyme induction. Potential side effects include risk of gallstone formation, drug interactions and emergence of resistant organisms. Long-term use has never been evaluated.

Other agents which have been utilised include methyltestosterone at a dose of 25 mg per day sublingually, which works within 7 days (Khandelwal and Malet 1994).

Strategies

When pruritus is severe a combination of generalised and local measures should be combined with systemic drug treatment. A strategy would be 4 g cholestyramine three times a day, followed by an antihistamine or phenothiazine. Cimetidine can be added if required. As itch can be worse at night, a sedative may be useful. Sedating antihistamines such as chlorpheniramine will be helpful. Other sedation should be commenced with caution, however, as encephalopathy may be precipitated. Any obstructive cause of jaundice should be treated and relieved. Other agents which have been tried in patients with jaundice include ursodeoxycholic acid, low dose propafol, and ondansetron (Khandelwal and Malet 1994).

As detailed above, opiate antagonists hold tremendous promise in the treatment of pruritus and are likely to come into greater use as trial data becomes available. Heroic efforts such as plasmapheresis have also been performed and found to be temporarily effective in some patients with intractable pruritus (Cohen *et al.* 1985). It is, however, both expensive and labour intensive and this may be excessive in an otherwise compromised patient.

Bleeding as a terminal event

One-third of deaths from cirrhosis occur as a result of upper gastrointestinal tract bleeding from oesphageal or gastric varices (Cutler and Mendeloff 1981; Gilbert 1990; Longstreth 1995). Mortality from this source, even from a first bleed, is approximately 30–40% despite therapeutic intervention, whereas for re-bleeds, mortality is even higher. This, when compared to mortality of 8% from bleeding unrelated to portal hypertension, gives an indication of the dramatic and torrential nature of bleeds from this source (Silverstein *et al.* 1981; Morgan and Clamp 1988). The patient will usually experience repeated bouts of massive haematemesis or maelena of several hundred ml of blood. The event will be distressing to both the patient and their family, and in many instances merits preparation, through a careful discussion with the patient and family of their thoughts and concerns.

While endoscopic treatment with banding ligation or sclerotherapy remains the treatment of choice in the therapeutic setting, intervention of this nature will not be appropriate in a dying patient. If bleeding from this source is untreated or unpalliated, death will result within a matter of one to two hours. If warning bleeds have occurred, an injection of diamorphine will be appropriate and go a long way to lessen the discomfort for both the patient and their relatives.

Depression and chronic liver disease

Recently it has been described that patients with depression (as assessed by the Beck Depression Inventory) while awaiting transplantation had a significantly poorer perceived quality of life, poorer adaptive coping, and lower Karnofsky performance scores as compared to non-depressed patients. Although patient survival was not different between depressed and non-depressed groups following liver transplantation, patients with depression were significantly more likely to die while awaiting transplantation than non-depressed patients (Singh *et al.* 1997a). It is clear therefore that the prevalence of depression is probably underestimated in patients with end-stage liver disease, even more so given that most patients with end-stage liver disease are ineligible for transplantation. It is therefore reasonable to treat patients with overt signs of depression.

Quality of life issues and chronic liver disease

Although no significant literature exists in relation to quality of life in the latter days of patients dying from the complications of end-stage liver disease, it was recognised early in the evolution of liver transplantation programmes that quality of life was important in the timing of transplantation. A recent meta-analysis found statistically significant pre- to post-transplant improvements in physical/functional quality of life, sexual functioning, daily activities, social functioning, and overall quality of life perceptions. The majority of these studies documented physical functional and global quality of life advantages for transplant recipients relative to ill comparison groups (Brauata *et al.* 1999).

Until recently, little consideration was given to patients with chronic liver disease who were not candidates for transplantation. It is increasingly recognised that even among patients awaiting liver transplantation, feelings of tension, anxiety, mood disturbance, and depression are common. What is equally interesting is that among subgroups of patients with chronic liver disease awaiting transplantation, patients with HCV infection tend to have a greater tendency towards depression. Moreover, even in the absence of cirrhosis, a reduction in quality of life scores is apparent (Foster *et al.* 1998; Singh *et al.* 1997b; Dew *et al.* 1997). It is clear that newer treatment modalities need assessing in relation to quality of life. This is supported by the description of enhanced quality of life following the introduction of the TIPS procedure (Nazarian *et al.* 1996), despite the 'unproven' categorisation of the procedure by the National Institutes of Health (Shiffman *et al.* 1995).

Conclusions

Chronic end-stage liver disease develops over many years and has a terminal phase highly relevant to palliative care. Although transplant programmes have done much to alter the course of disease, even in the UK at least four people die from the disease for every one transplanted. Common symptoms and signs include ascites, jaundice, itch, and encephepatopathy. Bleeding from varices in the oesophagus or stomach is the final cause of death in about one-third of those who die. The management of these symptoms and strategies to improve quality of life and support for the patient and their family (see Chapter 22) is not yet sufficiently evaluated in the terminal phases of illness and should be the focus of future research.

References

Anthony, P.P., Vogel, C.L., Sadikali, F., Barker, L.F., and Peterson, M.R. (1972). Hepatitis-associated antigen and antibody in Uganda: correlation of serological testing with histopathology. *British Medical Journal* 1: 403–6.

Arroyo, V., Claria, J., Salo, J., and Jimenez, W. (1994). Antidiuretic hormone and the pathogenesis of water retention in cirrhosis with ascites. *Seminars in Liver Disease* 14: 44–58.

Arroyo, V., Ginès, P., and Salo, J. (1994). A European survey on the treatment of ascites and cirrhosis. *Journal of Hepatology* **21**: 667–72.

Arroyo, V., Ginès, P., Gerbes, A.L., Dudley, F.J., Gentilini, P., Laffi, G. *et al.* (1996). Definition and diagnostic criteria of refractory ascites and hepatorenal syndrome in cirrhosis. *Hepatology* **23**: 164–76.

Arroyo, V., Ginès, P., Jimenez, W., and Rodes, J. (1991). Ascites, renal failure, and electrolyte disorders in cirrhosis. Pathogenesis, diagnosis and treatment. In McIntyre, N., Benhamou, J.P., Bircher, J., Rizetto, M., and Rodes, J. (eds), *Textbook of Clinical Hepatology*, Oxford: Oxford Medical Press, pp. 429–70.

Arroyo, V., Rodes, J., Gutierrz-Lizarraga, M.A., and Revert, L. (1996). Prognostic value of spontaneous hyponatraemia in cirrhosis with ascites. *American Journal of Digestive Diseases***21**: 249–56.

Beasley, R.P., Hwang, L., Lin, C., and Chien, C.C. (1981). Hepatocellular carcinoma and hepatitis B virus: a prospective study of 22,707 men in Taiwan. *Lancet* **2**: 1129–32.

Beasley, R.P., Hwang, L., Lin, C., Stevens, L.E., Wang, K.Y., and Sun, T.Y. *et al.* (1981). Hepatitis B immune globulin efficacy in the interruption of perinatal transmission of hepatitis B virus carrier state. *Lancet* **2**: 387–93.

Benoit, J.N. and Grainger, D.N. (1988). Intestinal microvascular adaptation to chronic portal hypertension in the rat. *Gastroenterology* **94**: 471–6.

Bergasa, N.V. and Jones, E.A. (1995). The pruritus of cholestasis: potential pathogenic and therapeutic implications of opioids. *Gastroenterology* **108**:1582–8.

Bergasa, N.V., Schmitt, J.M., Talbot, T.L., Alling, D.W., Swain, M.J., Turner, M.L., Jenkins, J.B., and Jones, E.A. (1998). Trial of oral nalmefene therapy for the pruritus of cholestasis. *Hepatology* **27**: 679–84.

Bergasa, N.V., Talbot, N.L., Alling, D.W., Schmitt, J.M., Walker, E.C., Baker, B.L., Korenman, J.C., *et al.* (1992). A controlled trial of naloxone infusions for the pruritus of chronic cholestasis. *Gastroenterology* **102**: 544–9.

Blanc, P., Daures, J.P., and Pierruges, R. (1990). Treatment of acute hepatic encephalopathy; lactulose-neomycin v placebo. Randomised bio equivalents assay. *Journal of Hepatology* **11** (Suppl. 2), S8.

Blanc, P., Daures, J.P., Rouillon, J.M., Peray, P., Pierrugues, R., Larrey, D. *et al.* (1992). Lactitol or lactulose in the treatment of chronic hepatic encephalopathy: the results of a meta-analysis. *Hepatology* **15**: 222–8.

Bories, P., Garcia-Compean, D., Michel, H., Bowel, M., Capran, J.P., Gauthier, A., *et al.* (1986). The treatment of refractory ascites by the Le Veen shunt: a multi-centre controlled trial (57 patients). *Journal of Hepatology* **3**: 212–18.

Brauata, D.M., Olkin, L., Barnato, A., Keeffe, E. and Owens, D. (1999) Health-related quality of life after liver transplantation: a meta-analysis. *Liver Transplantation & Survey* **5**: 318–31.

Brown, S.E., Howard, C.R., Zuckerman, A.J., and Steward, M.W. (1984). Affinity of antibody responses in man to hepatitis B vaccine determined with synthetic peptides. *Lancet* **1**: 184–7.

Capocaccia, R. and Farchi, G. (1988). Mortality from liver cirrhosis in Italy: proportion associated with consumption of alcohol. *Journal of Clinical Epidemiology* **41**: 347–57.

Carey, J.B. and Williams, G. (1961). Relief of pruritus of jaundice with a bile acid sequstring resin. *Journal of the American Medical Association* **176**: 432–5.

Cohen, L.B., Ambinder, E.P., Wolke, A.M., Field, S.P., and Schnaffner, F. (1985). Role of plasmapheresis in primary biliary cirrhosis. *Gut* **26**: 291–4.

Conn, H.O. (1977). Trail making and number-connection tests in the assessment of mental state in portal systemic encephalopathy. *American Journal of Digestive Diseases* 22: 541–50.

Conn, H.O., Levey, C.M., Vlahcevic, Z.R., Rodgers, J.B., Maddrey, W.C., Seeff, L., and Levy, L.L. (1977). Comparison of lactulose and neomysin in the treatment of chronic portal systemic encephalopathy: a double blind trial. *Gastroenterology* 72: 573–83.

Cutler, J.A. and Mendeloff, A.I. (1981). Upper gastrointestinal bleeding. Nature and magnitude of the problem in the US. *Digestive Diseases and Sciences* 26 (Suppl.): S90–S96.

Dew, M.A., Switzer, G.E., Goycoolea, J.M., Allen, A.S., DiMartini, A., Kormos, R.L., and Griffith, B.P. (1997). Does transplantation produce quality of liver benefits? A quantitative analysis of the literature. *Transplantation* 64: 1261–73.

Dufour, M.C., Stinson, F., and Caces, M. (1993). Trends in cirrhosis, morbidity and mortality: US, 1979–1988. *Seminars in Liver Disease* 13: 109–25.

Foster, G.R., Goldin, R.D., and Thomas, H.C. (1998). Chronic hepatitis C virus infection causes a significant reduction in quality of life in the absence of cirrhosis. *Hepatology* 27: 209–12.

Ghent, C.N., Bloomer, J.R., and Klatskin, G. (1977). Elevations in skin tissue levels of bile acids in human cholestasis: Relation to serum levels and pruritus. *Gastroenterology* 73: 1125–30.

Ghent, C.N. and Carruthers, S.G. (1988). Treatment of pruritus in primary biliary cirrhosis with rifampicin. Results of a double-blind crossover randomised trial. *Gastroenterology* 94: 488–93.

Ghent, C.N. (1987). Pruritus of cholestasis is related to effects of bile salts on the liver, not the skin. *American Journal of Gastroenterology* 82: 117–18.

Gilbert, D.A. (1990). Epidemiology of upper gastrointestinal bleeding. *GI Endoscopy* 36 (Suppl.): S8–S13.

Ginès, P., Arroyo, V., Quintero, E., Planas, R., Bory, F., Cabrera, J. *et al.* (1987). Comparison of paracentesis and diuretics in the treatment of cirrhotics with tense ascites: results of a randomized study. *Gastroenterology* 93: 234–41.

Ginès, P., Arroyo, V., and Vargas, V. (1991). Paracentesis with intravenous infusion of albumin as compared with peritoneovenous shunting in cirrhosis with refractory ascites. *New England Journal of Medicine* 325: 829–35.

Ginès, P., Fernandez-Esparrach, G., and Arroyo, V. (1997). Ascites and renal functional abnormalities in cirrhosis. pathogenesis and treatment. *Ballieres Clinical Gastroenterology* 11: 365–85.

Ginès, P., Teto, L., Arroyo, V., Planas, R., Panes, J., Vivier, J. *et al.* (1988). Randomised study of therapeutic paracentesis with and without intravenous albumin in cirrhosis. *Gastroenterology* 94: 1493–502.

Gregorio, G.V., Ball, C.S., Mowat, A.P., and Miele-Vergani, G. (1993). Effects of rifampicin in the treatment of pruritus in hepatic cholestasis. *Archives of Disease in Childhood* 69: 141–3.

Grippon, P., LePonchin-Laffite, M., Boschat, M., Wang, S., Faure, G., Dutertre, D., and Opolon, P. (1986). Evidence for the role of ammonia in the intra-cerebral transfer and metabolism of tryptophan. *Hepatology* 6: 682–6.

Guazzi, M., Polese, A., Magrini, F., Fiorentini, C., and Olivari, M.T. (1975). Negative influences of ascites on the cardiac function of cirrhotic patients. *American Journal of Medicine* 59: 165–70.

Hadziyannis, S.J., Merikas, G.E., Afroudakis, A.P. (1970). Hepatitis-associated antigen and chronic liver disease. *Lancet* 2: 100–1.

Hanid, M.A. and Levi, A.J. (1980). Phototherapy for pruritus in primary biliary cirrhosis. *Lancet* 2: 530.

Jalan, R., Simpson, K.J., Redhead, D.N., Chalmers, N., and Hayes, P.C. (1994). Transjugular intrahepatic portosystemic shunt (TIPSS): long-term follow up. *Quarterly Journal of Medicine* **87**: 567–73.

Khandelwal, M. and Malet, P.E. (1994). Pruritus associated with cholestasis. A review of pathogenesis and management. *Digestive Diseases and Sciences* **39**: 1–8.

Kleinknecht, D. (1992). Management of acute renal failure. In Cameron, S., Davison, A.M., Grunfeld, J.P. (eds), *Oxford Textbook of Clinical Nephrology* (1st edn). Oxford: Oxford University Press, pp. 1015–25.

La-Vecchia, C., Levi, F., Lucchini, F., Francheschi, S., and Negri, E. (1994). Worldwide patterns and trends in mortality from liver cirrhosis, 1955–1990. *Annals of Epidemiology* **4**: 480–6.

Lebrec, D., Giuily, N., Hadengue, A., Vilgrain, V., Moreau, R., Poynard, T., *et al.* (1996). Transjugular intrahepatic pruritus shunts: comparison with paracentesis in patients with cirrhosis and refractory ascites: a randomised trial. *Journal of Hepatology* **25**: 135–44.

Leevy, C.M. (1968). Cirrhosis in alcoholics. *Medical Clinics of North America* **52**: 1445–51.

Lelbach, W.K. (1976). Epidemiology of alcoholic liver disease. In Popper, H. and Schaffner, F. (eds), *Progress in Liver Diseases.* New York: Grune and Stratton, pp. 494–515.

Lockwood, A.H., Yap, E.W.H., and Wong, W.H. (1992). Cerebral amino metabolism in patients with severe liver disease and minimal hepatic encephalopathy. *Journal of Cerebral Blood Flow and Metabolism* **11**: 334–41.

Longstreth, F.G. (1995). Epidemiology of hospitalization for acute upper gastrointestinal haemorrhage. *American Journal of Gastroenterology* **90**: 206–10.

McHutchinson, J.G. and Runyon, B.A. (1994). Spontaneous bacterial peritonitis. In Surawicz, C.M. and Owen, R.L. (eds), *Gastrointestinal and Hepatic Infections.* Philadephia: WB Saunders, pp. 455–75.

Martensson, J., Svensson, H., and Tobiasson P. (1985). The influence of the bacterial flora of the gut on sulphur amino acid degradation. *Scandinavian Journal of Gastroenterology* **20**: 959.

Martin, P. (1990). Hepatitis C: from laboratory to bedside. *Mayo Clinic Proceedings* **65**: 1372–6.

Moore, K., Wendon, J., Frazer, M., Karani, J., Williams, R., and Badr, K. (1992). Plasma endothelin immunoreactivity in liver disease and the hepatorenal syndrome. *New England Journal of Medicine* **327**: 1774–8.

Morgan, A.G. and Clamp, S.E. (1988). OMGE International upper gastrointestinal bleeding study. *Scandinavian Journal of Gastroenterologyenterol* **23** (Suppl. 144): S51–S58.

Navasa, M., Follo, A., Llovet, J.M., Clemente, G., Vargas, V., Rimola, A. *et al.* (1996). Randomised, comparative study of oral ofloxacin versus intravenous cefotaxime in spontaneous bacterial peritonitis. *Gastroenterology* **111**: 1011–17.

Nazarian, G.K., Ferral, H., Bjarnason, H., Castaneda-Zuniga, W.R., Rank, J.M., Bernadas, C.A., and Hunter, D.W. (1996). Effect of transjugular intrahepatic shunt on quality of life. *American Journal of Roentgenology* **167**: 963–9.

Osborne, E.C., Wootten, I.D.P., DaSilva, L.C., and Sherlock, S. (1959) Serum bile acid levels in liver disease. *Lancet* **2**: 1049–53.

Pagliaro, L., D'Amico, G., and Pasta, L. (1994). Portal hypertension in cirrhosis: natural history. In Bosch, J. and Groszmann, R. (eds), *Portal Hypertension: Pathophysiology and Treatment.* Cambridge, MA: Blackwell Scientific, pp. 72–92.

Peltekian, K.M., Wong, F., Liu, P.P., Logan, A.G., Sherman, M., and Blendis, L.M. (1997). Cardiovascular, renal and neurohumoral responses to single large volume paracentesis in cirrhotic patients with diuretic resistant ascites. *American Journal of Gastroenterology* **92**: 394–9.

Pokross, P.J. and Reynolds, T.B. (1986). Rapid diuresis in patients' ascites from chronic liver disease: the importance of peripheral oedema. *Gastroenterology* **90**: 1827–33.

Raabe, W. and Onstad, G. (1985). Portocaval shunting changes neuronal sensitivity to ammonia. *Journal of the Neurological Sciences* **71**: 307–14.

Reed, W.D., Stern, R.B., Eddleston, A.L., Williams, R., Zuckerman, A.J., Bowes, A., and Earl, P.M. (1973). Detection of hepatitis B antigen by radio-immunoassay in chronic liver disease and hepatocellular carcinoma in Great Britain. *Lancet* **2**: 690–4.

Runyon, B.A. (1986). Paracentesis of ascitic fluid: a safe procedure. *Archives of Internal Medicine* **146**: 2259–61.

Runyon, B.A. (1988). Spontaneous bacterial peritonitis: an explosion of information. *Hepatology* **8**: 171–5.

Runyon, B.A. (1997). Patient selection is important in studying the impact of large-volume paracentesis on intravascular volume. *American Journal of Gastroenterology* **92**: 371–3.

Runyon, B.A. (1998). Management of adult patients with ascites caused by cirrhosis. *Hepatology* **27**: 264–72.

Runyon, B.A., Canawati, H.N., and Akriviadis, E.A. (1988). Optimisation of ascitic fluid culture technique. *Gastroenterology* **95**: 1351–5.

Saunders, J.B., Walters, J.R.F., Davies, B., and Patton, A. (1981). Twenty years prospective study of cirrhosis. *British Medical Journal* **282**: 263–6.

Schubert, G.E., Bethke-Bedurftig, B.A., Bujnoch, A.W., and Diem. A. (1982). Die Leberzirrhose in autopsiegut von 48 jahrn. I. Haufigkeitsanderungen regionale unterschiede. *Zeitschrift fur gastroenterologie* **20**: 213–30.

Sharp, H.L., Carey, J.B., White, J.B., and Krivit, W. (1967). Cholestyramine therapy in patients with a paucity of intrahepatic ducts. *Journal of Pediatrics* **71**: 723–36.

Shiffman, M.L., Jeffers, L., Hoofnagle, J.H., and Tralka, I.S. (1995). The role of transjugular intrahepatic portosystemic shunt for treatment of portal hypertension and its complications: a conference sponsored by the National Digestive Diseases Advisory Board. *Hepatology* **22**: 1591–7.

Sieber, C.C. and Groszmann, R.J. (1992). Nitric oxide mediates hyporeactivity to vasopressors in mesenteric vessels of portal hypertensive rats. *Gastroenterology* **103**. 235–9.

Silverstein, F.E., Gilbert, D.A., and Tedesco, F.J. (1981). The national ASGE survey on upper gastrointestinal bleeding. I. Study design and baseline data. II. Clinical prognostic factors. *GI Endoscopy* **27**: 73–93.

Singh, N., Gayowski, T., Wagener, M.M., and Marino, I.R. (1997a). Depression in patients with cirrhosis. Impact on outcome. *Digestive Diseases and Sciences* **42**: 1421–7.

Singh, N., Gayowski, T., Wagener, M.M., and Marino, I.R. (1997b). Vulnerability to psychologic distress and depression in patients with end stage liver disease due to hepatitis C virus. *Clinical Transplants* **11**: 406–11.

Stanley, M.M., Ochi, S., Lee, K.K., Nemchausky, B.A., Greenlec, H.B., Allen, J.I. *et al.* (1989). Peritoneovenous shunting as compared with medical treatment in patients with alcoholic cirrhosis and massive ascites. *New England Journal of Medicine* **321**: 1632–8.

Sushma, S., Dasarathy, S., Tanden, R.K., Jain, S., Gupta, S., and Bhist, M.S. (1992). Sodium benzoate in the treatment of acute hepatic encephalopathy: a double blind randomised trial. *Hepatology* **16**: 138–4.

Taylor-Robinson, S.D., Sargentoni, J., Marcus, C.D., Morgan, M.Y., and Bryant, D.J. (1994). Regional variations in cerebral proton spectroscopy in patients with chronic hepatic encephalopathy. *Metabolic Brain Disease* **9**: 347–59.

Thomas, D.A., Williams, G.W., Isata, K., Kenshalo, D.R. Jr, and Dubner, R. (1992). Effects of central administration of opioids on facial scratching in monkeys. *Brain Research* **585**: 315–17.

Thornton, J.R. and Losowsky, M.S. (1988). Opioid peptides and primary biliary cirrhosis. *British Medical Journal* **297**: 1501–4.

Thornton, J.R. and Losowsky, M.S. (1988). Plasma methionine enkephalin concentration and prognosis in primary biliary cirrhosis. *British Medical Journal* **297**: 1501–4.

Varadi, D.P. (1974). Pruritus induced by crude bile and purified bile acids: experimental production of pruritus in human skin. *Archives of Dermatology* **109**: 678–81.

Vince, A., Killingly, M., and Wrong, O.M. (1978). Effective of lactulose on ammonia production in a faecal incubation system. *Gastroenterology* **74**: 744–9.

Chapter 8

Renal palliative care

Lewis M. Cohen, Gary S. Reiter, David M. Poppel, and Michael J. Germain

Introduction

Organ transplantation (and) hemodialysis … altering the character and duration of dying, and expanding recognition of the mental hygienic value of open communication concerning dying and death with the fatally ill person are beginning to brush aside existing curtains of silence.

(Herman Feifel, Weisman 1972)

Ars moriendi is ars vivendi: The art of dying is the art of living.

(Sherwin Nuland 1993)

Nephrology and palliative medicine are on the verge of discovering each other, and when this occurs they will find several areas of commonality and mutual benefit. Nephrologists are now vigorously deliberating over issues related to discontinuation of dialysis. Retrospective and prospective research (Neu and Kjellstrand 1986; Cohen *et al.* 1995), community and panel discussions, and practice guidelines (RPA & ASN, 1999; Patient Services Committee, 1996) are resulting in a clinical model that should also be applicable to cessation of other types of life-support treatments. Palliative medicine has much to offer the end-stage renal disease (ESRD) population, which is increasingly elderly, suffers from multiple diseases and symptoms, and has a greatly reduced life expectancy (Levinsky and Rettig 1991).

This chapter will emphasise the practice of nephrology in the US, and will focus on patients who are maintained with either haemodialysis or peritoneal dialysis. While the chapter is hampered by the absence of a discrete medical literature that synthesises palliative care and nephrology, it is propelled by the growing convergence and potential synergy of these evolving specialties.

Why renal palliative care?

Renal failure results from various diseases irreversibly damaging both kidneys and leading to a decrease in the glomerular filtration rate (GFR). Once the GFR drops below 10 ml min uraemic symptoms ensue. Common uraemic symptoms are nausea and vomiting, anorexia, tiredness, itching, weakness, decreased sexual function and libido. Without dialysis or transplant the patient will become comatose and die as GFR decreases further.

Dialysis patients paradoxically witness both the miraculous benefits and the very real limitations of modern medicine. While dialysis sustains life by substituting for the kidneys, the underlying systemic diseases responsible for causing renal failure usually continue to progress. For example, a person with ESRD and diabetes may be sustained for years on dialysis, but may also experience blindness, amputations, painful neuropathies, and other severe complications. Under such circumstances dialysis supports life, but not necessarily what the individual considers quality of life. In some surveys almost two-thirds of ESRD patients rate their quality of life as being less than 'good' (Roberts and Kjellstrand 1988, Levy and Wynbrandt 1975). After a point, treatment can become a Sisyphean ordeal. This subgroup ought to be easy to identify (Ifudu *et al.* 1998), and could be targeted for specific palliative care interventions. There is, however, a growing awareness that patients benefit from palliative care throughout the spectrum of a life-threatening illness, and this opinion is reflected in portions of this chapter and its tables.

Who is affected?

The inception of the 1973 US Medicare ESRD Program resulted in nearly universal access to dialysis treatment. Subsequently, the population of patients receiving dialysis support has steadily grown and aged. The acceptance of sicker patients, whose renal disease results from or is associated with more severe co-morbid conditions, has also increased. These factors affect both the quality and length of patients' lives.

According to the 1997 and 1998 annual reports of the US Renal Data System (USRDS 1997; USRDS 1998), the prevalence of patients on haemodialysis and peritoneal dialysis at the end of 1996 was 283 932, with an annual incidence of 73 091 patients. The average age of the incident population has increased every year that data have been collected; in 1986 the mean age was 56 years while this increased to 60 years by 1995. The fastest growth has occurred among the oldest age groups; 46% of the incident patients in 1996 were 65 years old or greater and 20% were over 75 years of age. In 1996, co-morbid disorders of incident patients included: diabetes (42%), coronary artery disease (35–40%), congestive heart failure (30–40%), hypertension (25%), peripheral vascular disease (20–23%), and cerebrovascular disease (12–16%).

The annual mortality rate of patients on dialysis in the US is approximately 25%; this is higher than that of AIDS or of most cancers. Cardiovascular complications account for at least half of the deaths. The expected lifetime of a dialysis patient is between 16% and 37% that of age- and sex-matched general population. The risk of death for a 45-year-old patient is 20 times that of a person of the same age not receiving dialysis. Although the techniques of dialysis care have improved, the 5-year survival rate remains low. Only 27.5% of the 1980 incident cohort survived 5 years, while 29.4% of the 1990 cohort remained alive after 1995. Two-thirds of the haemodialysis population is 55 years of age or older; the five year survival rate for patients aged 55–64 is 33%, and the rate drops to 21% for ages 65–74.

The presence of congestive heart failure (CHF) is a serious risk factor in the ESRD population; the median survival of a Canadian cohort with CHF at baseline was 36 months, as compared to 62 months for patients without CHF (Hartnett *et al.* 1995). Both the patients referred for dialysis, and the physicians who refer them, are generally unaware of these dire statistics.

What are the problems?

ESRD symptoms can be divided into those which are directly related to dialysis or uraemia, and those which accompany the underlying systemic disorders that led to the renal failure. Hypotension, cramps, headaches, and a sense of impending doom occur in 30% of dialysis treatments, however 80% of these episodes involve only 20% of the patients. Patients on long-term dialysis complain of sleep disturbances, pruritis, fatigue, restless legs, memory impairment, and thirst.

Sexual dysfunction is common in both men and women; 65–70% of men experience impotence, 50–80% of women have decreased libido or delayed orgasm, and 90% of women have abnormal menses. It is rare for women on dialysis to be able to carry a pregnancy to term.

Calciphylaxis is a newly recognised complication of dialysis therapy. This condition has a small but increasing incidence, and it involves painful necrosis of skin and subcutaneous fat leading to expanding and deep ulcerations that are often impossible to control.

Patients receiving dialysis experience a variety of psychological and cognitive symptoms (Levy and Cohen 2000). Initiation of dialysis can be overwhelming. Dialysis sessions are long and boring, confining, and sometimes terrifying. Patients suffer intrusion into their personal lives in a variety of ways, including monitoring of food and fluid intake, a large and complicated medication regimen, changes in their capacity for employment, and major disruption to recreational activities and the person's usual daily routine. Many patients suffer a lack of self-esteem related to disfigurement from vascular access grafts in haemodialysis and abdominal distension in peritoneal dialysis. Impotence combined with cessation of urination further diminishes self-esteem in men.

Depression occurs in 5–25% of patients with ESRD. Many of the symptoms of renal failure, such as fatigue, sleep disturbance, anorexia, and sexual dysfunction, are also listed in the DSM IV criteria for major depression. Physicians risk failing to identify and treat depression in ESRD because of the significant overlap of symptoms. Depressive episodes or suicide attempts prior to the onset of renal disease, and a family history of affective disorders, are helpful clues for diagnosing depression in this population. It is also worthwhile to begin by asking patients, 'Are you depressed most of the time?' (Chochinov et al. 1997)

What are the treatment considerations?

Comprehensive palliative care of patients with ESRD requires continuous assessment of symptoms and quality of life through a collaborative relationship between the patient, his/her family, and the health care team. People with ESRD experience psychological, social, and spiritual discomfort. Recognition that one's life expectancy is significantly reduced by ESRD can precipitate an existential crisis. This life-crisis can be quite disturbing, yet when viewed from the perspective of a life-transition, it can provide people with the opportunity to complete the essential personal work of the last stages of life with friends and loved ones.

Treatment for the physical symptoms of ESRD needs to reflect the altered pharmacokinetics of some medications. These are reviewed in Tables 8.1 and 8.2.

Sleep disturbances are notoriously resistant to treatment. The usual hypnogogic agents should be combined with basic behavioural techniques that rely on an appreciation of good sleep hygiene (avoid reading and watching television in bed, get out of the bed if you do not fall asleep in 15 minutes, etc.). Identification and appropriate treatment for sleep apnoea is important.

Table 8.1 Drug regimes for symptoms of ESRD and reflecting altered pharmacokinetoes of some medications

Medication	Dose (normal renal function)	% usual dose in ESRD	Supplement (after HD?)	Addendum
Pain medications				
Narcotic analgesics				
Codeine	30–60 mg q4–6h	50%	unknown	
Fentanyl	25–300 mcgs q72h	50%	no	
Meperidine	50–100 mg q3–4h	50–75%	no	*Caution:* active metabolite, normeperidine accumulates in ESRD and may cause seizures. Avoid use in ESRD.
Morphine sulfate		50%	no	Active
Intravenous	1–20 mg IV q1–2h			metabolite
Immediate release oral	10–20 mg q2–4 h			accumulates
Sustained release oral	15–300 mg q12h		no	in ESRD
Non-narcotic analgesics				
Acetaminophen	650–1000 mg q6h	decrease dosing interval to q8h		1/2 dose
Ibuprofen	800 mg q8h	no change	no	* Most NSAIDS require no dose adjustment but should be used with caution because of increased risk of uraemic bleeding and gastro-intestinal side effects
Salsalate	1500 mg q8–12h	50%	500 mg	
Adjuvants: tricyclics, anti-arrythmics and anti-seizure agents				
Amitriptyline	10–100 mg qhs	no change	no	orthostatic hypotension seen in tricyclics
Carbamazepine	100–1200 mg q24h	no change	no	
Desipramine	12.5–150 mg qhs	no change	no	less sedating than amitriptyline
Doxepin	10–75 mg qhs	no change	no	
Gabapentin	300 mg q 8–24h	300mg qod	300 mg	
Mexiletine	100–300 mg q6–8h	no change	no	
Phenytoin	300–400 mg q24h	no change	no	
Glucocorticoids				
Dexamethasone	0.75–16 mg q24h	no change	no	
Hydrocortisone	20–500 mg qd	no change	no	
Prednisone	5–60 mg qd	no change	no	

Table 8.1 cont.

Medication	Dose (normal renal function)	% usual dose in ESRD	Supplement (after HD?)	Addendum
Gastrointestinal agents				
Anti-emetics				
Cisapride	5–10 mg qid	no change	no	
Haloperidol	0.5–1 mg qhs-bid	no change	no	may sedate
Metoclopramide	5–20 mg qid	50%	no	
Prochlorperazine	5–10 mg PO qid 25 mg PR bid	no change	no	
Medications for dyspepsia				
Cimetidine	400–800 mg qhs	25–50%	no	
Famotidine	20–40 mg qhs	10%	no	
Lansoprazole	30 mg qd	no change	no	
Omeprazole	20–40 mg qd	no change	no	
Ranitidine	150–300 mg qhs	25%	37.5–75 mg	
Sucralfate	1 gm qid	avoid use		contains aluminum
Psychotherapeutic agents				
Antidepressants (see above for tricyclics)				
Fluoxetine	20–60 mg qam	no change	no	
Lorazepam	0.5–2 mg bid-tid	no change	no	
Midazolam	1.25 mg sq/iv, titrate to response, 0.4–4 mg/hr	no change	no change	useful in terminal delirium
Phenobarbital	50–100 mg bid-tid	no change	dose after HD	
Thiopental	20–200 mg/hr IV	75%	no	for severe terminal delirium
Phenothiazines				
Chlorpromazine	300–800 mg q24h	no change	no	may use PO/PR or IV for terminal delirium
Promethazine	20–100 mg q24h	no change	no	
Agents for pruritis				
Antihistamines				
Astemizole	10mg qam	no change	no	
Diphenhydramine	25–50 mg qid	no change	no	
Hydroxyzine	25–100 mg qid	unknown	unknown	
Cardiac agents – angina and CHF				
Amlodipine	5–10 mg qam	no change	no	
Atenolol	50–100 mg q24h	25%	25–50 mg	accumulates in ESRD
Captopril	12.5–50 mg q8h	50% q 24h	dose after HD	increases serum digoxin levels
Digoxin	0.125–0.5 mg qam	10–25%		radioimmunoassay may overestimate levels
Diltiazem	90–300 mg qam	no change	no	
Enalapril	5–20 mg q12h	50%	dose after HD	

Table 8.1 cont.

Medication	Dose (normal renal function)	% usual dose in ESRD	Supplement (after HD?)	Addendum
Cardiac agents – angina and CHFf (cont.)				
Isosorbide	10–20 mg tid	no change	dose after HD	
Lisinopril	5–40 mg qam	25–50%	dose after HD	
Metoprolol	50–100 mg bid	no change	dose after HD	
Nadolol	80–320 mg q24h	25%	40 mg	
Nitroglycerin	many different doses and routes of administration	no change	no	follow routine doses depending on whether given PO, SL or transdermal
Propranolol	80–160 mg bid	no change	no	metabolites may accumulate, hypoglycemia reported in ESRD
Antibiotics, etc.				
Acyclovir	5 mg/kg q8h	2.5 mg/kg	dose after HD	neurotoxic in ESRD
Fluconazole	50–200 mg qam	25%	dose after HD	may use 150 mg stat dose for vulvovaginal candidiasis
Itraconazole	100–200 mg qam	no change	no	

All medications and doses are PO unless otherwise specified. q24h refers to total daily dose of medication, usually given in divided doses; qd refers to medication usually given once daily but is at times given in divided doses; PO, oral; SL, sublingual; qhs, at bedtime; qid, 4 times daily; tid, 3 times daily; bid, twice daily; sq, subcutaneously; IV, intravenously; PR, per rectum.

This table is taken in part from Swan, S. and Bennett, W. (1997). Use of drugs in patients with renal failure. In Schrier, R., Gottschalk, C. (eds), *Diseases of the Kidney*, Vol. I (6th edn). Boston, New York, Toronto, London: Little, Brown, pp. 2968–3005.

Sexual dysfunction has been a subject of considerable clinical interest. While men have low free testosterone, increased binding globulin, and increased clearance of testosterone, treatment with testosterone fails to restore normal sexual function. Occasional reversal of impotence has followed use of clomiphene, yohimbine, erythropoitin, and parathyroidectomy. Psychotherapy, behavioural therapy, and surgical techniques, including the use of a pumping apparatus or implantation of a silastic rod, are also employed. More recently, anecdotal reports suggest that sildenafil may be of considerable benefit to some of these patients.

There are some data that suggests longer, 'better' dialysis not only achieves increased clearances, but also improves survival (Parker *et al.* 1994; Hakim *et al.* 1994; Held *et al.* 1991). In one study the Kt/V, a measure of dialysis clearance, rose from 1.18 to 1.46, the urea reduction ratios shifted from 63% to 69.6%, and the crude mortality rate dropped from 22.5% to 18.1%. An even greater decrease was seen in another programme where the gross annual mortality fell from 22.8% to 9.1%, along with a proportionate decrease in hospital days.

Unfortunately, some of the known or suspected complications of dialysis treatment, e.g. the sleep disturbances, sexual dysfunction, cramps, and painful neuropathy that are so common among this population, are not well controlled by modifications of standard in-centre

Table 8.2 Suggestions for treatment of physical symptoms in ESRD

Symptom	Treatment	Dosage	Comment
Cramps	Quinine	260–325 mg PO prn	Give prior to symptoms. Limit to 3 doses/day
	Carnitine	1000–2000mg iv during dialysis	Also used for myopathy, cardiomyopathy, refractory anaemia
Restless leg syndrome	Clonazepam	0.5–2 mg Hs prn	
	Carbidopa-Levodopa	25/100 mg Hs prn	
	Pergolide	0.05–0.2 mg qd	
	Pramipexole	0.3 mg qd	
Pruritis	H1 antagonists— Clemastine	2.68 mg bid prn	Trial any H1 antagonist
	Skin moisturiser— Hydrourea cream		
	Activated charcoal	6 g qd×8 weeks	
	UVB light		
	IV Lidocaine	100 mg iv during dialysis	Potential seizures
	Ketotifen		Mast cell stabiliser
	Ondanstron	4 mg bid	High cost
	Plasmapheresis	3–4 exchanges	
Hypotension – intra-dialytic or persistent	Alterations to the dialysis bath, temperature, sodium, ultrafiltration		
	Midadrine	1–10 mg tid prn or pre-dialysis	Oral alpha adrenergic agonist
	Sertraline	25–50 mg pre-dialysis	

haemodialysis. Slow nocturnal haemodialysis and continuous peritoneal dialysis may eliminate most of the dialysis-specific symptoms; but many of the co-morbid disorders associated with ESRD are not reversed by dialysis and continue their inexorable course.

Dialysis discontinuation

The ESRD population in the US is composed of an increasing proportion of elderly, chronically ill patients, and many of these individual's medical problems are progressive and cannot be cured. This development has been paralleled by a greater regard for patient autonomy and a lowered threshold for medical decisions that hasten death (Cohen 1998). Not surprisingly, the decision to discontinue dialysis support has become an important option.

One in five patients withdrew from dialysis prior to their death, according to the 1994–96 USRDS data. This was the recent and well-publicised decision of Pulitzer Prize-winning novelist James Michener (Krebs 1997). Factors associated with dialysis cessation include diabetes, ethnicity (Caucasian), dementia, and cachexia. Age is another important factor, with 40% of those over 65 years having discontinued dialysis support. Rates as high as 66% have been reported in these subgroups (Port *et al.*1989, Cummins 1998, Nelson *et al.* 1994).

Neu and Kjellstrand (1986) conducted the seminal retrospective study on dialysis discontinuation. They reported withdrawal in 9% of 1766 patients in a large Minnesota programme between 1966 and 1983; this accounted for 22% of all ESRD deaths. Although at the time of its publication many were surprised at the high incidence of withdrawal, these statistics have now been nationally validated and exceeded by other centres (Port *et al.* 1989).

Eight states in the US and Canada were included in a more recent study of the psychosocial and ethical aspects of discontinuation, and the resulting quality of death (Cohen *et al.* 1995, Germain, Cohen and Poppel 1998). Median survival from the time of the last dialysis was 6 days: three-quarters died in 10 or fewer days.

Using a quality of dying measure that took into account the duration of survival time following discontinuation, the presence of pain and suffering, and the psychosocial factors, nearly half (48%) of the sample were judged to have had 'good' deaths, 38% were 'fair', and 14% were 'bad' deaths. The investigators concluded that many of the less than satisfactory deaths could have been ameliorated by the application of modern palliative care.

Dialysis withdrawal allows patients who are terminally ill to shorten the time of suffering, and also to bring their lives to a close in an orderly fashion. Dialysis withdrawal itself does not result in any pain or discomfort. While fluid gains could potentially produce pulmonary oedema and respiratory distress, in our experience this rarely occurs. In these uncommon cases, isolated ultrafiltration with fluid removal without toxin clearance can be performed. Alternatively, morphine and sedatives can be administered for respiratory distress.

An often overlooked intervention is not starting (withholding) dialysis in the chronically ill patient whose quality of life would likely not benefit from treatment (Lowance 1993). Some American nephrologists give almost all patients a discrete trial of dialysis, with the understanding that if there is no apparent benefit then the treatment can be withdrawn.

Initiation criteria restrict dialysis in England, Japan, and other countries, but are not in effect in the US. However, the Institute for Medicine has recognised the need for practice guidelines concerning appropriate initiation and withdrawal from dialysis (Rettig and Levinsky 1991). The National Kidney Foundation has published guidelines for initiation and withdrawal of dialysis with excellent checklists. The Renal Physicians Association with the American Society of Nephrology has published evidence based guidelines modeled on the Agency for Health Care Policy and Research Methodology.

Priorities for further research

It is time for nephrology to push aside its denial of death and to work collaboratively to incorporate palliative medical innovations into clinical practice. Although $11.13 billion dollars was spent in 1994 on the care of ESRD, few patients are able to maintain full-time work, and many suffer with potentially treatable physical and psychological symptoms. The same research protocols that have compared symptom management in cancer and AIDS could be applied to ESRD. More medications need to be systematically studied and codified for this population. While sleep disorders and sexual dysfunction are not linked to mortality, they fundamentally influence people's quality of life, are extraordinarily common in ESRD, and require further attention. We have had several patients decide to terminate dialysis after experiencing unremitting agony from calciphylaxis, and this condition needs to be further studied. Greater psychosocial input needs to occur in matching patients to haemodialysis or peritoneal dialysis, and this should be tested. Clinical guidelines are being developed, and these need be more rigorously examined and compared.

Implications for clinical management

When we first began studying dialysis cessation about 10 years ago, 10% of ESRD patient deaths in New England were preceded by termination of dialysis (Cohen *et al.* 1993). However, by 1996 over one-quarter of deaths reported to the ESRD Network of New England (1996) were preceded by the decision to discontinue treatment. This reflects an on-going change on the part of dialysis staff, who are increasingly willing to listen to their patients and acknowledge their right to make autonomous decisions. But, this also reflects the pressures of an ageing, chronically ill population that is facing the limitations of dialysis. These limitations need to be more energetically and honestly confronted.

Similarly, nephrology practices are dependent on protocols aimed at guiding and assuring quality assessment and quality improvement. In recognition of the several advances in dialysis care, e.g. better dialysers, medications to control anaemia and renal osteodystrophy, protocols have largely focused on optimising results in biochemical and physiological parameters. Use of such protocols has been widely accepted as a necessity in attaining improved medical outcomes, and efforts are on-going to improve older protocols and develop new ones as treatment options evolve. Dialysis care teams are accustomed to the use of protocol pathways.

New renal palliative care protocols need to be developed that will assure the education of staff in the principles and practices of advanced care planning, offer palliation of patients' physical and psychological symptoms, and provide assistance with bereavement and long-term support for families. Protocols that attend to patient and family needs can be implemented side by side with those protocols that already address biochemical and physiological quality assurance. Dialysis rounds can be altered by the inclusion of symptom assessment measures. Morbidity and mortality conferences do not have to be restricted to surgery programmes, but can be introduced to dialysis centres. These regular conferences can focus on the circumstances of each death, and will be greatly enriched if information concerning the family perspective of the end-of-life care were also presented. There is an opportunity for us to explore how to fulfil the promise of a good death (Emanuel and Emanuel 1998), and we are certain that ESRD will pose a mutually beneficial challenge to the art and science of palliative care.

We are extremely optimistic that palliative care will be rapidly incorporated into the dialysis setting, because of widespread use of interdisciplinary teams and the extensive reliance on treatment protocols. Dialysis is routinely delivered in a team based setting. Nephrologists, nurses, social workers, and dieticians collaborate in providing this care. The dialysis teams are perfectly situated to adopt the interdisciplinary team model that is common to palliative care; a model which provides excellent symptom management and quality of life assessment. The close working nature of the teams, and the intimate relationships that often form between staff, patients, and families, lend themselves to facilitating a mutual search for meaning in the life-transition that dialysis represents.

Acknowledgments

Nancy Jordan, PharmD, for assistance in developing the medication tables. Penelope Pekow, PhD, for statistical analysis. Anne Woods, LICSW, for editorial assistance and her collaboration in the research endeavours. The Project on Death in America, Faculty Scholar Program, for its support of Dr Cohen. The Greenwall Foundation, for its support of the Dialysis Discontinuation Study. The Open Society, for its support of the Dialysis Discontinuation Study. The Excellence in End of Life Program of The Robert Wood Johnson Foundation for its support of the Renal Palliative Care Initiative.

References

Chochinov, H.M., Wilson, K.G., Enns, M., and Lander, S (1997). 'Are you depressed?' Screening for depression in the terminally ill. *American Journal of Psychiatry* **154**: 674–6.

Cohen, L.M. (1998). Suicide, hastening death, and psychiatry. *Archives of Internal Medicine* **158**: 1973–6.

Cohen, L.M., Germain, M., Woods, A., Gilman, E.D., and McCue, J. (1993). Patient attitudes and psychological considerations in dialysis discontinuation. *Psychosomatics* **34**: 395–401.

Cohen, L.M., McCue, J., Germain, M., and Kjellstrand, C. (1995). Dialysis discontinuation: a 'good' death? *Archives of Internal Medicine* **155**: 42–7.

Cohen, L.M., McCue, J.D., Germain, M., and Woods, A. (1997). Denying the dying: advance directives and dialysis discontinuation. *Psychosomatics* **38**: 27–34.

Cummings, N.B. (1998). Withholding and withdrawing dialysis, *Mediguide to Nephrology* **6**(1): 1–6.

Emanuel, E.J. and Emanuel, L.L. (1998). The promise of a good death. *Lancet* **351**(II): 21–9.

ESRD Network of New England Inc. (1996). Annual Report, pp. 54–5.

Germain, M., Cohen, L.M., and Poppel, D. (1998). Termination of dialysis: a good death. Presentation to Annual Meeting of the American Society of Nephrology, Philadelphia, PA.

Hakim, R.H., Breyer, J., Ismail, N., and Schulman, G. (1994). Effects of dose of dialysis on morbidity and mortality. *American Journal of Kidney Diseases* **23**(5): 661–9.

Hartnett, J.D., Foley, R.N., Kent, G.M., Barre, P.E., Murray, D., and Parfrey, T.S. (1995). Congestive heart failure in dialysis patients: prevalence, incidence, prognosis and risk factors. *Kidney International* **47**: 884–90.

Held, P.J., Levin, N.W., Bovberg, R.R., Pauly, M.V., and Diamond, L.H. (1991). Mortality and duration of hemodialysis treatment. *Journal of the American Medical Association,* **265**(7): 871–5.

Ifudu, O., Paul, H.R., Homel, P., and Friedman, E.A. (1998). Predictive value of functional status for mortality in patients on maintenance hemodialysis. *American Journal of Nephrology* **18**: 109–16.

Krebs, A. (1997) James Michener, author of novels that sweep through the history of places, is dead. *New York Times*, Friday 17 October, p. C31.

Levinsky, N.G. and Rettig, R. (1991). Special report, the Medicare end-stage renal disease program: a report from the Institute of Medicine. *New England Journal of Medicine* **324**(14): 1143–8.

Levy, N.B. and Cohen, L.M. (2000). Central and peripheral nervous systems in uremia: psychiatric considerations. In Massry, S.G. and Glassock, R.J. (eds), *The Textbook of Nephrology* (4th edn). Philadelphia: Lippincott, Williams, and Wilkins.

Levy, W.B. and Wynbrandt, G.D. (1975). The quality of life on maintenance haemodialysis. *Lancet* **1**: 1328–30.

Lowance, D.L. (1993). The factors and guidelines to be considered in offering treatment to patients with end-stage renal disease: A personal opinion. *American Journal of Kidney Diseases* **21**(6): 679–83.

Nelson, C.B., Port, F.K., Wolfe, R.A., and Guire, K.E. (1994). The association of diabetic status, age, and race to withdrawal from dialysis. *Journal of the American Society of Nephrology* **4**:1608–14.

Neu, S. and Kjellstrand, C.M. (1986). Stopping long-term dialysis: an empirical study of withdrawal of life-supporting treatment. *New England Journal of Medicine* **314**: 14–20.

Nuland, S.B. (1993). *How We Die: Reflections on Life's Final Chapter*, New York: Alfred A. Knopf, p. 268.

Parker, T.F., Husni, L., Huang, W., Welew, N., and Lowrie, E.G. (1994). Survival of hemodialysis patients in the US is improved with greater quantity of dialysis. *American Journal of Kidney Diseases* 23(5): 670–80.

Patient Services Committee of the National Kidney Foundation, The (1996). *Initiation or Withdrawal of Dialysis in End Stage Renal Disease: Guidelines for the Health Care Team.* New York: National Kidney Foundation.

Port, W.K., Wolf, R.A., Hawthorne, V.M., *et al.* (1989). Discontinuation of dialysis therapy as a cause of death. *American Journal of Nephrology* 9: 145–9.

RPA & ASN (1999). *Clinical Practice Guidelines on shared decision making in the appropriate initiation and withdrawal from dialysis.* Washington, DC.

Roberts, J.C. and Kjellstrand, C.M. (1988). Choosing death: withdrawal from chronic dialysis without medical reason. *Acta Medica Scandinavica* 223: 181–6.

United States Renal Data System 1998 Annual Report, The. Excerpts. *American Journal of Kidney Diseases* 32(2) (Suppl. 1) August 1998: S1–213.

United States Renal Data System 1997 Annual Report, The. Excerpts. *American Journal of Kidney Diseases* 30(2) (Suppl. 1) August 1997: S1–213.

Weisman, A.D. (1972). Introduction. *On Dying and Denying: A Psychiatric Study of Terminality*, New York: Behavioural Publications.

Chapter 9

Palliative care for patients with dementia

Patricia Hanrahan, Daniel J. Luchins, and Kathleen Murphy

Introduction

This chapter discusses the epidemiology of dementia and the need for palliative care, followed by a description of common problems among patients with dementia and their caregivers. We argue that palliative care is an important alternative to conventional care in the terminal phase of dementia. We establish that professional and family caregivers view palliative care as appropriate for the end-stages of dementia, and review related research on access to hospice for dementia patients as well as the findings of pilot studies on providing palliative care and hospice to this vulnerable population. The research is primarily from a US perspective, with other work referenced when appropriate.

Extent of the need for palliative care

As a consequence of increasing life spans, the incidence and prevalence of dementia has increased. Although some patients with dementia will die from other causes, researchers have estimated that dementia is the fourth leading cause of death (Katzman 1979). It is difficult to determine the exact prevalence of deaths due to dementia because death certificates often list complications of the disease as the cause of death, rather than the dementia itself. Nevertheless, information about the prevalence of dementia gives us fairly good estimates of how many patients are likely to need palliative care in the end stages of the disease.

Epidemiology

The striking feature of the dementias is their almost exponential increase in incidence and corresponding prevalence with age. The annual incidence of dementia doubles nearly every 5 years from age 65 to 89, from 7 per 1000 in the group aged 65 to 69 to 118 per1000 in the group aged 86 to 89 (Bachman *et al.* 1993). Prevalence figures show a similar doubling from age 65 through age 95, with approximately one-third of individuals over 85 years (Skoog *et al.* 1993) and about one-half of those over 95 years being demented (Wernicke and Reisches 1994).

As our population ages, dying with dementia will become one of the most common ways in which older people end their final years of life. Often not recognised as a terminal illness and seriously under-reported as a cause of death, dementia may already be one of the leading causes of death of older people. Alzheimer's disease, for instance, is understated on death certificates; deaths attributable to Alzheimer's disease are estimated to be about 5 times the number of cases identified through death certificates (Hoyert 1996). Recent estimates suggest that 7% of all deaths are caused by Alzheimer's disease (Ewbank 1999). Since dementia due to vascular disease is also likely to be a frequent cause of death, the extent of mortality due to dementia is even greater. Given the ageing population in industrialised countries, this suggests a substantial need for palliative care among those in the terminal phase of dementia. Because this population has not traditionally been served by hospice programmes, hospices need to become more knowledgeable about the care of end-stage dementia patients.

Problems in patients with severe dementia

Several types of problems emerge as dementia progresses, including deficits due to dementia, medical complications arising from functional impairments, behavioural problems, and caregiver burden.

Impairment due to dementia

These include functional impairments in all or most activities of daily living, severe cognitive decline and a loss of the ability to engage in purposeful activities. A more extensive description of these problems can be found in the Global Deterioration Scale (Reisberg et al. 1982).

Common medical complications

Common medical problems related to the functional impairments of dementia were assessed in a study of 47 patients who were enrolled in hospice (Luchins, Hanrahan and Murphy 1997). At intake, 86% had more than one complication: the majority had swallowing problems (72%); decubitus ulcers also occured frequently (70%); aspiration pneumonia was common (55%); as were dehydration (57%), malnutrition (50%), and urinary tract infections (37%). Other conditions associated with old age are also likely to be present, such as osteoarthritis and cardiovascular problems. These findings are similar to those reported in a retrospective study of care for people in the last year of life which included 170 dementia patients (McCarthy, Addington-Hall and Altmann 1997). Common symptoms included mental confusion (83%), urinary incontinence (72%), pain (64%), low mood (61%), constipation and loss of appetite (57%). Although similar problems were reported for cancer patients, dementia patients experienced these difficulties for a longer duration.

Behavioural problems

These are also quite common in dementia and increase with the severity of the disease. Frequently reported behavioural problems include apathy, disinhibition, wandering, agitation, aggression, and binge eating (Burns et al. 1990; Mega et al. 1996; Teri et al. 1988). These problems are pervasive in institutional settings: 65% of the demented patients in long-term care institutions had behavioural syndromes (Nasman et al. 1993). Delusions and depression were found in 40% of nursing home patients with dementia (Rovner et al. 1990).

Delusions have been reported in up to 73% of dementia patients (Wragg and Jeste 1989). Hallucinations and delusions may occur throughout the course of the dementing disorder and are likely to be associated with other behavioural problems, such as aggression, agitation and wandering (Teri *et al.* 1988; Lachs *et al.* 1992). As the dementia progresses, apathy and disinhibited behaviours become more prevalent. The combination of psychoactive medications and behavioural interventions are helpful in managing these disorders (Luchins, Hanrahan and Ovsiew 1999; Pinkston and Linsk 1984; Schneider *et al.* 1990; Meco *et al.* 1994; Engel *et al.* 1990; Teri and Uomoto 1991).

Caring for the caregivers

A multitude of studies have established that family caregivers deal with considerable burdens in their caregiving role and are themselves at risk for psychiatric disorders, particularly depression (Gallagher *et al.* 1989; Goldman and Luchins 1984; Pruchno and Resch 1989). Because the course of dementia can last from two to ten years, families in the US often experience economic problems in securing needed services such as home care and respite care as a consequence of having exhausted the limited benefits provided by public and private insurance. In a case study of family caregivers of dementia patients, one husband described himself as in need of hospice services for himself as well as for his severely demented wife because he was 'desperate, financially and physically drained' (Luchins, Hanrahan and Litzenberg 1998). Hospice services, which focus on the needs of the caregiver–patient dyad, are especially important to the families of end-stage dementia patients. The Carers' Checklist is a useful instrument for assessing the objective and subjective burden involved in caring for dementia patients (Hodgson, Higginson and Jefferys 1998).

Appropriate health care for end-stage dementia patients

Palliative care?

The benefits of palliative care, which concern easing the dying process, apply to end-stage dementia patients just as they do to patients with other terminal illnesses. These patients usually die of medical complications of the disease, such as aspiration pneumonia. Although some end-stage dementia patients are in a vegetative state, others are at least intermittently aware of their environment, as well as of pain and discomfort from complications of their dementia. The most severely deteriorated patients are at Stage 7 of the Global Deterioration Scale (GDS) (Reisberg *et al.* 1982). At this point patients are dependent in all or most of their activities of daily living; they are unable to engage in purposeful activities; and speech is limited to a few words a day. Typically, they are no longer able to recognise their loved ones.

Despite being incurably ill, severely demented patients in the US often receive aggressive rather than palliative care at the end of life in acute care hospital settings (Ahronheim *et al.* 1996). Also, although many dementia patients die in nursing homes, there is very little provision of grief and bereavement services in these settings (Murphy, Hanrahan and Luchins 1997).

In an effort to determine whether palliative care and hospice are viewed as beneficial for end-stage dementia patients, we surveyed physicians, family members of dementia patients, and gerontologists in the US (Luchins and Hanrahan 1993). In all, over 1400 of those surveyed responded, a response rate of 61%. A continuum of care from most aggressive, at level 1, to palliative care only, at level 5, was presented. Level 5 was described as focusing on comfort and control of pain while excluding the use of resuscitation, medication for acute illness, and tube feeding. This least aggressive level was preferred by the majority of physicians who were gerontologists (61%), other gerontologists (55%), and family members (71%). A very small minority, ranging from 1.6% to 4.1%, favoured highly aggressive care in which everything would be done to prolong life. Family and professional caregivers were also quite positive about the role of hospice in end-stage dementia. Hospice care was viewed as appropriate for the end stages of dementia by 90% of the family members and 91% of the professional respondents. These findings are consistent with related research on other types of samples, a substantial proportion preferring palliative care in the event of a seriously dementing illness (see, for example, Danis et al. 1991; Diamond et al. 1989; Michelson et al. 1991; Payne et al. 1996).

Another important finding from the study was that relatively few respondents were aware of hospice programmes that served dementia patients. Ninety-one per cent of professionals and 68% of family members were aware of hospice programmes for cancer patients, while only 22% of professionals and 15% of families knew of hospice programmes that included patients with dementia. This combination of positive attitudes towards hospice and lack of knowledge of available hospice programmes suggests un-met need. Reasons for this problem are discussed later in the chapter.

Feasibility of providing palliative care and hospice services

A series of pilot studies suggest that the provision of palliative care through hospice programmes is a feasible alternative for severely demented patients (Volicer et al. 1986; Brechling et al. 1989; Hanrahan and Luchins 1995a; Volicer et al. 1994). For example, in collaboration with Meridian Hospice, we established a small pilot programme for end-stage dementia patients (Hanrahan and Luchins 1995a). This programme provided home care to 11 patients over a 2-year period. During this time 8 of the 11 patients died. The median survival time was 5 months with an average of 7 months. The deceased patients had an average survival time of 3 months with a range of 2 days to 1 year. Among the 3 surviving patients, the average length of stay was 16 months. The existence of a small subgroup of 'long stay' patients with end-stage dementia is consistent with findings from a study of an institutional hospice (Volicer et al. 1986) and a hospice solely for dementia patients (Brechling et al. 1989).

Five case studies of Meridian Hospice patients suggested that there was a good fit between the kinds of services provided and the needs of both patients and family caregivers (Luchins, Hanrahan and Litzenberg 1998). In general, the caregivers were very satisfied with the care provided by hospice. Services that were especially important to the family caregivers themselves included respite, education, counselling, and bereavement services. In addition, it is apparent from the caregivers' reports that the patients themselves benefited from skilled and individualised palliative care provided at home. Benefits that were mentioned included home visits by the hospice physician and nurses, palliative care, case-managed home health care, service provision in the home environment, and the high quality of staff care.

The provision of palliative care in Dementia Special Care Units (DSCUs, n = 68) was compared to traditional long-term care units (TLTCs, n = 35) at two Department of Veterans Affairs Hospitals in the US (Volicer et al. 1994). The focus of the DSCUs was on maintaining the patients' comfort rather than on trying to prolong life. In most cases, advance proxy planning limited medical interventions (Volicer *et al.* 1986). No such systematic planning programme was in place at the TLTCs. Levels of observed patient discomfort were lower in the DSCU patients than in the TLTC patients. The average three-month costs were $1477 lower in DSCUs than in TLTCs. Cost analysis focused on components of medical care that were likely to vary according to whether palliative versus aggressive care was provided, such as the costs of medication, radiology, and laboratory procedures. As one might expect, a higher proportion of the patients who received palliative care in the DSCUs died during this time (n = 53, 78%) than in the TLTC group (n = 12, 34%).

Access to hospice care

Although the available research supports the feasibility of palliative care and hospice for end-stage dementia patients, the fact that very few of the professional and family caregivers in our survey were aware of hospice programmes that serve dementia patients suggests unmet need (Luchins and Hanrahan 1993). In order to examine this issue further, we conducted a national census survey of all 1694 hospices belonging to the National Hospice Organization in the US; 70% responded (or 1184 programmes) (Hanrahan and Luchins 1995b). Our main question concerned the number of dementia patients in hospices who did not have some other terminal illness, such as cancer. In other words, their primary diagnosis was dementia. Although the responding hospices served 138 503 patients in 1990, less than 1% had a primary diagnosis of dementia and no other terminal illness. Within this group, 80% were in the end stages of dementia. This appears to be a major gap in the service delivery system.

Hospice staff were asked what problems had occurred in their efforts to serve dementia patients relative to other patients. In their view, the main obstacle was the difficulty in predicting the survival time of dementia patients. In the US, enrolment criteria for the Medicare hospice benefit requires a prognosis of death within six months. Because survival time in dementia ranges from two to ten years, it is difficult to predict a prognosis of six months until death. This problem highlights the need to study factors which will predict death in end-stage dementia.

Criteria for enrolling patients with dementia in hospice

Apart from the pioneering efforts of Dr Volicer and his colleagues in studying institutional hospices (1993), very little is known about factors influencing survival time in end-stage dementia. In order to address the need for guidelines we established and tested a set of enrolment criteria for the admission of end-stage dementia patients to hospice care which consisted of the characteristics of advanced dementia and the presence of medical complications of the disease (Table 9.1). These criteria were tested in a small pilot programme with Meridian Hospice (Hanrahan and Luchins 1995a), followed by a replication in eight additional hospices (Luchins, Hanrahan and Murphy 1997). Additionally, because the National Hospice Organization (NHO) developed its own guidelines while the study was in progress, we retrospectively examined the application of these guidelines to our sample (Stuart *et al.* 1996; Table 9.2). The NHO guidelines paralleled our own but with the addition of a more detailed description of medical complications and the suggestion that Stage 7C of Functional Assessment Staging (FAST) may be an appropriate cut-off point for enrolment (Reisberg 1988; Appendix). Using our experience with the 47 patients in our study, we have examined the implications of these refinements.

Table 9.1 Hospice enrolment criteria for end-stage dementia patients

I   Signs of very severe cognitive decline

A May have the following (if known):

Low mental status scores (MSQ or MMSE less than or equal to 1)

B All of the following impairments due to severe cognitive decline:

Incontinent
Needs assistance with eating
Needs assistance with walking
Needs assistance with bathing and grooming
Very limited speech or cannot communicate meaningfully
Unable to engage in purposeful activities

II Serious complications

Patient should have a current or recent history of one or more of the following impairments:

Difficulty swallowing food
Aspiration pneumonia
Dehydration
Malnutrition
Severe urinary tract infection
Decubitus ulcers
Septicaemia
Other serious complications

Predictors of survival time

Our hospice enrolment criteria predicted a median survival time of 4 months and a mean survival time of 7 months; 38% of patients survived for more than 6 months. These results are similar to the median survival of 2.5 months, with 35% living past 6 months, reported in a national study of Medicare hospice beneficiaries with a primary diagnosis of dementia (Christakis and Escarce 1996).

Scores on Functional Assessment Staging (Reisberg 1988) and mobility ratings were significantly related to survival time. However, 41% could not be scored on the FAST, as their disease progression did not fit the ordinal requirements of the measure. Among patients who could be scored on the FAST and who had reached Stage 7C, their mean survival time was 3.2 months compared with 18 months among those who could be scored and had not reached this stage, and 8.6 months among patients whose disease progression was not ordinal. This suggests that using NHO criteria relying on the FAST can identify a subgroup with very high mortality and a short time until death. Although the FAST can identify a subgroup of appropriate candidates for hospice, sole reliance on this measure might decrease access to hospice care for many severely demented patients.

Elements of palliative care and survival

Less aggressive care plans appeared to result in shorter survival times; patients whose care plans called for the use of medication for acute illness had longer survival times than those without this provision (Luchins, Hanrahan and Murphy 1997). However, the use of antibiotics did not make a difference in a replication study, involving 45 patients (Hanrahan *et al.*

Table 9.2 NHO medical guidelines for determining prognosis in dementia (Stuart *et al.* 1996)

I Functional assessment staging

A Patients who have reached the level of severity of dementia described here may have a prognosis of up to two years.

B At or beyond Stage 7 of the Functional Assessment Staging Scale.

C All of the following characteristics:

1 Unable to dress without assistance
2 Unable to bathe properly
3 Urinary and faecal incontinence
4 Unable to speak or communicate meaningfully
5 Unable to ambulate without assistance.

II Presence of medical complications

A Co-morbid conditions of sufficient severity to warrant medical treatment, documented within the past year.

B Co-morbid conditions associated with dementia:

1 Aspiration pneumonia
2 Pyelonephritis or other upper urinary tract infection
3 Septicaemia
4 Decubitus ulcers.

C Difficulty swallowing food or refusal to eat, sufficiently severe that patient cannot maintain sufficient fluid and calorie intake to sustain life. (Patients who are receiving tube feeding must have documented Impaired Nutritional Status.)

III Stage 7C of the FAST may be an appropriate enrolment cut-off (Appendix 9.1)

At this stage, patients are usually:

A Either mute or limited to a single intelligible word in the course of the day,

B Dependent in all activities of daily living, including mobility.

1999). It may be that a plan to use antibiotics was part of a generally aggressive approach to care, which could explain the inconsistency. On the other hand, feeding tubes prolonged life among those patients who had not reached Stage 7C, but not among more severely impaired patients. Lastly, the use of Foley catheters appeared to shorten survival time, perhaps because of the increased likelihood of urinary tract infections.

These findings suggest the need to examine more fully clinical choice points in dealing with complications of advanced dementia. For example, the presence of fever in advanced dementia has been linked with shorter survival times among slightly less impaired patients, although there was no difference among the most severely impaired (Volicer *et al.* 1993). Table 9.3 illustrates the options available in the US when patients with dementia present with fever, together with the information which needs to be considered when making a decision. Fever may be caused by a wide range of infections, such as pneumonia and urinary tract infections. The treatment of fever can also range from aggressive, including an extensive emergency room work up, to a limited home work up, accompanied by palliative treatment. The value of examining clinical choice points in this way is that it clarifies the available treatment/options – and the consequences of these options.

Table 9.3 An illustration of clinical choice point: FEVER

Possible causes:

Respiratory tract infections, including pneumonia	Less common infections (endocarditis, CNS)
Genitourinary tract infection	Infected pressure sores
Intra-abdominal process	Drug reaction
(gastroenteritis, diverticulitis, appendicitis, etc.)	Other non-infectious causes (cancer, vasculitis)

Phone assessment (vital signs, associated symptoms, interventions already tried, etc.)

Current event: severity, need for particular resources
Goals of care under current care plan
Dementia severity (stage)
Co-morbid conditions: number, severity, impact on prognosis, and QOL
Patient/family preferences

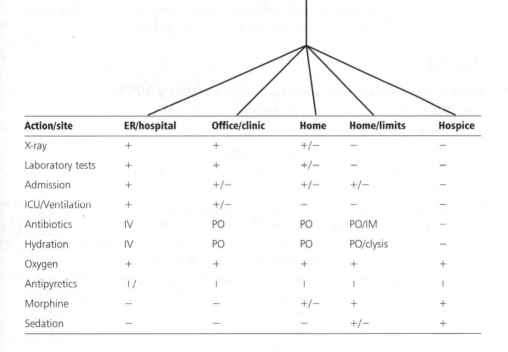

Action/site	ER/hospital	Office/clinic	Home	Home/limits	Hospice
X-ray	+	+	+/−	−	−
Laboratory tests	+	+	+/−	−	−
Admission	+	+/−	+/−	+/−	−
ICU/Ventilation	+	+/−	−	−	−
Antibiotics	IV	PO	PO	PO/IM	−
Hydration	IV	PO	PO	PO/clysis	−
Oxygen	+	+	+	+	+
Antipyretics	I/−	I	I	I	I
Morphine	−	−	+/−	+	+
Sedation	−	−	−	+/−	+

Priorities for future research

There is a compelling need to develop and evaluate ways of providing hospice and palliative care to patients who have not reached a terminal state as defined by Stage 7 of FAST. This may include patients earlier in Stage 7, as well as patients whose disease does not progress in linear fashion and some Stage 6 patients. At Stage 6 severe cognitive decline is present and significant impairments in functioning occur (Reisberg *et al.* 1982). Measures of mental status show considerable decline. Problems in performing activities of daily living include difficulties with dressing and bathing, as well as urinary and faecal incontinence. Family members and the patient's advance directive can provide important information as to the patient's quality of life at this stage. We have not systematically examined attitudes towards palliative care at Stage 6, however, anecdotal evidence suggests that many family members view their relative's quality of life at this stage as being quite poor. This raises questions about the wisdom of prolonging life in the presence of such severe deterioration. As in Stage 7, death is likely to arise from complications of the dementia.

Because the provision of palliative care and hospice for dementia patients is so rare there has been little opportunity for studies of its effectiveness, yet such studies need to be conducted. Also, other palliative care modalities need to be developed and evaluated in addition to hospice care, such as developing palliative care wards in nursing homes and hospitals, and palliative care programmes within home health care agencies. This would create the ability to integrate a palliative approach into the mainstream of medicine. Lastly, clinical choice points need to be developed and evaluated for the palliative treatment of other co-morbid conditions in advanced dementia, such as diabetes, cardiovascular problems, and cancer, as well as preventive care, such as mammograms and flu shots (Sachs 1994).

Appendix 9.1

Functional assessment staging (FAST, Reisberg 1988)

(Check highest consecutive level of disability)

1 No difficulty either subjectively or objectively.

2 Complains of forgetting location of objects. Subjective work difficulties.

3 Decreased job functioning evident to co-workers. Difficulty in travelling to new locations. Decreased organisational capacity.*

4 Decreased ability to perform complex tasks, e.g. planning dinner for guests, handling personal finances (such as forgetting to pay bills), difficulty marketing, etc.

5 Requires assistance in choosing proper clothing to wear for the day, season or occasion, e.g. patients may wear the same clothing repeatedly, unless supervised.*

6 A Improperly putting on clothes without assistance or cuing (e.g. may put street clothes on over night clothes, or put shoes on wrong feet, or have difficulty buttoning clothing) occasionally or more frequently over the past weeks.*

  B Unable to bathe properly (e.g. difficulty adjusting bathwater temperature) occasionally or more frequently over the past weeks.*

  C Inability to handle mechanics of toileting (e.g. forgets to flush the toilet, does not wipe properly, or properly dispose of toilet tissue) occasionally or more frequently over the past weeks.*

  D Urinary incontinence (occasionally or more frequently over the past weeks).*

  E Faecal incontinence (occasionally or more frequently over the past weeks).*

7 A Ability to speak limited to approximately a half a dozen intelligible different words or fewer, in the course of an average day or in the course of an intensive interview.

  B Speech ability is limited to the use of a single intelligible word in an average day or in the course of an intensive interview (the person may repeat the word over and over).

C Ambulatory ability is lost (cannot walk without personal assistance).

D Cannot sit up without assistance (e.g. the individual will fall over if there are not lateral rests (arms) on the chair).

E Loss of ability to smile.

F Loss of ability to hold up head independently.

*Scored primarily on the basis of information obtained from a knowledgeable informant and/or category.

References

Ahronheim, J.C., Morrison, R.S., Baskin, S.A., Morris, J., and Meier, D.E. (1996). Treatment of the dying in the acute care hospital. *Archives of Internal Medicine* **156**(18): 2094–100.

Bachman, D.L., Wolf, P.A., Linn, R.T., Knoefel, J.E., Cobb, J.Z., Belanger, A.J., White, C.R., and DiAgostino, R.B. (1993). Incidence of dementia and probable Alzheimer's disease in a general population. *Neurology* **43**: 515–19.

Brechling, B.G., Heyworth, J., Kuhn, D., and Peranteau, M.F. (1989). Extending hospice care to end-stage dementia patients and families. *The American Journal of Alzheimer's Care and Related Disorders and Research*: 21–9.

Burns, A., Jacoby, R., and Levy, R. (1990). Psychiatric phenomena in Alzheimer's disease. IV: Disorders of behaviours. *British Journal of Psychiatry* **157**: 86–94.

Christakis, N.A. and Escarce, J.J. (1996). Survival of Medicare patients after enrollment in hospice programs. *New England Journal of Medicine* **335**(3): 172–8.

Danis, M., Southerland, L.I., Garrett, J.M., *et al.* (1991). A prospective study of advance directives for life-sustaining care. *New England Journal of Medicine* **324**: 882–8.

Diamond, E.L., Jernigan, J.A., Moseley, R.A., *et al.* (1989). Decision-making ability and advance directive preferences in nursing home patients and proxies. *Gerontologist* **29**: 622–6.

Engel, B.T., Burgio, L.D., and McCormick, K.S. (1990). Behavioral treatment of incontinence in the long-term care setting. *Journal of the American Geriatrics Society* **38**: 361–3.

Ewbank, DC. (1999). Deaths attributable to Alzheimer's disease in the United States. *American Journal of Public Health* **89**(1): 90–2.

Gallagher, D., Rose, J., Rivera, P., *et al.* 1989. Prevalence of depression in family caregivers. *Gerontologist* **24**: 449–56.

Goldman, L.S. and Luchins, D.J. (1984). Depression in the spouses of demented patients. *American Journal of Psychiatry* **141**: 1467–8.

Hanrahan, P. and Luchins, D.J. (1995a). Feasible criteria for enrolling end-stage dementia patients in home hospice care. *The Hospice Journal* **10**(3): 47–54.

Hanrahan, P. and Luchins, D.J. (1995b). Access to hospice care for end-stage dementia patients: a national survey of hospice programs. *Journal of the American Geriatrics Society* **42**(1): 56–9.

Hanrahan, P., Raymond, M., McGowan, E., and Luchins, D.J. (1999). Criteria for enrolling dementia patients in hospice: a replication. *American Journal of Hospice and Palliative Care* **16**(1): 395–440.

Hodgson, C., Higginson, I., and Jefferys, P. (1998). *Carers' Checklist: An Outcome Measure for People with Dementia and their Carers*. London: The Mental Health Foundation.

Hoyert, D.L. (1996). Mortality trends for Alzheimer's disease: 1979–1991. *Vital Health Statistics* **28**: 1–23.

Katzman, R. (1979). The prevalence and malignancy of Alzheimer's disease. *Archives of Neurology* **33**: 217–18.

Lachs, M.S., Becker, M., Siegal, A.P., *et al.* (1992). Delusions and behavioral disturbances in cognitively impaired elderly persons. *Journal of the American Geriatrics Society* **40**: 768–73.

Luchins, D.J. and Hanrahan, P. (1993). What is the appropriate level of health care for end-stage dementia patients? *Journal of the American Geriatrics Society* **41**: 25–30.

Luchins, D.J., Hanrahan, P., and Litzenberg, K. (1998). Acceptance of hospice care for dementia patients by health care professionals and family members. In Volicer, L. and Hurley, A. (eds), *Hospice Care for Patients with Advanced Progressive Dementia*. New York: Springer.

Luchins, D.J., Hanrahan, .P, and Murphy, K. (1997). Criteria for enrolling dementia patients in hospice. *Journal of the American Geriatrics Society* **45(9)**: 1054–9.

Luchins, D.J., Hanrahan, P., and Osview, F. (1999). In Osview, F. (ed.), *Dementia in Public Mental Health Settings. Neuropsychiatry and Mental Health Services*. Washington: DC: American Psychiatric Press.

McCarthy, M., Addington-Hall, J., and Altmann, D. (1997). The experience of dying with dementia a retrospective study. *International Journal of Geriatric Psychiatry* **12**: 404–9.

Meco, G., Alessandria, A., Bonifati, V., *et al.* (1994). Risperidone for hallucinations in levo-dopa treated Parkinson's disease patients. *Lancet* **343**: 1320–71.

Mega, M.S., Cummings, J.L., Fiorello, T., and Gornbein, J. (1996). The spectrum of behavioral changes in Alzheimer's disease. *Neurology* **46(1)**: 130–5.

Michelson, C., Mulvihill, M., Hsu, M.A., *et al.* (1991). Eliciting medical care preferences from nursing home residents. *Gerontologist* **31**: 358–63.

Murphy, K., Hanrahan, P., and Luchins, D.J. (1997). A survey of grief and bereavement in nursing homes: the importance of hospice grief and bereavement for the end-stage Alzheimer's disease patient and family. *Journal of the American Geriatrics Society* **45(9)**: 1104–7.

Nasman, F., Bucht, G., and Eriksson, S. (1993). Behavioural symptoms in the institutionalized elderly: relationship to dementia. *International Journal of Geriatrics Psychiatry* **8**: 843–9.

Payne, K., Taylor, R.M., Stocking, C., and Sachs, G.A. (1996). Physicians' attitudes about the care of patients in the persistent vegetative state: a national survey. *Annals of Internal Medicine* **125(2)**: 104–10.

Pinkston, E.M. and Linsk, N. (1984). *Care of the Elderly: A Family Approach*. New York: Pergamon Press.

Pruchno, R.A. and Resch, N.L. (1989). Aberrant behaviours and Alzheimer's disease: mental health effects on spouse caregivers. *Journal of Gerontology* **44(5)**: S177–S182.

Reisberg, B. (1988). Functional assessment staging (FAST). *Psychopharmacology Bulletin* **24(4)**: 653–9.

Reisberg, B., Ferris, S.H., DeLeon, M.J., *et al.* (1982). The global deterioration scale for assessment of primary degenerative dementia. *American Journal of Psychiatry* **139**: 1136–9.

Rovner, B.W., German, P.S., and Broadhead, J. (1990). The prevalence and management of dementia and other psychiatric disorders in nursing homes. *International Psychogeriatrics* **2**: 13–24.

Sachs, G.A. (1994). Flu shots, mammograms, and Alzheimer's disease: ethics of preventative medicine and dementia. *Alzheimer's Disease and Associated Disorders* **8(1)**: 8–14.

Schneider, L.S., Pollack, V.E., and Lyness, S.A. (1990). A meta-analysis of controlled trials of neuroleptic treatment in dementia. *Journal of the American Geriatrics Society* **38**: 553–63.

Skoog, I., Nielson, L., Palmertz, B., *et al.* (1993). A population based study of dementia in 85 year olds. *New England Journal of Medicine* **328**: 153–8.

Stuart, B., Herbst, L., Kinzbrunner, B., *et al.* (1996). Medical guidelines for determining prognosis in selected non-cancer diseases. *Hospice Journal* **11**: 47–63.

Teri, L., Larson, E.B., and Reifler, B.V. (1988). Behavioral disturbance in dementia of the Alzheimer's type. *Journal of the American Geriatrics Society* **36**: 1–6.

Teri, L. and Uomoto, J.M. (1991). Reducing excess disability in dementia patients: training caregivers to manage patient depression. *Clinical Gerontologist* **10**: 49–63.

Volicer, B.J., Hurley, A., Fabiszewski, K.J., *et al.* (1993). Predicting short-term survival for patients with advanced Alzheimer's disease. *Journal of the American Geriatrics Society* **41**: 535–40.

Volicer, L., Collard, A., Hurley, A., *et al.* (1994). Impact of special care unit for patients with advanced Alzheimer's disease on patients' discomfort and costs. *Journal of the American Geriatrics Society* **42**: 597–603.

Volicer, L., Rheaume, Y., Brown, J., *et al.* (1986). Hospice approach to the treatment of patients with advanced dementia of the Alzheimer's type. *Journal of the American Medical Association* **256**: 2210–13.

Wernicke, T.F. and Reisches, F.M. (1994). Prevalence of dementia in old age: clinical diagnoses in subjects aged 95 years and older. *Neurology* **44**: 250–3.

Wragg, R.E. and Jeste, D.V. (1989). Overview of depression and psychosis in Alzheimer's disease. *American Journal of Psychiatry* **146**(5): 577–87.

Chapter 10

Sickle cell disease

Polly Edmonds

Introduction

Sickle cell disease (SCD) is a family of haemoglobin disorders characterised by chronic haemolysis (destruction of red blood cells), intermittent vaso-occlusion (occlusion of blood vessels), and marked variations in the character and severity of symptoms among individuals. SCD is now the second most common inherited disorder in the UK, with a prevalence of 0.23 per thousand births (Layton and Mufti 1998), and is associated with significant morbidity and mortality. This chapter will review pathophysiology and current management strategies for SCD, the identification of patients with a poorer prognosis, and the role of palliative care in the management of these patients.

Pathophysiology

SCD is a group of closely related conditions having in common abnormalities involving the β globin gene locus on chromosome 11. Normal adult haemoglobin consists of two α globin chains, two β globin chains, and an iron-containing haem group. In SCD a point mutation in the β globin gene results in the substitution of valine for glutamine at position 6. When this abnormality is inherited from each parent, homozygous SCD results (HbSS), no normal adult haemoglobin can be made, and only foetal and sickle haemoglobin are found. If a single sickle gene is inherited and the other is normal, the sickle cell carrier state (HbS trait) results and the individual is healthy under all normal circumstances. The frequency of sickle cell carriers in the UK is up to 1:4 in West Africans and 1:10 in Afro Caribbeans (Department of Health 1993). Other clinically significant conditions include compound heterozygous states with the sickle β globin gene and haemoglobin C (haemoglobin SC) or sickle β thalassaemia (Reed and Vichinsky 1998).

The substitution of valine for glutamine creates a hydrophobic area on the surface of the haemoglobin molecule that encourages polymerisation when the molecule is in the deoxygenated state. As a result, the red cell loses its softness and flexibility, causing damage to the red cell membrane and development of an abnormal and irreversible sickle shape (Juneja *et al.*1995). In addition, a partially compensated chronic haemolytic anaemia is found.

Which patients might benefit from palliative care in SCD?

It is estimated that the number of patients in the UK with sickle cell disease will be more than 10 000 by the year 2000 (Streetly *et al.* 1997). The median life expectancy for men and women with homozygous sickle cell anaemia in the US is 42 and 48 years respectively, a reduction of 25 to 30 years (Platt *et al.* 1994). In one UK centre, the mortality rate was 1 death per 128 years of follow-up (Gray *et al.* 1991). The most common causes of death from SCD are pulmonary complications, cerebrovascular accidents, causes related to infection, acute splenic sequestration, and chronic organ damage and failure (Platt *et al.* 1994; Gray *et al.* 1991). Factors predictive of early death are low foetal haemoglobin (HbF), renal insufficiency, acute chest syndrome (ACS), fits, and an elevated white cell count (Platt *et al.* 1994). In patients over 20 years old, more frequent (more than 3 per year) episodes of painful crisis are associated with an increased mortality (Platt *et al.* 1991.)

In the Co-operative Study of Sickle Cell Disease (CSSCD) only 18% of deaths occurred in chronically ill patients with clinically obvious organ failure, such as renal failure, congestive heart failure, or chronic stroke. A third (33%) of patients died acutely during sickle crisis, most commonly pain crisis, ACS, or acute stroke (Platt *et al.* 1994). The CSSCD also reported that only 5.2% of patients with SCD experience 3–10 episodes of pain each year. The number of patients that may be appropriate for intervention from a specialist palliative care service, therefore, may be relatively small.

Clinical complications of SCD

There is extreme variability in the clinical expression of SCD; the reasons for this are poorly understood. The clinical consequences of SCD are primarily associated with either haemolysis or vaso-occlusion. The pattern of organ involvement in SCD is shown in Table 10.1.

Table 10.1 Patterns of organ involvment in SCD by age group

Age group	Organ involvement: Vaso-occlusion	Chronic haemolysis
Children < 5 years	Dactylitis Acute splenic sequestration	
Children > 5 years	Painful crises affecting trunk Acquired asplenia— pneumococcal infection Stroke	Aplastic episodes— parvovirus infection Delayed growth
Adults	Painful crises affecting long bones Hepatic sequestration Acute chest syndrome Mesenteric syndrome Priapism Subarachnoid haemorrhage Retinopathy Avasular necrosis femoral head Chronic renal failure Chronic sickle lung	Anaemia Jaundice Gallstones

Management of clinical complications of SCD

Infection

Patients with SCD are particularly prone to infection as a result of hyposplenism (pneumococcus, salmonella species, and haemophilus) and parvovirus B19 infection. The CSSCD demonstrated in a randomised prospective trial that daily oral penicillin could prevent 84% of septic episodes when compared with placebo (Gaston *et al.* 1986). The introduction of prophylaxis with daily oral penicillin has reduced both the rate of infection and mortality related to pneumococcal infection. Childhood vaccinations against pneumococci and haemophilus influenza type B (Hib) have now been adopted in the UK (Davies and Oni 1997). Infection with human parvovirus B19 is the main cause of hypoplastic crisis in patients with SCD, causing a sudden and catastrophic fall in haemoglobin. A vaccine is under development (Davies and Oni 1997).

Acute chest syndrome

Acute chest syndrome is an important cause of morbidity and mortality in SCD. The CSSCD prospectively followed 3751 patients, identifying 1722 ACS episodes in 939 patients (Vichinsky *et al.* 1997). The presentation and clinical course of ACS was more severe in adults. Adults presented with shortness of breath, fever, and severe pain, and were more likely to have multi-focal lobar disease and severe hypoxia. The overall death rate was 1.8% (32 deaths in 1741 events), with the death rate 4 times higher in adults than children (4.3%, 18 deaths in 419 events in 271 patients compared to 1.1%, 14 deaths in 695 patients, 1322 events). Fatal cases generally developed rapid pulmonary failure, and the presence of pulmonary fat embolism (PFE) has been suggested to be associated with a greater severity of disease and risk of death (Reed and Vichinsky 1998).

ACS has also been a common and severe post-operative complication. Preventive factors include the use of a warm operating theatre, adequate pain control, early post surgical ambulation and avoidance of over hydration. The use of exchange transfusion in the immediate post-operative phase offers no advantage over standard transfusion (Reed and Vichinsky 1998).

Cerebrovascular disease and stroke

Stroke is a common complication of SCD and is a frequent cause of morbidity and death. The CSSCD demonstrated a prevalence of 4% (incidence 0.61 per 100 patient years) in HbSS patients, but stroke occurred in all common genotypes (Ohene-Frempong *et al.* 1998). Children and older patients were at highest risk of an infarctive stroke, whereas haemorrhagic stroke was commonest in the 20–29 age group. Across all ages the mortality rate was 26% in the two weeks following haemorrhagic stroke; no deaths occurred after infarctive stroke. In children with infarctive stroke intensive rehabilitation and transfusion are standard therapy; motor function may be recovered, but severe cognitive impairment is usually lasting. Most episodes of recurrent stroke can be prevented with chronic transfusions, although the optimal frequency has not been established. The role of transfusion in haemorrhagic stroke remains unclear (Reed and Vichinsky 1998).

Avascular necrosis of the hip

SCD is the most common cause of avascular necrosis of the hip in childhood, resulting in significant physical impairment and chronic pain, often progressing to require hip replacement. Conservative therapy is generally ineffective. Core decompression has been reported to improve pain control and slow progression in early avascular necrosis (Styles and Vichinsky 1996).

Management of painful crises

Pain is the most common clinical problem encountered in the care of the patient with SCD. The CSSCD report on pain and SCD observed that 39% of patients experienced no pain but 1% had more than 6 episodes per year. In this study the 5.2% of patients who averaged 3–10 pain episodes per year accounted for a third of all pain episodes; the frequency of pain crises was a marker of disease severity and predictive of other complications, thereby identifying patients at risk of early death. (Platt *et al.* 1991).

Psychosocial implications of pain in SCD

Pain in vaso-occlusive sickle crisis results from oxygen deprivation of tissues and avascular necrosis of the bone marrow. Although over 90% of hospital admissions in SCD are for painful crises, nearly all sickle pain is managed in the community (Fuggle *et al.* 1996, Westerman *et al.* 1997). In one study pain was reported by children and adolescents on 30% of days, and patients were absent from school as a result of pain on 21% of school days (Shapiro *et al.* 1995). Fuggle *et al.* (1996) reported that sickle pain resulted in over 7 times an increased risk of not attending school and was highly disruptive of social and recreational activities. Work in adults suggests that this group have major adjustment difficulties, including increased anxiety about death, disruption of social support networks, disability, dependence on pain medication, and conflict with health care providers (Butler and Beltran 1993).

Non-pharmacological management

Patients with SCD manage the majority of pain crises at home with a variety of non-pharmacological approaches including relaxation, local warmth, and hydration. McCrae and Lumley (1998) suggest factors such as negative thinking, passive coping, and somatic awareness are related to higher reporting of pain. Patients using self-hypnosis (Dinges 1997) and cognitive behavioural therapy (Thomas 1998; Gill 1997) may have lower levels of psychological distress and fewer hospital admissions than other patients.

Non-opioid and weak opioid analgesia

Many patients manage pain crises at home using simple analgesics, such as paracetamol, non-steroidal anti-inflammatory drugs (NSAIDs), and weak opioid analgesics. A logical, step-wise approach to the use of analgesics in this patient group is suggested, based on that advocated by the WHO for cancer pain (WHO 1986). It is crucial that these patients use non-opioid and weak opioid analgesics regularly rather than as required for optimal analgesia.

There has been interest in the use of co-analgesics in pain crises, particularly in relation to a potential opioid-sparing effect. One randomised, double-blind study of intravenous high dose methylprednisolone in children and adolescents demonstrated that a short course of methylprednisolone could decrease the duration of severe pain and in-patient analgesic use (Griffin *et al.* 1994). The long-term risks of high dose corticosteroids in this patient population are unknown, but potentiation of osteoporosis and avascular necrosis of the femoral head is a concern. In one randomised controlled trial of ketorolac in 21 patients with pain crisis, the ketorolac group required 33% less strong opioid than the placebo group, and analgesia was superior compared to opioid alone (Perlin *et al.* 1994). These results have not been reproduced. Care must be taken using NSAIDs, as they can exacerbate nephropathy in hypovolaemic patients.

Strong opioid analgesics: factors limiting use

Strong opioid analgesics are commonly used for in-patient management of painful crises in the UK, but their use is controversial. There is an incorrect perception that significant numbers of patients with SCD and pain are addicted to drugs such as pethidine and morphine. Shapiro (1997) reported that 9% of American haematologists and 22% of emergency department physicians thought that more than 50% of adult sickle cell patients were addicted to strong opioids; Waldrop and Mandry (1995) also demonstrated that health care professionals overestimate opioid dependence in sickle patients. In studies of large numbers of patients requiring strong opioids for pain, addiction occurs in less than 1% of patients with no prior history of substance abuse (Porter and Jick 1980; Perry and Heidrich 1982; Medina and Diamond 1977). In the Caribbean and Africa there appears to be less use of strong opioids in sickle crisis than in the UK or US (Konotey-Ahulu 1998; Serjeant and Serjeant 1996). The reasons for this are unclear, but the population of patients treated may be different (Bevan 1998; Brozovic *et al.* 1986). For example, patients with sickle cell haemoglobinopathy and mild phenotype sickle cell anaemia are more likely to have survived to adulthood in West Africa; these patients rarely require strong opioid analgesic in the UK (Bevan 1998). Whilst it is not uncommon for crises involving the limbs to be managed with mild analgesics at home, clinical experience with an older patient population in the UK suggests crises more frequently involve the trunk, liver, lungs, and gut and require hospitalisation for severe pain (Brozovic 1986). There is evidence that pain in SCD is underestimated and under-treated by health care professionals (Walters and Thomas 1995; Alleyne and Thomas 1994; Black and Laws 1996; Forbes and Forbes 1997; Murray and May 1988).

Health care professionals' fears of drug-seeking behaviour and their lack of awareness of optimal pain management strategies can lead to delays in treatment and inadequate analgesia for patients with painful sickle crises (Forbes and Forbes 1997; Murray and May 1988.)

Parenteral strong opioid analgesics in pain crisis

The use of management protocols for sickle pain, initiated in the accident and emergency department and maintained on the ward, are becoming more common in the UK. Standard management for patients admitted with painful sickle crises should be the regular, or continuous, administration of a strong opioid, usually by intravenous infusion. Morphine is the strong opioid of choice, and when administered by patient controlled analgesia (PCA), has been shown to provide better analgesia than intermittent opioid therapy in painful sickle crises (Robieux *et al.* 1992; Perlin *et al.* 1993). PCA has been increasingly widely adopted in the UK and appears safe and well tolerated. There are case reports of clinically significant respiratory depression occurring with the use of morphine in sickle crises (Gerber and Apseloff 1993), but these are extremely rare and should not occur with appropriate pre-scribing and monitoring.

In the UK there has been a move away from the use of pethidine for the management of pain crises. Pethidine offers no advantages over morphine. The onset of action and side effect profile of the two drugs is similar, and pethidine has a shorter duration of action (Simini 1996). Accumulation of the metabolite norpethidine can lead to central nervous system excitation, including fits in 1–12% of patients (Ballas 1997). There is one reported case of a death of sickle cell patient during a fit after high dose pethidine (Mitchell *et al.* 1991). In addition, subcutaneous or intramuscular administration of pethidine causes local irritation and fibrosis with repeated doses. There is a consensus in the UK that pethidine is less safe and effective than morphine for sickle pain.

Oral strong opioids in pain crisis

There are increasing reports on the use of oral morphine regimens in pain crises, with the potential for these to be either initiated or continued as an out-patient. In one study of nine patients, the use of an oral morphine regimen was associated with a significant reduction in the number of emergency department visits, total numbers of hours spent in the emergency department, and proportion of visits that resulted in admission to hospital (Conti 1996). Brookoff and Polomano (1992) reported on a strategy to manage sickle pain like cancer pain. Patients presenting with pain crises were given intravenous morphine in the emergency room; those achieving substantial pain relief within four to six hours were given a one- to two-week supply of oral controlled release morphine (with immediate release morphine for breakthrough analgesia) and discharged home. This policy resulted in a reduction in the number of admissions for sickle pain by 44%, a reduction in total in-patient days by 57%, length of hospital stay by 23%, and number of emergency department visits by 67%. Although this study was not controlled, there were no reported cases of drug addiction, or drug-seeking behaviour, and the out-patient morphine regimen appeared safe. Some authors commented that this policy resulted in patients seeking parenteral opioids in other local hospitals (Ballas *et al.* 1992). A randomised trial of oral controlled release morphine following an intravenous loading dose for pain crisis in children demonstrated no difference in pain scores and use of breakthrough analgesia for oral and intravenous morphine (Jacobson *et al.* 1997). In a pilot project in South West London, 12 patients with severe pain due to SCD were referred to a community palliative care team for review of analgesic use for sickle pain and community support for self-administered oral opioids at home in crisis. Twenty-three episodes of the pain crises were successfully managed in the community with strong opioid analgesia. The number of hospital admissions with pain crisis was reduced from 26 in the year preceding the intervention to 15, and in-patient bed-days from 346 to 177. The median number of admissions for pain crisis per patient per year was reduced from 3 to 1. No drug-seeking behaviour was identified in these highly selected patients, and the out-patient regimen, with daily monitoring from the community palliative care team, appeared safe (Edmonds *et al.* 1999).

Therapeutic advances in the management of SCD

Transfusion

Transfusion is used in SCD for the prevention of stroke and ACS. Stroke, growth failure, pain, and ACS may all be improved by transfusion (Reed and Vichinsky 1998). Haemachromatosis may occur when transfusions are continued over years, and may be managed by the use of desferrioxamine and apheresis.

Chemotherapy

In a large double-blind, randomised study of adult patients with SCD, hydroxyurea significantly reduced the number of sickle crises per year, episodes of ACS, and requirement for transfusion (Charache *et al.* 1995). Hydroxyurea increases HbF synthesis; HbF has an inhibitory effect on polymerisation of sickle cell haemoglobin. The long-term safety of this drug in SCD is unknown.

Stem cell transplantation

Stem cell or bone marrow transplantation offers the opportunity for a cure for patients with SCD and has been reported in over 100 children to date (Davies and Roberts 1996). Overall survival following transplantation is 90–95%, with 10–15% graft rejection. Identification of appropriate children is limited by lack of HLA matched siblings. Placental (umbilical cord) blood may prove to be an alternative source of stem cells for transplantation (Reid and Vichinsky 1998).

Palliative care services in SCD

Although the development of multi-professional teams for managing in-patients with sickle cell disease has long been advocated (Davies and Wonke 1991), there is a lack of evidence of efficacy. Yang *et al.* (1995) reported significantly less emergency room and in-patient use and lower health costs for patients enrolled in a comprehensive care clinic for SCD in the US. Butler and Beltran (1993) demonstrated that a community based, adult sickle cell support group enhanced participant's knowledge about SCD, improved the physician–patient relationship and helped resolve psychosocial adjustment problems. Sergeant and Sergeant (1996) also suggest that a day care centre with sympathetic and knowledgeable staff, able to administer both non-pharmacological and pharmacological therapies, is beneficial in terms of patient outcomes. Although the majority of patients with SCD spend most of their time in the community, few teams cross the community–hospital interface. This is surprising given that SCD is a chronic disease that has a major impact on lifestyle, in terms of school attendance, job opportunities, and finances.

A systematic review of specialist palliative care for cancer patients concluded that such services improved satisfaction and identified and dealt with more patient and family needs when compared to conventional care. In addition, multi-professional working in palliative care reduced the overall cost of care by reducing the amount of time patients spent in hospital (Hearn and Higginson 1998). To date, the experience of palliative care for patients with SCD is limited to anecdotal reports of involvement with patients predominantly with complex physical pain and psychosocial issues. Whilst these factors are not unusual in a palliative care setting, the chronicity of SCD, albeit with a limited life expectancy, means that existing palliative care services may not be best placed to meet those needs. There is an urgent need to develop and evaluate services for patients with SCD. These could initially be targeted at those patients who are high service users with more severe disease and shorter prognosis. Several options, either building on existing services or developing new services, are discussed below:

1 *Development of generic sickle cell services*, based on multi-professional team working, e.g. comprising doctors, specialist nurses, social worker, occupational therapist, physiotherapist, chaplain, and orthopaedic surgeon. The specific complications that occur in sickle cell disease, associated with the complex physical and psychosocial needs of these patients, suggest that the development of teams spanning the primary and secondary care interface and focusing on whole patient care are to be encouraged.

2 The *development of sickle cell nurse specialists*, a model previously developed in specialties such as palliative care, oncology, chest medicine, and diabetes. Their role could include improving communication between patient and medical team and providing education. Lorenzi (1993) demonstrated that education and the implementation of nursing guidelines for pain crisis could improve nurses' knowledge, although this intervention did not improve job satisfaction. Sickle nurse specialists could work closely with specialist palliative care teams to develop expertise in symptom control and psychosocial support for patients with complex needs.

3 The *development of effective management protocols* for pain in hospital and community. Managing all episodes of sickle crises in the community is clearly unrealistic and potentially unsafe. Although the majority of episodes of painful crises are already managed in the community, a small proportion of patients with frequent crises and complex pain use a large number of in-patient resources. There may be a subgroup of patients here who are highly motivated and who would benefit from more pro-active management of sickle pain in the community. The use of sickle management plans, or care pathways, similar to those developed in many in-patient units, could be transferred into the community, and procedures implemented to ensure that analgesic use was appropriate and potential life-threatening events such as ACS identified.

4 *Expansion of existing palliative care services* to care for patients with SCD at risk of early death. In the majority of patients with SCD there is no clearly defined advanced progressive phase. Adult patients with more symptoms are at increased risk of early death, but it is difficult to identify those patients who would benefit most from intervention by palliative care services. There is undoubtedly a subgroup of patients with complex pain and psychosocial needs, or chronic organ failure, who may benefit from short-term intervention, but it is unlikely that existing palliative care services could continue to manage this group of patients on an on-going basis as there are no clearly identified end points.

Conclusions

SCD is a common condition, affecting patients of predominantly Afro-Caribbean origin. Painful crises are the most frequent complication, but their management is often suboptimal as a result of fears relating to analgesic use and inadequate prescribing. The palliative care needs of this group of patients have not been clearly defined, but there is undoubtedly a subgroup with a poor prognosis and frequent pain crises who may benefit from some form of specialist palliative care intervention. Research is urgently needed to more clearly define the needs of this group, and the type of services that would most effectively meet them.

References

Alleyne, J. and Thomas, V.J. (1994). The management of sickle cell crisis pain as experienced by patients and their carers. *Journal of Advanced Nursing* 19: 725–32.

Ballas, S.K. (1997). Management of sickle pain. *Current Opinion in Haematology* 4: 104–11.

Ballas, S.K., Rubin, R.N., and Gabuzda, T.C. (1992). Treating sickle cell pain like cancer pain (letter). *Annals of Internal Medicine* 117(3): 263.

Bevan, D.H. (1998). Opiates for sickle crisis? (letter). *The Lancet* 352: 1632.

Black, J. and Laws, S. (1986). Pain relief and staff attitudes in hospital. In *Living with Sickle Cell Disease*. London: Sickle Cell Society, pp. 112–31.

Brookoff, D. and Polomano, R. (1992). Treating sickle cell pain like cancer pain. *Annals of Internal Medicine* 116: 364–8.

Brozovic, M., Davies, S.C., Yardumian, A., Bellingham, A., Marsh, G. and Stephens, A. (1986). Pain relief in sickle cell crisis (letter). *The Lancet* 2: 624–5.

Butler D.J. and Beltran, L.R. (1993). Functions of an adult sickle cell group: education, task orientation, and support. *Health & Social Work* 18(1): 49–56.

Charache, S., Terrnin, M., and Moore, R. (1995). Effect of hydroxyurea on the frequency of painful crisis in sickle cell disease. *New England Journal of Medicine* 322: 1317–22.

Conti, C., Tso, E., and Browne, B. (1996). Oral morphine protocol for sickle crisis pain. *Maryland Medical Journal* 45(1): 33–5.

Davies, S. and Oni, L. (1997). Management of patients with sickle cell disease. *British Medical Journal* 315: 656–60.

Davies, S.C. and Roberts, I.A.E. (1996). Bone marrow transplant for sickle cell disease – an update. *Archives of Diseases of Childhood* 75: 3–6.

Davies S.C. and Wonke, B. (1991). The management of haemoglobinopathies. In Hann, I. (ed.), *Clinical Haematology* 4(2): 361–89.

Department of Health (1993). *Report of a Working Party of the Standing Advisory Committee on Sickle Cell, Thalassaemia, and Other Haemoglobinopathies.* London: HMSO.

Dinges, D.F., Whitehouse, W.G., Orne, E.C., Bloom, P.B., Carlin, M.M., Bauer, N.K., Gillen, K.A., Shapiro, B.S., Ohene-Frempong, K., Dampier, C., and Orne, M.T. (1997). Self-hypnosis as an adjunctive treatment in the management of pain associated with sickle cell disease. *International Journal of Clinical and Experimental Hypnosis* 45(4): 417–32.

Edmonds, P., Todd, J., Hay, N., Baynham J., Chamberlain J., and Bevan, D.H. (1999). Management of patients with sickle cell pain in the community. *Journal of Royal College of Physicians* 33(6): 587–8.

Forbes, K. and Forbes, B. (1998). Sickle cell related pain: perceptions of medical practitioners (letter). *Journal of Pain and Symptom Management* 15(6): 333–4.

Fuggle, P., Shand, P.A., Gill, L. J., and Davies, S.C. (1996). Pain, quality of life and coping in sickle cell disease. *Archives of Diseases in Childhood* 75: 199–203.

Gaston, M., Verter, J., and Woods, G. (1986). Prophylaxis with oral penicillin in children with sickle cell anaemia. *New England Journal of Medicine* 314: 1594–9.

Gerber, N. and Apseloff, G. (1993). Death from morphine infusion during sickle cell crisis. *Journal of Paediatrics* 123: 322–5.

Gil, K.M., Edens, J.L., Wilson, J.J., Raezer, L.B., Kinney, T.R., Schultz, W.H., and Daeschner, C. (1997).

Coping strategies and laboratory pain in children with sickle cell disease. *Annals of Behavioural Medicine* **19**(1): 22–9.

Gray, A., Anionwu, E.N., Davies, S.C., and Brozovic, M. (1991). Patterns of mortality in sickle cell disease in the UK. *Journal of Clinical Pathology* **44**: 459–63.

Griffin, T.C., McIntire, D., and Buchanan, G.R. (1994). High dose intravenous methylprednisolone therapy for pain in children and adolescents with sickle cell disease. *New England Journal of Medicine* **330**(11): 733–7.

Hearn J. and Higginson, I.J. (1998). Do specialist palliative care teams improve outcomes for cancer patients? A systematic literature review. *Palliative Medicine* **12**: 317–32.

Jacobsen, S.J., Kopecky, E.A., Joshi, P., and Babul, N. (1997). Randomised trial of oral morphine for painful episodes of sickle cell disease in children. *The Lancet* **350**: 1358–61.

Juneja, H.S., Shulman, E., Reed, K., McIntire, L.V., and Natarajan, M. (1995). Pathophysiology and management of sickle cell pain crisis. Report of a meeting of physicians and scientists, University of Texas Health Science Centre at Houston, Texas. *The Lancet* **346**: 1408–11.

Konotey-Ahulu, F.I.D. (1998). Opiates for sickle crisis? (letter). *The Lancet* **351**: 1438.

Layton, D.M. and Mufti, G.J. (1998). Opiates for sickle crisis? (letter). *The Lancet* **352**: 1632.

Lorenzi, E.A. (1993). The effects of comprehensive guidelines for the care of sickle-cell patients in crisis on the nurses' knowledge base and job satisfaction for care given. *Journal of Advanced Nursing* **18**(12): 1923–1930.

McCrae, J.D. and Lumley, M.A. (1998). Health status in sickle cell disease: examining the roles of pain coping strategies, somatic awareness and negative affectivity. *Journal of Behavioural Medicine* **21**(1): 35–55.

Medina, J.L. and Diamond, S. (1977). Drug dependency in patients with chronic headache. *Headache* **17**: 12–14.

Mitchell, A., Fisher, A.P., Brunner, M., Ware, R.G., and Hanna, M. (1991). Pethidine for painful crisis in sickle cell disease. *British Medical Journal* **303**: 249.

Murray, N. and May, A. (1988). Painful crises in sickle cell disease – patients' perspectives. *British Medical Journal* **297**: 452–4.

Ohene-Frempong, K., Weiner, S.J., Sleeper, L.A., Miller, S.T., Embury, S., Moohr, J.W., Wethers, D.L., Pegelow, C.H., and Gill, F.M. (1998). Cerebrovascular accidents in sickle cell disease: rates and risk factors. *Blood* **91**(1): 288–94.

Perlin, E., Fincke, H., and Castro, O. (1993). Infusional/patient controlled analgesia in sickle cell vaso-occlusive crisis. *The Pain Clinic* **6**: 113–19.

Perlin, E., Fincke, H., Castro, O., Rana, S., Pittman, J., Burt, R., Ruff, C., and McHugh, D. (1994). Enhancement of pain control with ketorolac tromethamine in patients with sickle cell vaso-occlusive crisis. *American Journal of Haematology* **46**(1): 43–7.

Perry, S. and Heidrich, G. (1982). Management of pain during debridement: a survey of US burn units. *Pain* **13**: 267–80.

Platt, O.S., Brambilla, D.J., Rosse, W.F., Milner, P.F., Castro, O., Steinberg, M.H., and Klug, P.P. (1994). Mortality in sickle cell disease. Life expectancy and risk factors for early death. *New England Journal of Medicine* **330**: 1639–44.

Platt, O.S., Thorington, B.D., Brambilla, D.J., Milner, P.F., Rosse, W.F., Vichinsky, E., and Kinney, T.R. (1991). Pain in sickle cell disease: rates and risk factors. *New England Journal of Medicine* **325**: 11–16.

Porter, J. and Jick, H. (1980). Addiction rare in patients treated with narcotics (letter). *New England Journal of Medicine* **302**(2): 123.

Reed, W. and Vichinsky, E.P. (1998). New considerations in the treatment of sickle cell disease. *Annual Review of Medicine* **49**: 461–74.

Robieux, I.C., Kellner, J.D., Coppes, M.J., Shaw, D., Brown, E., Good, C., O'Brodovich, H., Manson, D., Olivieri, N.F., Zipursky, A., *et al.* (1992). Analgesia in children with sickle cell crisis: comparison of intermittent opioids vs. continuous intravenous infusion of morphine and placebo-controlled study of oxygen inhalation. *Paediatric Haematology and Oncology* 9(4): 317–26.

Serjeant G. and Sergeant, B. (1996). Painful crises in sickle cell disease (letter). *The Lancet* 346: 1190–1.

Shapiro, B.S., Dinges, D.F., Orne, E. C., Bauer, N., Reilly, L.B., Whitehouse, W.G., Ohene-Frempong, K., and Orne, M.T. (1995). Home management of sickle cell related pain in children and adolescents: natural history and impact on school attendance. *Pain* 61(1): 139–44.

Shapiro, B.S., Benjamin, L.J., Payne, R., and Heidrich, G. (1997). Sickle cell related pain: perceptions of medical practitioners. *Journal of Pain and Symptom Management* 14(3): 168–74.

Simini, B. (1996). Sickle cell pain crisis (letter). *The Lancet* 347: 262.

Streetly, A., Maxwell, K., and Mejia, A. (1997). *Sickle Cell Disorders in Greater London: a needs assessment of screening and care services.* London: Bexley and Greenwich Health Authority.

Styles, L.A. and Vichinsky, E.P. (1996). Core decompression in avascular necrosis of the hip in sickle cell disease. *American Journal of Haematology* 52(2): 103–7.

Vichinsky, E.P., Styles, L.A., Colangelo, L.H., Wright, E.C., Castro, O., and Nickerson, B. (1997). Acute chest syndrome in sickle cell disease: clinical presentation and course. Cooperative Study of Sickle Cell Disease. *Blood* 89(5): 1787–92.

Waldrop, R.D. and Mandry, C. (1995). Health professional perceptions of opioid dependence among patients with pain. *American Journal of Emergency Medicine* 13(5): 529–31.

Waters, J. and Thomas, V. (1995). Pain from sickle cell crisis. *Nursing Times* 91(16): 29–31.

Westerman, M.P., Bailey, K., Freels, S., Schlegel, R., and Williamson, P. (1997). Assessment of painful episode frequency in sickle cell disease. *American Journal of Haematology* 54: 183–8.

World Health Organisation (1986). *Cancer Pain Relief.* Geneva: WHO.

Yang, Y.M., Shah, A.K., Watson, M., and Mankad, V.N. (1995). Comparison of costs to the health sector of comprehensive and episodic health care for sickle cell disease patients. *Public Health Reports* 110(1): 80–6.

Chapter 11

HIV /AIDS

Gabi Brogan and Rob George

Doubt it seems to me, is the central condition of a human being in the 20th century. One of the things that has happened to us … is to learn how certainty crumbles in your hand.

Salman Rushdie (1989), *Following the instigation of a fatwa*

Introduction

In this chapter we focus on the care of people with HIV/AIDS in the UK, and assume that, for the foreseeable future, AIDS will be fatal and HIV will be transmissible only through certain body fluids or sexually. We do not discuss the situation in developing countries, where the problem is assuming the biblical proportions foreseen: at least 33.4 million living with HIV/AIDS; over 1.7 million young people being infected with HIV every year in Africa, and 700 000 in Asia and the Pacific (UNAIDS Global data, www.unaids.org). In these societies, where disease continues unmodified by therapeutic advance, the only treatment is care, and palliation is a pressing need. The debate about the appropriate role of palliative care that is central to this chapter is therefore irrelevant as far as the developing world is concerned.

We contend that in the industrialised world specialist palliative care is still relevant to HIV disease, although the context and character of its practice will vary over time. We also argue that the lessons palliative care specialists have learnt from the care of patients with HIV/AIDS give valuable insights into our involvement in other diseases.

Changes in HIV/AIDS

We begin by looking at the changes of the last decade, first in patterns of spread and second the effect of new treatments.

Epidemiology

AIDS emerged in the early 1980s. By 1988 palliative care services for people with the disease had been established in the UK, with the first community HIV palliative care team at the Middlesex Hospital (George and Hart 1989) and the first AIDS hospice at the Mildmay Mission Hospital in East London. By 1994 there were six in-patient units solely treating patients dying with AIDS and a significant number of other hospice and specialist palliative care services willing to take referrals (Hospice Information Service 1994). Although it has often taken much political skill and persuasion, and many units have been shamed into it, over 80% of services will now care for people with HIV/AIDS. In high incidence areas at least, these patients now enjoy the privileges of access to the full range of specialist palliative care services traditionally afforded cancer patients.

The HIV population in this country, as in the rest of Europe, is not large and, primarily through good health education, has not reached the proportions predicted. At the end of 1997 15 074 people in the UK were known to be living with HIV and receiving care. Those infected tend to live in urban areas, particularly London. However, behind these figures is a population that has changed in character over time (PHLS 1998; MRC Collaborative Study Group 1996; Kelleher, Cox and McKeogh 1997).

Initially, HIV/AIDS was a disease affecting homosexual men, those infected by contaminated blood, and some intravenous drug users. For example, in 1986 94% of AIDS cases in the UK were in gay men. This had fallen to 58% in 1997. In the same period, the proportion of injecting drug users with AIDS had only increased from 2% to 8% and heterosexual transmission had increased from 3% to 31% of the total cases.

The majority of these new cases are black Africans, mostly using the UK as refuge. This ethnic group makes up 18% of new infections and is the largest after gay men. The UK may well follow the US and find AIDS becoming a disease of destitution affecting those from lower socio-economic classes, refugees, drug addicts and workers in the sex industry. If this is the case the service needs of patients will change too. African refugee women, for example, are radically different from middle-class gay men: services in metropolitan London reflect this with some areas employing HIV midwives, health visitors, ethnic workers, etc. Of societal concern, the stigma associated with HIV infection may also become generally attached to these minorities.

Other research on social habits may indicate another disturbing trend. It suggests that the fear of HIV/AIDS that led to safer sexual practices in the early 1990s has diminished in some groups. Gay men in their late teens are once again a growing population of newly infected people. Anonymous seroprevalence data suggest also that the incidence in metropolitan STD clinics has begun to rise after a nadir in 1991–5, and, in some parts of London, antenatal screening has given an asymptomatic seroprevalence of 1:200. The universal introduction of voluntary antenatal testing in London is now seen as cost effective (Postma *et al.* 1999). In short, HIV infection may rise across society, not just in marginalised groups. We simply do not know.

Therapeutics

Therapeutic advances have had an enormous impact on the clinical course of HIV infection. When HIV/AIDS first emerged, it was a disease characterised by 'highs' and 'lows'. As immunity gradually faded patients repeatedly faced death from successive, variably treatable opportunistic infections and malignancies as part of a fairly rapid mortality. No one survived. Although obvious, the need for palliation was generally not easily accepted by acute clinicians who basically viewed HIV as an infection and therefore curable. Nevertheless, it became seen as a necessity. At the turn of the 1990s, although we could treat some of the complications of AIDS but could only *hope* for a cure, the introduction of the reverse transcriptase inhibitor Zidovudine meant it was possible to prevent viral replication. The possibility of control was in sight. However, although some patients responded dramatically, the effects turned out to be time limited as viral resistance emerged. Side effects from the drug were also significant. By this time it was also clear that HIV had a significant neuro-pathic effect in the central nervous system (CNS) and dementia was being seen as a threat for the future. So death and dying still had to be faced, although prognosis was improving with increasingly effective prophylaxis for opportunistic infections.

From 1996, however, the clinical landscape changed radically with the widespread intro-duction of combination therapies of reverse transcriptase and protease inhibitors, and improved prophylactics. The greater the viral load suppression by antiviral treatment, the lower the likelihood of disease progression (Montaner *et al.* 1998). Survival now increased dramatically and in-patient bed use declined (Aalen *et al.* 1999). Recorded AIDS deaths fell 44% in the UK between 1996 and 1997 (Alcorn 1998/9). Whilst the cost of Highly Active Antiretroviral Therapy (HAART) is considerable, it is now conceivable that new treatments can re-establish immunity and even achieve control or 'cure'. Clinicians and patients are able now to expect long-term survival with more optimistic treatment centres seeing HIV as a predominantly out-patient problem. By 2001 the number of individuals on treatment is likely to increase by 50–100% compared with the pre-1996 levels. Clinicians involved with treating HIV/AIDS are once again uneasy about 'giving up' on curative approaches in the individual. Nevertheless, the future remains uncertain for patients currently doing well on treatment, particularly as viral resistance continues to develop (Sherer 1998). As treatments fail there may be a reversion to the early presentation of the disease, or even the develop-ment of more aggressive strains.

These new drugs could also be a mixed blessing. They have significant short- and long-term side effects and do not penetrate the CNS well; compliance is also an issue. We could conceivably find ourselves 'producing' a population of patients increasingly disabled by neurodegenerative sequelae and iatrogenic disease (Sherer 1998).

To summarise, we are now seeing a variable and unpredictable course of HIV in the UK. Some patients remain free of serious symptoms and complications until late in the illness; some appear to remain asymptomatic for years or even decades with preserved immunity, whereas others may suffer debilitating malaise or frequent acute events. HIV is not yet another out-patient disease. Patients must continue to have access to a full spectrum of care. Those most in need of palliation, such as late presenters, are usually those in the greatest and most complex general need, which likely as not involves other family members.

Palliative care in AIDS/HIV: a continuing need

We now come to the change in palliative care. The clinical details are not reviewed, as they are covered in detail elsewhere (Butters *et al.* 1992; George 1995; Adler 2000; Walsh 1991).

Symptom control

Maintaining quality of life with a minimum symptomatic load is essential for patients cop-ing with uncertainty. The main symptom control issues highlighted in studies are around pain (Breitbart 1996; Hewitt *et al.* 1997). Other symptoms include breathlessness, nausea, gastrointestinal disturbance, fatigue, and weight loss. These are not that different than in other diseases. There are four areas where HIV/AIDS presents particular challenges:

1 New symptoms may warrant investigation even for patients with end-stage disease because many easily treatable conditions can present atypically in this group.

2 Some distressing symptoms may be controlled effectively only by specific treatment of the underlying conditions.

3 For symptomatic reasons, many drugs used for prophylaxis may be continued to the end of life.

4 Combination therapies may place a heavy symptomatic load upon the individual.

Specialist palliative care must continue to be accessible to HIV clinicians, at the very least in a consultative capacity, for all patients once they are on some form of therapy.

Late presenters

Some patients continue to present late in the disease course, with opportunistic infections and tuberculosis sealing their poor prognosis (MRC Collaborative Study Group 1996; Del Amo *et al.* 1996). Clients from the African subcontinent make up a large majority of these late presenters. Their disease course and prognosis remain disturbingly similar to those of AIDS patients in the 1980s. Their requirements for palliative care are equally high.

Long-term survivors

The improved survival of patients with AIDS has allowed long-term complications including malignancies and neurodegenerative conditions such as dementia to emerge as significant clinical problems (Royal Free/Chelsea and Westminster Hospitals Collaborative Group 1997). There is little research yet to guide clinicians on the best way to manage the long-term problems, but the concept of late complications of 'treated' disease is not unique to HIV/ AIDS. It is comparable to children and adolescents with haematological malignancies 'cured' by chemotherapy and/or radiotherapy who develop second tumours in early adult life.

Neurodegeneration

The incidence of progressive multi-focal leucoencephalopathy (caused by the opportunistic JC virus) may be up to 8% (Sadler *et al.* 1998). HIV encephalopathy is now the most common CNS complication in patients with HIV/AIDS and has far reaching implications for the patient, their carers/family, and the cost to society. In-patient days per person-year in AIDS subjects with neurological complications are almost double those for AIDS subjects without neurological complications (Starace *et al.* 1998). The problems they face are those suffered by anyone with progressive neurological dysfunction. They need high levels of nursing care during an unpredictable course of increasing disability and dependency that may last years (McKeogh 1995). The challenge for palliative care services, as with all dying patients, is to demonstrate that quality of life, dignity, and peace is possible. HIV may offer us a test bed for examining models of care for such groups.

Malignancy

There is a growing spectrum of malignancies, which differ widely in disease course and response to treatment. Some, for example Kaposi's sarcoma, have declined in incidence as a direct result of combination antiretroviral therapy while others, such as lymphoma, have increased. Interestingly, the development of lymphoma and the higher incidence of squamous carcinomas appear not to be related to our current markers of immunity (Jacobson 1998).

Hepatitis C

It has become clear that a large and hitherto hidden epidemic of hepatitis C (HCV) infection is also taking place amongst some groups of people already seriously affected by HIV infection, especially injecting drug users. Patients who are HIV and HCV positive have a reduced prognosis. These patients have more severe liver damage and faster progression of liver disease with increased fibrosis and cirrhosis than HCV alone. Many HIV drug treatments carry a risk of liver inflammation and can exacerbate the problem (Coutinho 1998). HCV could well be an important factor in the excessively unpredictable clinical course that drug users with HIV seem to have.

Long-term antiretroviral treatment

Many patients have been on antiretrovirals for some years now and with the discovery of new treatments and improved prognosis it is likely that patients could be on regimes that span decades. Side effects are numerous and can be severe. As well as hepatitis, pancreatitis, and painful peripheral neuropathies as acute side effects, protease inhibitors tend to cause non-insulin diabetes mellitus along with massively elevated triglycerides and peripheral lipodystrophy. This disfiguring side effect occurs in up to 50% of patients and is characterised by fat loss from the face, limbs, and upper trunk along with central adiposity (Carr et al. 1998). This is often marked and can have a considerable impact on body image. As a result of these metabolic effects, there have already been reports of angiographically proven coronary artery disease (Henry et al. 1998). Survival from HIV may prove to be at the expense of diabetes and coronary heart disease in the medium- to long-term, psychological, social, and spiritual issues.

Specialist palliative care for AIDS/HIV patients involves caring for dying in the young. The average age of an AIDS patient is 37.5 years against 66 years in patients with cancer (Butters et al. 1991). HIV is a sexually transmissible disease: it will therefore always be an uncomfortably symbolic disease of the young with major psycho-emotional, spiritual, and social fallout (George 1998). These are largely matters of uncertainty as much as they are of mortality and will always be part of HIV management.

White middle-class groups, typified by the gay community, tend to be assertive and informed, demanding autonomy and partnership in their care. Difficulty coping with physical deterioration is often a central feature and patients often opt for active treatment till death. There is, we suggest, a reduced sense of 'fatality' and a desire to live on the one hand, but an intolerance of the consequences of illness on the other, hence a patient may suddenly shift from an aggressively curative mentality to a paradoxical request for euthanasia (George and Spittle 1998). The extremely uncomfortable conversations that these may entail need the skilled interdisciplinary work familiar to specialist palliative care.

Patients with HIV are also often plagued by existential questions. The nature of this disease frequently leaves patients who have religious beliefs in doubt, confusion, and fear around dying. Understandably, one study suggests that fear of death was more common in those who felt guilty about their infection or considered it as a punishment (from God or in general) (Kaldjian, Jekel and Friedland 1998). These patients were also less likely to discuss resuscitation status or have a living will.

Patients from Africa present wholly different problems that reflect as much as anything our inability to accommodate unfamiliar world views. In its starkest form one may see perfectly rational patients who are expressing distress using spiritual language (talk of spirits, the devil, etc.) being referred to psychiatric services with a diagnosis of psychosis (King and George 1999). These are issues familiar to specialist palliative care rather than late twentieth-century scientific medicine. They are of course as much general problems of dying young; HIV just expresses them in stark ways.

This brings us to the next section: what HIV has to teach us.

Lessons from managing HIV/AIDS

Handling uncertainty

HIV disease constantly challenges the definition of palliative treatment and the acute/palliative interface with clinical constellations in which 'curable' and palliative elements co-exist. HIV is itself now partially treatable, and this has brought into question whether palliative care has a role at all. In its most extreme expression, this view argues that specialist palliative care was very helpful in the early years of HIV, but is no longer relevant as HIV is now arguably a chronic, stable, or possibly even curable problem. Talk of death and dying is therefore unduly negative; if anything, palliative care should move to focus primarily on psychological support, compliance, and management of the symptomatic side effects of antiviral therapies.

We consider this view to be wishful thinking rather than evident fact. Nevertheless, it does illustrate the need for specialist palliative care to work alongside patients and their clinicians as they manage clinical uncertainty in the face of potentially attainable cure. Similar tensions between cure and palliation are becoming a feature of cancer care and have always been an issue in, for example, haematology, nephrology, and cardiology.

This is an important area for the specialty to address. There is a strong case for palliative care to own its areas of expertise and apply them broadly, not least because society's preoccupation with the war on disease is inclined to marginalise holistic measures linked to death and dying. Seeing and presenting specialists in palliative care as managers of uncertainty rather than just of death may be a more fruitful and more honest future for the specialty.

Apart from gay men, patients with HIV/AIDS tend to come from marginalised groups in society: those working in the sex industry (and those using them), injecting drug users, and refugees from areas where HIV/AIDS is endemic and is transmitted heterosexually. Characteristically, these minorities take up services late and sit uneasily with conventional care. HIV has taught us that we cannot assume that all patients have the same health beliefs or commitment to treatment or cure.

Consequently, we cannot approach them all in the same way, and we cannot assume what makes a good death or what comprises a family or close social group. However, we can be fairly sure that multidisciplinary palliative care is better equipped for this task than curative medicine.

Through these experiences, AIDS has also made us face up to the practicalities of confidentiality, consent, autonomy, and justice, and the ways in which they have influenced resource allocation and how palliative and curative care work together. There is no doubt for example that the vocal way in which users demanded services led to their needs being met. There is a lesson here for patient groups from other diseases to lobby for charitable and statutory resources going into service development or research rather than just into science.

In summary, we maintain that specialist palliative care has a continued role in the management of patients with HIV/AIDS, but that the challenges of caring for these patients will continue to make their mark on the development and maturation of specialist palliative care. The same issues of handling uncertainty, of meeting the needs of those dying prematurely, and of ensuring social and cultural equity arise for other groups needing palliation.

The future

The impact of uncertainty on resources

HIV/AIDS presents major difficulties in policy making, resource allocation and care provision. Uncertainty and change have and continue to apply to the clinical manifestations of HIV infections. The influences of lifestyle, ethnicity, and social stigmatisation, the anathema of deaths in the young, and expensive therapeutic advances that promise a cure-all contribute to the challenges of providing appropriate and effective care. This is as true in palliative as in acute care.

In many ways, we see HIV as paradigmatic of late twentieth-century medicine. The consumerist baby boomer generation brought up to believe science would eradicate disease is now beginning to develop fatal disease. Its god is failing, but still promising success provided money is devoted to research and new treatments—the 1999–2000 allocation for treatment and cure in the UK is just over £233 million (Bellis *et al.* 1999). There are huge funding issues as the drug armamentarium increases, and therapeutics competes with care for the same monies.

Improved survival and reduced numbers of in-patients have led in England and Wales to cuts in central funding for HIV services by 7.7% between 1996–7. However, this has been achieved through the new combination therapies which have their own cost consequences: the cost of combination therapy *alone* is of the order of £12 300 per patient-year and the lifetime cost of a child infected with HIV was estimated recently to be £178 300 (Montaner *et al.* 1998).

Despite the vast HIV budget, at the time of writing, Health Authorities are expected to fund increased drug costs within existing resources and the fall in mortality from combination therapies means that there is pressure to make this a high priority. However, there is now a rise in infected patients seen in centres (9% between 1995 and 1997) (Wilkins *et al.*, in preparation) and money for them has to come from somewhere. It seems clear that financial support for these new treatments will take priority over palliative care.

The impact of uncertainty on palliative care services

As resources are limited, HIV/AIDS services that fail to show that they meet an overt need will find themselves very vulnerable. For example, in 1998 a major residential and hospice unit closed due to the rapid decrease in numbers of people needing that type of care (*see* chapter 18). Palliative care services must be flexible and adaptive to survive. A good example of this is the Mildmay, the original HIV hospice, which, in response to the rising numbers of women and children with HIV, has opened a unit catering for the needs of parents and children with AIDS and a family care centre.

In our own unit in central London, we provide specialist palliative care to one of the major HIV centres in the UK, and serve a local community with many refugees, drug users and sex workers. In the mid-1980s we developed a dedicated HIV palliative care service. Over time it became clear that this was less necessary and now HIV needs are met amply by an HIV clinical nurse specialist attached to the specialist palliative care team who advises and supports generic and specialist staff whose patients have intermediate disease. For symptomatic or advanced disease, we provide a consultative presence in the in- and out-patient services, and community work is integrated into our generic palliative care load. Five years ago HIV/AIDS made up 40% of the case load, which has since reduced to 10%: this is not over burdensome, although the patients present more complex and pressing psycholog-ical and social needs (Wilkins *et al.* in preparation). We anticipate that viral resistance and iatrogenic problems will filter through over time, but our configuration will be able to cope.

The last decade has shown that specialist palliative care has an important role in symp-tom control, psychosocial support, spiritual issues, and care of those dying with HIV/AIDS. That will continue with patients who present late. We think that we may also be involved with more 'complex' cases earlier on: patients with difficult symptom control problems, immigrants with different spiritual and cultural beliefs, and patients with complicated psy-chosocial backgrounds. This can be done by providing a consultative service to other health professionals, rather than by providing full multidisciplinary team involvement. In certain areas, specialist HIV/AIDS palliative care services may be justified (for instance, the work of Mildmay with women and children). Elsewhere specialist palliative care services should be able to assimilate any increasing numbers unless there is a genuinely unexpected change in the epidemic.

Some patients with HIV/AIDS will, we believe, continue to require in-patient hospice care. Most patients prefer to be treated in their own homes (Singh *et al.* 1991) but poor housing and support facilities, rapidly changing illness, and emotional and physical exhaus-tion can make this difficult (Goldstone *et al.* 1995). Thus, there is still a place for hospice units to offer 24-hour nursing care, symptom control and respite for carers and patients. Future demand for these services is difficult to predict. It is very easy to close services as needs fall, but it would be quite another case to resuscitate them should the need re-emerge (Downey 1997).

Palliative care services will need to continue to adapt to changing circumstances. It seems highly probable, for example, that we will see a rise in long-term manifestations of the disease, in complications of medical treatments, and consequently in the numbers of chronically ill or disabled patients who require extensive care and resources. The impact of this on the patients, their carers, and society will not go unnoticed indefinitely as inequities in resourcing are already being highlighted (National Aids Trust 1999). In the short term, care can be subsumed into generic palliative care services, in the longer term this may not be the case.

Conclusions

HIV/AIDS in the UK has surprised us all. It is not the epidemic we expected and is not elu-sive to treatment. The field is changing rapidly and the rate and direction of this change is uncertain and unpredictable. This has brought with it a degree of confusion for both the health professionals and those affected by the disease. Working in this field is therefore chal-lenging and exciting but also filled with insecurity. HIV/AIDS can now be considered a chronically fatal disease with acute treatable complications. This has an impact on the patient, the family and friends, the clinicians, and society.

The role of specialist palliative care in the care of patients with HIV has gradually changed. Currently we need to:

1 support colleagues in difficult therapeutic decisions around the benefits and burdens of treatment and withdrawal;

2 to ensure that drug treatment and viral control are not bought at an unacceptable loss of quality of life; and

3 to continue assisting with the complex problems of different cultures, patients presenting late in their disease and their palliative and terminal care.

This is best done through collaborative models of care, which must reflect local conditions.

Specialist palliative care must maintain a meaningful presence in HIV/AIDS of interdisciplinary skill to help with conflict resolution, breaking bad news, and the tensions that arise in managing uncertainty. We have no doubt that in the fullness of time conventional specialist palliative care focusing on end-of-life issues will be called upon once again to help. Let's try to make it easier by marketing our skills as those of managing uncertainty, suffering, and conflict, not just managing death. Let's also ensure that the lessons we have learned translate into practice and are used to the advantage of other patients not enjoying the benefits of decent palliation.

References

Aalen, O., Farewell, V., De Angelis, D., Day, N., and Gill, O. (1999). New therapy explains the fall in AIDS incidence with a substantial rise in number of persons on treatment expected. *AIDS* **13**: 103–8.

Adler, M. (ed.) (2000). *ABC of AIDS*. London: BMJ Publications.

Alcorn, K. (ed.) (1998/9). *National AIDS Manual*. (21st edn.). London: NAM Publications, p. 68.

Bellis, M., McVeigh, J., Thomson, R., and Syed Q. (1999). AIDS funding, the national lottery. *Health Services Journal*, June: 22–3.

Breitbart, W. (1996). Pain management and psychosocial issues in HIV and AIDS. *The American Journal of Hospice and Palliative Care*, January/February 1996: 21–9.

Butters, E., Higginson, I., Wade, A., *et al.* (1991). AIDS models of care: community HIV/AIDS teams. *Health Trends* **23**(2): 59–62.

Butters, E., Higginson, I., George, R., Smits, A., and McCarthy, M. (1992). Assessing the symptoms, anxiety and practical needs of HIV/AIDS patients receiving palliative care. *Quality of Life Research* **1**: 47–51.

Carr, A., Samaras, K., Burton, S., *et al.* (1998). A syndrome of peripheral lipodystrophy, hyperlipidaemia and insulin resistance in patients receiving HIV protease inhibitors. *AIDS* **351**:1881–3.

Coutinho, A. (1998). HIV and hepatitis C among injecting drug users. *British Medical Journal* **317**: 424–5.

Del Amo, J., Petruckevitch, A., Phillips, A., Johnson, A., *et al.* (1996). Spectrum of disease in Africans with AIDS in London. *AIDS* **10**: 1563–9.

Downey, M. (1997). Developing palliative care services for patients with AIDS. *European Journal of Palliative Care* **4**(4): 121–3.

George, R.J.D. (1995). Palliative and terminal care. In Mindel, A. and Miller, R. (eds), *AIDS: A Pocket Book of Diagnosis and Management*. London: Edward Arnold.

George, R.J.D. (1998). An anatomy of suffering. In *Horizons in Medicine*. London: Royal College of Physicians.

George, R.J.D. and Hart, G. (1989). The Bloomsbury response to AIDS. In Pye, M. *et al.* (eds), *Responding to the AIDS Challenge*. London: Longman, pp. 41–68.

George, R.J.D. and Spittle, M. (1998). AIDS and the young dying. In Karim, A.B.M.F. *et al.* (eds), *Death: Medical, Spiritual and Social Care of the* Dying. Amsterdam: V.U. University Press, pp. 55–73.

Goldstone, I., Kuhl, D., Johnson, A., Le, R., and Macleod, A. (1995). Patterns of care in advanced HIV disease in a tertiary treatment centre. *AIDS Care* 7(1): S47–S57.

Henry, K., Melroe, H., Huebsch, J., *et al.* (1998). Severe premature coronary artery disease with protease inhibitors. *The Lancet* 251: 1328.

Hewitt, D., McDonald, M., Portenoy, R., Rosenfeld, B., Passik, S., and Breitbart, W. (1997). Pain syndromes and etiologies in ambulatory AIDS patients. *Pain* 70: 117–23.

Hospice Information Service (1994). *Directory of Hospice Services*. London: St Christopher's Hospice.

Jacobson, L.P. (1998). Impact of HAART on incidence of malignancies among HIV infected individuals. Second National AIDS Malignancy Conference, Bethesda.

Kaldjian, L.C., Jekel, J.F. and Friedland, G. (1998). End of life decisions in HIV-positive patients: the role of spiritual beliefs. *AIDS* 12: 103–7.

Kelleher, P., Cox, S., and McKeogh, M. (1997). HIV infection: the spectrum of symptoms and disease in male and female patients attending a London hospice. *Palliative Medicine* 11: 152–8.

King, B. and George, R.J.D. (1999). Providing palliative care for African clients with HIV disease. *Journal of Nursing Management* (in press).

McKeogh, M. (1995). Dementia in HIV disease—a challenge for palliative care? *Journal of Palliative Care* 11: 30–3.

Montaner, J., Hogg, R., Raoud, J., Harrigan, R., and O'Shaughnessy, M. (1998). Antiretroviral treatment in 1998. *The Lancet* 352: 1919–22.

MRC Collaborative Study Group (1996). Ethnic differences in women with HIV infection in Britain and Ireland. *AIDS* 10: 89–93.

National AIDS Trust (1999). *1999–2000 HIV/AIDS Budget Allocation*. Briefing Paper.

Postma, M.J., Beck, E.J., *et al.* (1999). Universal HIV screening of pregnant women in England: cost effectiveness analysis. *British Medical Journal* 318:1656–60.

Public Health Laboratory Service AIDS Centre and Scottish Centre for Infection and Environmental Health (1998). *AIDS/HIV Quarterly Surveillance Tables*. London: PHLS: December.

Royal Free/Chelsea and Westminster Hospitals Collaborative Group (1997). Survival after diagnosis of AIDS: a prospective observational study of 2625 patients. *British Medical Journal* 314: 4094–13

Sadler, M., Chinn. R., Healy, J., *et al.* (1998). New treatments for progressive multifocal leukoencephalopathy in HIV-1 infected patients. *AIDS* 12(5): 533–5.

Sherer, R. (1998). Current antiretroviral therapy and its impact on Human Immunodeficiency virus-related wasting. *Seminars in Oncology* 25: no. 2 (Suppl 6): 92–7.

Singh, S., Hawkins, D., Connolly, M., and Gazzard, B. (1991). Model of care for the hospital treatment of individuals with HIV infection. *Health Trends* 23: 55–9.

Starace, F., Dijkgraaf, M., Houweling, H., Postma, M., and Tramarin, A. (1998). HIV associated dementia: clinical, epidemiological and resource utilisation issues. *AIDS Care* 10(2): S113–S121.

UNAIDS Global data available from www.unaids.org

Walsh, T.D. (1991). An overview of palliative care in cancer and AIDS. *Oncology* 5(9): 7–11.

Wilkins, P., King, B., Robinson, V., and George, R.J.D. (in preparation) Changing patterns of HIV palliative care practice in a specialist centre.

Chapter 12

Palliative care in nursing homes

Ian Maddocks and Deborah Parker

Introduction

In populations in nearly every part of the world, the proportion of older people is increasing, and traditional ways of providing support within their families are beginning to fail. In the developed countries, family support increasingly has been replaced by institutional care, and the number of nursing home beds has burgeoned to an extent where governments seek to constrain them. Even in Asia, where traditional family values demand a powerful duty of care for elderly members, it is proving difficult or impossible to maintain adequate care, particularly in chaotic overcrowded cities. In this chapter we review the current role of nursing homes, with particular reference to Australia: we consider the differences between the clients of and the care provided in nursing homes and palliative care services; we discuss the palliative care needs of nursing home residents; and we consider new and emerging models of care.

New roles for nursing homes

The nursing home is where many of us will spend our last months or years, and increasingly it is the place where we shall die. The role of the nursing home has continued to evolve in more recent decades, as greater awareness and concern about the costs of in-patient health care have constrained the numbers of hospital beds, and have encouraged hospitals to decrease lengths of stay, reserving their expensive care for acute cases, and zealously transferring to other sites of care those for whom the intensive investigation and active specialist treatment which major hospitals practice is deemed to be inappropriate.

The increasing number of nursing home beds has caused many governments concern as health costs steadily increase, and measures to slow that increase have been sought. The result has been that progressively over the last two decades it has become more difficult to gain admission to a nursing home. Potential nursing home patients now need to be sicker or more frail than formerly. Along with hospices, therefore, nursing homes have been led to assume a greater responsibility for dying persons, with the additional demands for supportive and medical care which that entails (Hunt and Maddocks 1994). Introduction of case mix funding or other techniques for counting cost and restricting expenditure—well established in the US and now part of medical life in Australia—has further encouraged both public and private hospitals to transfer out those patients with chronic, progressive, or terminal illnesses and to recommend their placement in hospices and nursing homes.

Of all the deaths in South Australia, the proportion occurring in nursing homes increased from 1% in 1960 to 20% in 1990 (Hunt and Maddocks 1997). In the UK, the proportion increased from 5% in 1969 to 14% in 1987 (Cartwright 1991). Over the same time, the pattern of illness in those admitted to nursing homes began to change, with degenerative and chronic diseases being supplanted by more active pathologies, such as cancer. The proportion of cancer patients among referrals in South Australia from nursing homes to hospice agencies was 20% in 1990 and 45% in 1993 (Hunt and Maddocks 1997).

Concurrently, also, a greater awareness of the value of a palliative care approach to illnesses other than cancer has occurred, with more hospice programmes ready to admit persons with non-malignant conditions. In 1992–3, 58 cases of chronic lung disease, renal failure, and chronic heart failure formed 7.7% of referrals to the Southern Community Hospice Programme in Adelaide and in 1995–6 there were 113 such cases, constituting 12.6% of all referrals (Maddocks 1998). A closer sharing between hospice and nursing home of responsibility for the care of the dying elderly is encouraged by these changes.

Important differences between nursing homes and hospices

Although hospices and nursing homes both offer care for the dying, there remain major differences in the services and resources available in the two settings and in the populations they serve. In hospices the predominant diagnosis is cancer, occurring in any age group. Hospice care is seen to demand the skills and knowledge of registered nurses, who consti-tute a high proportion of the staff; the 'unit of care' involves relatives and friends, and care extends into the bereavement period.

The nursing home focuses on custodial care for the elderly (there is often an age criterion for admission) together with encouragement and assistance with activities of daily living. The commonest nursing home diagnoses are dementia, cardiovascular, and haematological and musculoskeletal conditions. Care is given by a mix of registered nurses and nursing care assistants, the 'unit of care' is the resident and little provision is made for support of rela-tives or for bereavement care (Maddocks et al. 1996; Munley et al. 1982, Murphy et al. 1997).

Abbey (1998) described nursing homes as being influenced by a philosophy she termed 'normalisation', one which encourages continued activity and rejects unnecessary limitation of function. This has led to dilemmas for nursing home staff in their everyday practice of care. For example, should the frail old resident with dementia who is close to death continue to be 'normalised' by being showered daily and sat up in a chair? Abbey claimed that a major change in culture and policy was required before adequate palliative care for residents in nursing homes would be possible.

The contribution by nursing homes to palliative care delivery

The amount of care properly called 'palliative', and calling for special expertise in nursing homes, is difficult to quantify. In a survey in 1990, directors of nursing homes in South Australia estimated that 3% of their residents were requiring what they understood as palliative care (Hunt and Bond 1990). More recent South Australian surveys have suggested a higher level of need. Directors of nursing participating in an Australia-wide survey by Maddocks et al. (1996) estimated that 6% of residents had palliative care needs, and Clare and DeBellis (1997) concluded that this may be as high as 9.5%.

Client comparisons

There is relatively little published data comparing clients of a palliative care service with those resident in nursing homes. Studies of palliative care clients have focused primarily on clinical and socio-demographic characteristics which influence admission to different types of palliative care services (Addington-Hall *et al.*1998; Bradshaw 1993; Dunlop *et al.* 1989; Dunphy and Amesbury 1990; Komesaroff *et al.* 1989).

Amar (1994) compared a random sample of 50 hospice patients and 50 nursing home patients in the US. The hospice patients were younger, alert and orientated, and had a diagnosis of cancer. Only 4% of the nursing home patients were alert and orientated on admission; most had diagnoses of cardiac disease, lung disease or dementia. The author argued that hospice programmes in the US derive two benefits from involvement with nursing homes. First, they generate a large number of referrals to the hospice programme of patients who make a minimal demand on its services. Second, nursing homes receive continuing support from the hospice service for patients who are transferred into their care. The link with a hospice assists nursing home marketing, and helps to increase expertise among the nursing home staff. Costs such as medication related to a terminal diagnosis, medical and wound supplies, and allied therapies are taken up by the hospice contract (Watt 1997). In Australia, where there is no financial incentive for nursing homes to provide palliative care, the move to an increased liaison with palliative care teams is driven more by issues of equity and quality of life than by financial considerations. This is also true of the UK.

Maddocks *et al.* (1996) studied the utilisation of health services by 104 clients aged 70 years and over who had been referred to a comprehensive palliative care service in southern Adelaide, Australia, comparing it with that of 87 persons admitted to nursing homes in the same geographical region. Nursing home residents tended to be widowed and were older; only 1% had a diagnosis of cancer but 22% had a diagnosis of dementia. Only 3% of these new admissions were known to a palliative care service. The health services they had been receiving focused on maintenance care such as physiotherapy, podiatry, and occupational therapy. In comparison, the clients of the palliative care service were younger, more likely to be male, and used a wide variety of community health services. None had a diagnosis of dementia and 79% had a diagnosis of cancer. Of the 10 most common documented symptoms, both groups experienced pain and confusion (Table 12.1). Pain was the most common symptom for palliative care clients and the fourth most common symptom for nursing home residents. The ranking of confusion was reversed, being first for nursing home residents and fourth for palliative care clients. Palliative care symptoms were weakness, dyspnoea, anorexia, weight loss, nausea, cough, vomiting, and drowsiness. Nursing home residents suffered from urinary incontinence, loss of skin integrity, behavioural problems, anxiety, immobility, restlessness, impaired motor co-ordination, and constipation.

Particularly important for palliative care services in this listing of differences were the relative absence of a cancer diagnosis and frequency of dementia among nursing home residents. However, this work would need to be replicated more widely, before further conclusions can be drawn. We concluded that palliative care providers should be cautious in assuming that knowledge and skills accrued in providing care for those dying from cancer can be directly transposed to the care of elderly people dying in nursing homes.

Table 12.1 The 10 common symptoms of Southern Community Hospice (SCHP) clients and nursing home residents, as documented in clinical records

SCHP clients n = 104	Symptom (%)	Nursing home residents n = 87	Symptom (%)
Pain	70	Confusion	81
Weakness	64	Urinary incontinence	79
Dyspnoea	43	Loss of skin integrity	71
Confusion	34	Pain	69
Anorexia	28	Behavioural problems	67
Weight loss	21	Anxiety	48
Nausea	18	Immobility	46
Cough	17	Restlessness	41
Vomiting	16	Impaired motor co-ordination	40
Drowsiness	16	Constipation	35

Source: Maddocks et al. (1996).

Nursing home residents requiring palliative care

The predominant diagnoses of 45 residents identified by staff in these nursing homes as requiring palliative care were neurological (56%), haematological/cardiovascular (42%) and musculoskeletal conditions (40%) (Maddocks et al. 1996). Approximately half (53%) had a diagnosis of dementia and 27% were known to have cancer. These residents were highly dependent—most were bed-bound and requiring total assistance, were incontinent of urine and faeces, and were drowsy and disorientated. Behavioural problems such as unco-operativeness or resistive behaviour and aggression were present, although the difficulty caused by such symptoms lessened as death approached.

Many of the symptoms described for these residents were similar to those expected of hospice patients. Weakness, fatigue, anorexia, anxiety, constipation, dysphagia, and pain were commonly reported. Opioids had been administered to 80% of those residents identified as experiencing pain. Opioids were ordered regularly and with breakthrough doses for 47%, regularly but without breakthrough orders for 19%, and on an 'as required' basis in 34%. Residents with a diagnosis of dementia were less likely to have been prescribed opioids and were less likely to be ordered breakthrough opioids. The difficulty inherent in pain assessment or evaluation of response to treatment in demented individuals may have contributed to these differences (Maddocks et al. 1996).

The nursing home residents included in this study lived in institutions in the same geographical region as the palliative care service. However only limited consultative palliative care services had been extended to nursing homes up to the time of this study. Of the 45 residents identified, only 9 (20%) were already known to the palliative care service; 6 of these had a diagnosis of cancer, and 1 a diagnosis of dementia. Of the residents who had been palliative care clients, only 1 was visited by the palliative care service after nursing home admission.

The hospice patient differed from the dying nursing home resident in being generally more independent until close to the time of death, and evidencing fewer behavioural problems as well as less cognitive decline and incontinence. Opioid prescribing practices differed in the two locations. Less than half of the nursing home residents were ordered regular opioids with breakthrough doses, as is advocated for good clinical practice. In the nursing home intramuscular administration of morphine was common, a route which hospice practice generally avoids as causing more pain than a subcutaneous injection. Other studies have indicated that opioids are less likely to be prescribed in the nursing home (Lloyd-Williams 1996) or that large doses of opioids are regarded as not indicated for residents with dementia (Wilson *et al.* 1996). However, in the US, analysis of nursing home reports has recently indicated that only a minority of those patients recorded as experiencing pain were receiving appropriate analgesics (Bernabei *et al.* 1998). Palliative care services may be considered by nursing home staff as appropriate primarily for residents who have cancer, but not for individuals with dementia.

Provision of palliative care in the nursing home setting

Understanding of palliative care

When asked to define palliative care registered and enrolled nurses in Australian nursing homes associated it with end of life, death and dying, comfort care, terminal care, or easing people out of life. Nursing home staff in the UK appear to have a less clear understanding of the term (Katz *et al.* 1999). A difficulty for nursing home care, given the association of palliative care with the end of life, is the question of prognosis. Some nursing home staff suggested that all their residents would be classified as requiring palliative care; others limited the designation to those likely to die within a fixed (and short) period of time (Maddocks *et al.* 1996). This matter is focused by the issue of costs of care. In the US, an arbitrary estimate of prognosis of less than six months is used to qualify a patient for reimbursement for hospice service involvement within a nursing home. A cancer diagnosis facilitates prediction (though it is still usually wildly inaccurate), but other diseases can have a very uncertain and protracted terminal period (Watt 1996). In Australia this dilemma has not needed to be addressed, since no extra funding provision has been made available to nursing homes for delivery of palliative care.

Medical management in the nursing home

In Australia, and in the UK, the medical management of nursing home residents is the responsibility of the general practitioner or family doctor. The resident may have been known to the general practitioner for many years or, if newly arrived in that area of residence, be a new patient to that medical practice. The general practitioner remains the primary carer even after referral to a palliative care team. General practitioners therefore need to be skilled in palliative care and to have a good working relationship with both the nursing home staff and the palliative care team. In the Adelaide study the main issue highlighted by registered nurses in regard to general practitioners was conflict regarding pain management (Maddock *et al.* 1996). Inadequate pain relief, administration of opioids by an inappropriate route, or medical disregard for the assessment by nurses of pain (particularly for those residents with dementia) were criticisms frequently raised. The most satisfactory relationship reported was in a nursing home where one general practitioner conducted a regular daily clinic on site, and was therefore readily contacted by the nursing staff, who had a high measure of confidence in him. Similar findings have been reported in a recent UK study of nursing homes (Katz *et al.* 1999).

Time to provide care for patients and for relatives

Nursing homes are funded at a level which must be regarded as basic and frugal. In Australia the accepted hospice standard for hours of registered nursing is 45.5 hours per patient per week. In nursing homes this may vary from 9 to 27 hours per week, calculated on the basis of the dependency of the resident and employing a tool known as the Resident Classification Instrument (Hunt and Bond 1990). In 1997 a new system of nursing home funding in Australia was introduced—the Resident Classification Scale. The underlying principle of funding has not changed, but new categories have been introduced which identify residents requiring palliative care and make allowance for the time required in counselling relatives. Whether the new system of funding offers opportunity for better care requires study.

Further constraints on the time available for care in the nursing home stem from the shorter lengths of stay and a greater proportion of acute illness among residents now being met with. Nursing homes are increasingly being expected to admit patients who previously spent a period of convalescence in a private or public hospital. To be admitted to a nursing home requires a high level of dependency. This trend is also reported in the UK where greater numbers of dying persons are admitted to nursing homes who previously were cared for by other agencies of the National Health Service (Avis *et al.* 1997).

What is necessary for the satisfactory delivery of palliative care?

In the study by Maddocks *et al.* (1996), focus groups of nursing home staff raised many key issues relevant to the provision of good palliative care. Many hospices are purpose-built, or have undergone major modification to encourage patient and family privacy. In nursing homes, space is limited and no more than a single room may have been allocated for palliative care. This risks being stigmatised as 'the death room' and can cope with only one dying resident at any one time. Families sometimes wish to be involved in care and to stay with their relative; this is encouraged in hospices but may be difficult in the nursing home. Care of the dying in multiple bed rooms has raised issues regarding the counselling and debriefing of other residents' some of whom may have been sharing that room for many years. Residents with dementia present additional challenges for staff in communicating the death of one resident to the others.

Counselling and attachment issues for staff

Staff often have been involved in the care of a particular resident for years. Useful strategies to deal with grief include attendance at funerals and maintaining contact with families following a death. Nursing staff also form special attachments to residents, including those with advanced dementia, sustaining rapport with touch and intimacy over a period of many years. Formal counselling for nursing home staff following the death of a resident is unusual; it is handover time, tea breaks or after hours social gatherings which are more likely to provide opportunity for mutual debriefing and support. Personal care workers, who are less trained and often younger, seem to receive less help from these informal networks than the more mature trained staff. Access to formal counselling should be considered by the management of nursing homes.

Advance directives and 'good palliative care' orders

In South Australia the *Consent to Medical Treatment and Palliative Care Act*, proclaimed in 1996, enables individuals to write instructions concerning their care at the end of life or to appoint an agent to decide appropriate care in the event of their incapacity with a terminal illness. The writing of *Good Palliative Care* orders was a recommendation of the Parliamentary Select Committee which prepared the *Consent to Medical Treatment and Palliative Care Act*. This suggests that instead of writing a negative instruction—'Do Not Resuscitate' (or some coded form of that), medical staff should be encouraged to prefer a positive openly-shared plan with a focus on the relief of discomfort and on good palliative care. The recommendation has been widely implemented in South Australian hospitals. Few nursing home residents have taken up the provision to write instructions about their care at the end of life, or to appoint agents. One of the difficulties is that the individual must be mentally competent to complete either schedule. This effactually precludes residents who have dementia or other cognitive difficulties. The general practitioner and the nursing home need to promote these provisions earlier, prior to or immediately on admission to a nursing home. Informal advance directives (having no legal force) continue to be common. The nursing home staff or general practitioner write 'no active treatment', 'comfort care only' or 'for palliative care'.

Education

Postgraduate awards in palliative care are available for Registered Nurses in Australia and some other countries. Education for personal care workers (who have minimal basic training) is more problematic. Nursing home staff in Australia commented on the time and cost of attending educational programmes and the lack of relevance of many to the nursing home setting. Palliative care education, like palliative care practice, has often focused on cancer care. Education needs identified by staff in Australian nursing homes were: pain and symptom management, counselling skills, the physiology of death, and knowing when to withhold routine care. Nursing home staff also raised the need for further education of some general practitioners (Maddocks *et al.* 1996). That need is being partly met in Australia through the introduction of Divisions of General Practice, funded to support in-service education of general practitioners. The Divisions have undertaken many education projects in palliative care, involving both theoretical content and practical experience through hospice attachment. In the UK and other countries, further training for general practitioners may be partly met by developments in continuing education, short courses, and diploma and masters programmes.

Bereavement care

Formal bereavement care for family members of residents who die in a nursing home is uncommon (Murphy *et al.* 1997). Nursing homes are funded for the care that the resident requires, with no specific allowance for the needs of the family. Following a death, a nursing home will receive no funding for bereavement support for a relative. However where an elderly spouse survives a resident of many years standing, staff may accept responsibility for bereavement care in their own time and without having had any training. In a care setting where death is a universal outcome and the population is elderly, the necessity for bereavement care similar to that offered by a palliative care service seems obvious. It might be argued that acceptance of death is more likely among family members who have visited their aged relative in a nursing home over many years. But nursing homes are becoming providers of care for residents who remain for relatively short periods before death and who may otherwise have received palliative care in a hospice where bereavement care is usually offered.

New models of care

The roles for hospices in many countries continue to evolve. They are now less geared to long-stay clients than before, and increasingly are used for short-term crisis interventions or terminal care for the last few days (or, at most, weeks) of life. This is not necessarily how the public or other professionals view hospice care (Maccabee 1994). Within the community, hospices have a much more positive image than nursing homes. Neither patients nor their carers readily accept the suggestion of transfer from a hospice to a nursing home. But if nursing homes recognise the importance of their role in terminal illness, and strive to improve the care of dying residents, that transition may be viewed more positively. Maccabee (1994), followed the transfer of 10 families from a hospice to nursing home. For 3 families this experience was rated positively, for 6 the experience was described as traumatic, and for 1 good care and a peaceful death counterbalanced an initial negative experience. The care given in the nursing home was regarded as less specialised than the hospice. The provision of nursing home annexes to palliative care units was suggested as offering continuity of care and raising the standards of nursing homes through sharing skills with the specialised units.

A nursing home annexe of this kind was established by the Southern Community Hospice Programme, Adelaide, in 1997. A nursing home situated very close to Daw House hospice, the in-patient unit of the programme, agreed to give priority for admission to clients of the palliative care programme who qualified for nursing home placement. All staff in this nursing home received training in palliative care, and a general practitioner experienced in palliative care agreed to accept responsibility for residents who did not have a general practitioner in the area. Following transfer, regular contact is maintained with the staff, the resident and the family by the palliative care team.

Such an arrangement between hospice and nursing home can lessen the stress felt by individuals and their families when relocation from a specialised level of care in the hospice or hospital to the general nursing care of the nursing home is suggested. A further advantage is that other residents of the nursing home may benefit from the training and support that the staff receive. Many nursing homes are far removed from any hospice, however, and cannot avail themselves of such advantages.

In the UK, nursing home palliative care liaison positions have been appointed to provide consultative support and education for nursing homes within a specified region. To assist the consultant nurse in providing palliative care, 'link nurses' have been established in these nursing homes. 'Link nurses' undergo an initial intensive training in palliative care and are released to attend support meetings on a regular (often monthly) basis. Their responsibility is to co-ordinate palliative care within each facility and to ensure palliative care standards are maintained, under the supervision of and with the regular encouragement of the consultant nurse.

In Adelaide, South Australia, two palliative care nurse practitioners employed for 12 months provided a consultancy and education service to 33 of the 49 aged care facilities (nursing homes and hostels) in the southern region of the city. As part of this project 84 'link nurses', who were members of staff from these participating facilities, underwent a 3-day training course to address organisation and palliative care issues in aged care. A regular monthly meeting also provided on-going education and support to the 'link nurses'. Evaluation of the project indicated that 'link nurses' increased their knowledge, skills and confidence in providing palliative care. Care became more resident-focused, based on assessment rather than traditional nursing routines, institutional policies or funding considerations. Interest in palliative care and morale in the participating facilities was judged to have increased during the project period. Although no continued funding was available to support the palliative care nurse practitioner positions, 'link nurses' continue to attend a monthly special interest group co-ordinated by palliative care community nurses. The existing community hospice programme also provides on-going clinical support (Maddocks *et al.* 1999).

Avis *et al.* (1997) conducted a project to extend hospice standards of palliative care to nursing homes that were registered for palliative care with the Nottingham Health Authority in the UK. A nurse adviser with the assistance of a peer support group of district nurses provided training, support and advice for staff concerning palliative care issues, facilitated access to specialist advice, and provided support and advice for patients and relatives, including bereavement care and psychological support. Evaluation of the project indicated a significant impact, with a decrease in the sense of isolation experienced by nursing home staff through building collegial relationships with the district nurses and the palliative care service. Patients were also positive about the effect of the project, noting the opportunity to talk to someone outside the nursing homes and for families to have access to bereavement care.

The provision of palliative care in nursing homes in the US is very different. Castle *et al.* (1997) discussed the emergence of special care hospice units in nursing homes; the number of these increased by 100% from 1992 to 1995. The authors attributed this increase to the availability of Medicare reimbursement for hospice care and also saw it as a response to the competitiveness of the market. The need to attract private paying residents means that nursing homes have to offer services outside those normally expected of them. Profit and economic survival may not be the most desirable motivation for providing quality palliative care, but most nursing homes are unable to provide the 'extra care' inherent in offering a quality service without access to some form of government subsidy or additional private input.

Conclusion

Palliative care services will increasingly face the challenge of determining their responsibility in the provision of care for persons dying from illnesses other than cancer, particularly for the degenerative conditions which accompany old age. This cohort will become larger, and more of a problem within busy urban societies. If activities are restricted to those special areas of cancer, HIV, or motor neurone disease, palliative care risks criticism as elitist, discriminatory, or irrelevant. Cold pragmatic costings of the care necessary to meet adequately the needs of the frail and uncomfortable elderly, particularly when they are undergoing a slow terminal decline, may encourage those voices urging legislation of medical assistance of suicide when quality of life is seen to be irremediably poor. Palliative care has offered a humanising and loving example to society. But it should not be permitted to remain sequestered from this challenge of wider care.

Three challenges exist:

1 To research the models of care that work best for terminally ill patients in nursing homes and their families. The model of link nurses requires further exploration, although it may need to involve wider groups in medicine, nursing, and social care. There is natural concern that extending palliative care to all who are dying may require a large increase in resources.

2 To learn more about the needs of frail and elderly dying people, so that better education can be provided for staff working in nursing homes.

3 For palliative care and nursing home staff to liaise and co-operate to provide the optimal care, education, and research.

References

Abbey, J. (1998). Breaking the silence: Palliation for people with dementia. In Parker, J. and Aranda, S. (eds), *Palliative Care—Explorations and Challenges*. Australia: MacLennon and Petty, pp. 172–83.

Addington-Hall, J.M., Altmann, D., and McMarthy, M. (1998). Which terminally ill cancer patients receive hospice in-patient care? *Social Science and Medicine* **46**: 1011–16.

Amar, D.F. (1994). The role of the hospice social worker in the nursing home setting. *American Journal of Hospice and Palliative Care* **11**(3):18–23.

Avis, M., Greening-Jackson, J., Cox, K., and Miskella, C. (1997). Evaluating the community palliative care project. Report for the Nottingham Community NHS Trust, Nottingham.

Bernabei, R., Gambassi, G., Lapane, K., Landi, F., Gatsonis, C., Dunlop, R., Lipsitz, L., Steel, K., and Mor, V. (1998). Management of pain in elderly patients with cancer. *Journal of the American Medical Association* **279**: 1877–82.

Bradshaw, P.J. (1993). Characteristics of clients referred to home, hospice and hospital palliative care services in Western Australia. *Palliative Medicine* **7**:101–7.

Cartwright, A. (1991). Changes in life and care in the year before death 1969–1987. *Journal of Public Health Medicine* **13**: 81–7.

Castle, N.G., Mor, V., and Banaszak-Holl, J. (1997). Special care hospice units in nursing homes. *The Hospice Journal* **12**(3): 59–69.

Clare, J. and DeBellis, A. (1997). Palliative care in South Australian nursing homes. *Australian Journal of Advanced Nursing* **14**(4): 20–8.

Dunlop, R.J., Davies, R.J., and Hockley, J.M. (1989). Preferred versus actual place of death: a hospital palliative care support team experience. *Palliative Medicine* **3**: 197–201.

Dunphy, K.P. and Amesbury, B.D.W. (1990). A comparison of hospice and home care patients: patterns of referral, patient characteristics and predictors of place of death. *Palliative Medicine* **4**: 105–11.

Hunt, R. and Bond, M. (1990). Terminal care in nursing homes: a survey of South Australian directors of nursing. *Geriaction* **9**(1): 7–8.

Hunt, R. and Maddocks, I. (1994). Review of nursing home term care. *Geriaction* **13**(1): 23–5.

Hunt, R. and Maddocks, I. (1997). Terminal care in South Australia: historical aspects and equity issues. In Clark, D., Hockley, J., and Ahmedzai, S. (eds), *Facing Death—New Themes in Palliative Care*. Buckingham: Open University Press, pp. 101–5.

Katz, J., Komaromy, C., and Sidell, M. (1999). Understanding palliative care in residential and nursing homes. *International Journal of Palliative Nursing* **5**(2): 58–64.

Komesaroff, P.A., Moss, C.K., and Fox, R.M. (1989). Patients' socioeconomic background: influence on selection of in-patient or domiciliary hospice terminal care programmes. *The Medical Journal of Australia* **151**: 196–200.

Lloyd-Williams, M. (1996). An audit of palliative care in dementia. *European Journal of Cancer Care* **5**(1): 53–5.

Maccabee, J. (1994). The effect of transfer from a palliative care unit to nursing homes—are patients' and relatives' needs met? *Palliative Medicine* **8**: 211–14.

Maddocks, I. (1998). Chronic heart failure: a malignant condition. *Medical Journal of Australia* **168**: 200.

Maddocks, I., Abbey, J., Pickhaver, A., Parker, D., DeBellis, A., and Beck, K. (1996) *Palliative Care in Nursing Homes*. Report to the Commonwealth Department of Health and Family Services. Adelaide: Flinders University of South Australia.

Maddocks, I., Parker, D., McLeod, A., and Jenkin, P. (1999). *Palliative Care Nurse Practitioners in Aged Care Facilities—Report to the Department of Human Services*. Adelaide: Flinders University of South Australia.

Munley, A., Powers, C.S., and Williamson, J.B. (1982). Humanising nursing home environments: the relevance of hospice principles. *International Journal of Ageing and Human Development* **15**(4): 263–84.

Murphy, K., Hanrahan, P., and Luchins, D. (1997). A survey of grief and bereavement in nursing homes: The importance of hospice grief and bereavement for the end-stage Alzheimer's disease patient and family. *Journal of the American Geriatrics Society* **45**: 1104–7.

Watt, K. (1996). Hospice and the elderly: a changing perspective. *The American Journal of Hospice and Palliative Care*, November/December: 47–8.

Watt, K. (1997). Hospices within nursing homes: should a long term care facility wear both hats? *The American Journal of Hospice and Palliative Care*, March/April: 63–5.

Wilson, S., Kovach, C., and Stearns, S. (1996). Hospice concepts in the care for end-stage dementia. *Geriatric Nursing* **17**(1): 6–10.

Chapter 13

Palliative care in the hospital setting for patients with non-malignant disease

Peter Pitcher and Carol Davis

Introduction

This chapter aims to address the needs of patients dying from progressive non-malignant diseases and those of patients living with non-malignant diseases in the acute hospital setting, and to discuss the challenges that these patients present. Throughout we have tried to suggest appropriate responses to these challenges and in conclusion, to define the agenda for future research and development. Three perspectives run as vertical threads through the chapter, that of the patient and the family, that of non-specialist staff, and that of specialist palliative care staff. Our work is limited by the lack of formal trials of palliative care for patients with non-malignant disease in the acute hospital setting. We have therefore also reflected on our experiences as members of an interdisciplinary hospital palliative care team (HPCT). Where necessary, we have made considered extrapolations from the literature on palliative care for cancer patients in the acute hospital and other settings.

Historical context

Balfour Mount (Mount 1976) claimed that, 'the general hospital as a setting for terminal care has disturbing deficiencies: particularly the medical, emotional and spiritual needs of their patients are generally neglected'. He used this argument, backed up by research into patients' attitudes to dying (Mount et al. 1974), to support the integration of palliative care units in general hospitals. The pattern of service delivery that he and others developed at the Royal Victoria Hospital, Montreal, comprised an in-patient specialist palliative care unit, a domiciliary service, and a hospital-wide consultative service as well as research, teaching, and administrative functions. Thus specialist palliative care services were based in an acute hospital rather than in, 'separate institutions with special expertise in treating terminally ill patients' (Mount 1976).

In England the first hospital palliative care team, the St Thomas' terminal care support team, was established in 1976 (Bates et al. 1981). In parts of the country prior to that, and indeed subsequently in some hospitals, specialist palliative care advice for in-patients in the acute hospital setting was provided on a 'grace and favour' basis.

Deficiencies in the care of the dying in acute hospitals

Despite the development of such services, deficiencies in the care of those dying in the acute hospital setting have continued to be documented. Prospective research has demonstrated unmet symptom control and psychological and spiritual needs in those dying in hospital (Hinton 1963; Hockley et al.1988; Brescia et al. 1990; Simpson 1991). Several retrospective studies have collected data from the relatives of patients who died in the hospital and have reported similar findings (Hinton 1979; Parkes and Parkes 1984; Addington-Hall et al. 1991; Seale 1991). Relatives of those dying in hospital also have psychological, social, or physical needs. Fatigue is commonly experienced by relatives (Hockley et al. 1988). Many of these problems may be compounded by perceived lack of information and explanation.

Some of the most thought provoking and worrying incidents and problems were highlighted in a non-participant observation study of 50 dying patients in 4 large teaching hospitals (Mills et al. 1994). The observer found that the care of many of these patients was poor. In particular, contact between nurses and dying patients was minimal and basic interventions to maintain patient comfort were often not provided. Several short case reports are described in the paper. In one, a multidisciplinary ward round visited a patient in a side room but failed to notice she was dead. Other incidents are described which prompted the observer to abandon her non-participant role. Such reports are upsetting but, it is hoped, likely to catalyse change.

Specialist palliative care in hospitals

In many developed countries the number of people who die in hospital is increasing. In England and Wales in 1992 almost half of deaths from all causes and 60% of deaths from cancer occurred in hospital (HIS, Hospice Facts and Figures 1996). At that time there were 163 HPCTs or single palliative care nurse specialists in the UK (Eve and Smith 1994). By 1996, the number had grown to 275. Of these, 173 (62%) specialist palliative care support services were provided by a lone palliative care nurse specialist. The trend, however, is towards the appointment of interdisciplinary teams. In the 1995 Hospice Information Service Directory of Hospice and Palliative Care Services in the UK and Republic of Ireland, most HPCTs were identified as willing to accept patients with a range of non-malignant diseases as well as those with a diagnosis of cancer.

'Palliative Care in the Hospital Setting' (National Council for Hospice and Specialist Palliative Care Services 1996), recommended that:

◆ The palliative care approach should be an integral part of all clinical practice, available to all patients with life threatening illness;

◆ The HPCT should be a multidisciplinary group of full-time, part-time and attached staff with a range of complimentary skills;

◆ There should be clear understanding between the HPCT and referring clinicians, and with patients, as to the advisory nature of the relationship between the team and the primary hospital carers.

In this chapter, we assume that these principles underpin the provision of specialist palliative care services in acute hospitals.

Which patients with non-malignant disease require specialist palliative care?

It is very difficult to identify which patients with non-malignant disease in the acute hospital setting require specialist palliative care input. An important aim of hospital based palliative care services is to improve the level of generic palliative care skills throughout the hospital by example and education. Even if such a service is restricted to patients with malignant disease, it would be hoped that staff would translate some of the experience and skills learned through their interaction with that HPCT to patients with non-malignant disease. This is probably happening but it would be extremely difficult to prove. It has been said that the success and relevance of palliative care will be judged not by the number of specialist teams but by the capacity to influence the care offered to all patients irrespective of diagnosis and place of care (O'Brien *et al.* 1998).

Until recently our team did not provide a service to the medical oncology and clinical oncology wards, only to the general surgery, general medicine, and elderly care wards where the patient population is usually a mixture of those with malignant and those with non-malignant diseases; often the majority of patients on a ward will not have cancer. Despite this unusual situation, patients with non-malignant disease still only constituted 18% of our referrals. In a survey of 50 randomly selected HPCTs listed in the 1997 Directory of Hospice and Specialist Palliative Care Services, 19 teams responded. The proportion of patients they saw with non-malignant disease varied from 0% to 12%, median 5% (National Council for Hospice and Specialist Palliative Care Services and Scottish Partnership Agency for Palliative Care and Cancer Care 1998). These figures need to be viewed in the context of the low response rate. Moreover, these services probably evolved in very different ways. It can therefore be very difficult to compare services in different parts of the country and different parts of the world.

Determinants of referrals to hospital palliative care team

A variety of factors may influence the likelihood of a patient with non-malignant disease being referred to a HPCT. For example, in a study of 26 patients referred to a hospital palliative care team, 15 were dying of cancer and 11 of non-malignant disease (Hockley *et al.* 1988). This might be accounted for, at least in part, by the fact that one of the authors of the paper, who was intimately involved in the setting up of that team, was a respiratory physician. On the other hand, until the relatively recent development of specialist registrar training in palliative medicine in the UK, many doctors working in palliative care would have trained in oncology and would be most comfortable caring for patients with cancer. Colleagues in other parts of the hospital may still see them as cancer experts and may be less likely to refer patients with non-malignant disease. Just as every patient and his/her family is different so too every team has its own personality and relationship with its parent hospital and local specialist palliative care unit. World-wide, epidemiological and cultural influences and the way in which health services have developed locally, will be relevant.

Using our own hospital based team as an example, it is obvious that the history of the development of the team is an important influence. Until the inception of the team, specialist palliative care advice for patients in the acute hospitals was provided, on request, by a consultant from the local palliative care unit, Countess Mountbatten House in Southampton, UK. All aspects of this specialist palliative care service, which was established in 1977, were available for patients with cancer, but not for those with non-malignant disease. In 1995 an interdisciplinary hospital palliative care team was set up to provide a specialist palliative care consultancy service to patients with cancer and non-malignant disease according to need rather the medical diagnosis. The team is part of Countess Mountbatten House, but is based in the acute hospital which is seven miles away. It remains the only part of the Southampton specialist palliative care services which provides care for patients with non-malignant disease. This could cause confusion and it means that we cannot facilitate referral of patients with non-malignant disease to local community based specialist palliative care services because they do not see patients with non-malignant disease. The pattern of referrals to our team in Southampton has probably been influenced by several factors (Table 13.1).

Other less tangible but nonetheless important factors may influence our perceptions and those of others of the role of the specialist palliative care team in the acute hospital setting. For example two of the five members of the team are funded by Macmillan Cancer Relief. Their work is not restricted to cancer patients and, on occasions, this has caused problems. After spending a long time with one such member of the HPCT, the wife of a patient with severe peripheral vascular disease, angina, and heart failure on the coronary care unit, stood up to return to his bedside and froze. Staring at the health professional's name badge, and seeing the word 'Macmillan' she said, 'Oh no, has he got cancer too?'

Who we are as people is significant too: one day over coffee we shared our personal experiences of illness and death. There were a higher than expected number of major losses in such a small group. Most of us had experienced care of our loved ones in the acute hospital setting which we felt could, and should, have been better. We acknowledged that this must have had an influence on how our careers evolved. It wasn't surprising that we were all trying to improve the quality of care for patients dying in hospital.

The hospital challenge

Part, but by no means all, of our work as a palliative care service in a hospital is supporting doctors and nurses in their care of patients who are expected to die on this admission. Recently the Study to Understand Prognosis and Preferences for Outcomes and Risks of

Table 13.1 Perceived factors influencing referral pattern

- Success rate. Improve the situation for one patient and get another referral!
- Hospital staff may associate specialist palliative care in Southampton with malignant rather than non-malignant disease.
- Whether or not staff had attended teaching sessions run by members of the team and/or spent some time visiting the team.
- Those referring to the team soon got to know our individual interests, experience, skills, and, no doubt, our shortcomings.
- Office moves: when based on the surgical unit we saw more of their patients, when based in the infectious diseases unit we saw more patients with HIV disease.
- Our current research interests and projects. For example, when a medical student attached to the team carried out a study of breathlessness in lung cancer and COPD patients, we noted a rise in referrals for COPD.
- Personal experiences of ward staff. For example, after a senior nurse in the hospital had cancer herself we noticed that she referred more patients to our team.

Treatments (SUPPORT) looked at all patients who were hospitalised at one of five participating American teaching hospitals over four years and who were also in the advanced stages
of at least one of nine medical conditions (acute respiratory failure, coma, chronic obstructive pulmonary disease, chronic heart failure, cirrhosis, colon cancer, lung cancer, multi-
system failure, multi-system failure and cancer) (Lynn *et al.* 1997).

A total of 9105 patients were enrolled in the study. Of the 4124 patients who died on
that admission, 55% were conscious in the last 3 days of life and two-fifths of them suffered severe pain most of the time. At least a quarter had moderate or severe breathlessness. Three-fifths (63%) of them had difficulty tolerating physical or emotional
symptoms. Of the 263 patients with chronic heart failure, 42% had severe pain and 65%
were breathless in the last 3 days of life. Two-fifths (40%) of these patients received a
major treatment intervention in the last 3 days of their life. Whilst there is no doubt that
an important symptom control measure is optimisation of treatment of the underlying
disease, such measures may not be efficacious in patients with advanced disease; furthermore they may not be appropriate. The appropriateness of any intervention varies
between individuals and, in any one individual, it varies over time. Practitioners of
specialist palliative care need to use data such as that from the SUPPORT to argue for
the judicious, simultaneous use of disease orientated and palliative approaches to treatment. The challenge is to strike the right balance between the two and recognise that the
appropriateness and acceptability of these approaches fluctuates over time. Readers will
be familiar with a variety of diagrams that have been used to illustrate the relationship
between curative disease orientated approaches and palliative approaches to patient care
(Figures 13.1 and 13.2). An alternative model emphasises the fluctuating nature of this
relationship (Figure 13.3).

It is over-simplistic to assert that, for example, as chronic heart failure worsens, symptom control measures take precedence over disease orientated measures. Sometimes the
most appropriate intervention could be heart transplantation! The situation is further
complicated by the fact that it is very difficult to judge prognosis in these patients (Lynn

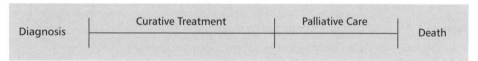

Fig 13.1 Curative care then move to palliative care.

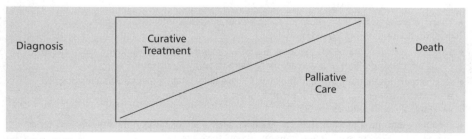

Fig 13.2 Palliative care an increasingly important component of care.

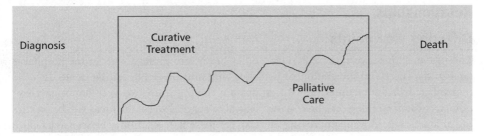

Fig 13.3 Palliative and curative care run alongside each other.

et al. 1997). They may appear close to death on a number of occasions but make good recoveries. The treatment for hospitalised patients with severe heart failure, or indeed other non-malignant diseases, demands skill and really good team work. The acute team need to be open to ideas about different approaches to treatment. The palliative care team need to be aware that, usually, their expertise is not specific to patients with heart disease and that it may not be appropriate to simply extrapolate their experience of patients dying of cancer to those dying of chronic, non-malignant disease. Rather, the two teams need to learn from each other and work alongside each other as well as the patient and their family. To us, this is one of the most rewarding aspects of our work as part of a hospital palliative care team.

Assessing whether patients have specialist palliative care needs

Whenever we are asked to see a patient, we try to assess whether they have specialist palliative care needs. Questions we may ask ourselves and those who referred the patient include:

1 Does the patient have a life-threatening illness for which curative treatment is no longer available?

2 What is the role of the ward doctors and nurses? Would the patient's essential care be better provided by the ward team with the hospital palliative care team's role being one of support for them in doing this, rather than that of becoming involved with the patient?

3 Do our skills match the patient's needs? For instance, would referral to the hospital discharge facilitator or chronic pain team be more appropriate?

Frequently, the answers to these questions are not straightforward.

We aim to follow up an initial visit with further visits at appropriate intervals, if necessary, and to discharge the patient from our service once the problems have resolved. On these occasions, we offer to see the patients again if new problems arise which are within the remit of palliative care. It is not unusual for the patient to be re-referred on the same admission. Sometimes this is appropriate but on other occasions, we still do not think we have a role. In these instances, the problems are more often social problems than health problems. We feel that the proportion of re-referred patients with non-malignant disease is similar to that of patients with malignant disease but this may vary over time and the experience of other teams may be different.

Relationships

Differing viewpoints

The relationship between the HPCT and other heath care professionals in the hospital is vital to the successful integration of palliative care into the acute setting. It needs to be remembered that sometimes the two groups are coming from two very opposing viewpoints. For staff working on a busy acute medical or surgical ward, the focus will be on curing or at least significantly improving survival. For these staff death may be seen as a failure or inappropriate outcome. For palliative care professionals, death is seen as normal and acceptable much of the time. At times these two viewpoints may result in different views about when patients should be referred for specialist palliative care advice and indeed about the focus of care once the referral has been made. Not infrequently this results in ethical debate. The issue of whether to hydrate or not is familiar to us in palliative care. It is much more likely to be regarded as a big issue in the acute hospital setting.

> An elderly lady, unconscious and dying of advanced cancer on the elderly care ward, was being intravenously hydrated. There was much discussion between the family and professionals as to whether this should continue. The lady's son made a very useful observation, 'If she had been at home none of this would have ever come up.' The fluids were stopped soon after.

Palliative care professionals need to help hospital staff explore some of the ethical frameworks which are perhaps more familiar to us but nonetheless still difficult.

Advising and facilitating

The other important aspect of our relationship with hospital staff is that of our advisory and facilitative role. We must always remember that the patient has often, though not always, been admitted to hospital for some sort of acute intervention rather than for specialist palliative care support. They are invariably under the care of doctors and nurses who are accountable for the patient's care 24 hours a day which we are not. We must not make ourselves indispensable through being the key decision makers, or indeed appearing to be so to the patient or family. In a survey of French physicians in a Paris teaching hospital, the notion of specific palliative care units in the hospital was rejected. Instead the option of improved training in palliative care and the input of a palliative care support team was favoured (Vidal-Trecan 1997). This preference has been reflected in our own environment. A busy surgical ward in Southampton made many referrals to the team. Over a period of a couple of years referrals decreased. When a patient was referred recently one of the staff nurses greeted us by saying 'we don't see much of you these days … mind you that's how it should be I suppose. You've taught us how to do it ourselves and now we only need to call you for the really difficult ones …' This was, for us, a real measure of our effectiveness.

Education

A recent editorial in the *British Medical Journal* (Gibbs *et al.* 1998) discussed issues about the care of patients dying from heart failure and highlighted that many would benefit from palliative care at the end of their lives. The challenge for all health professionals involved in the care of patients dying from heart failure and indeed any other non-malignant disease, is to provide best possible palliative care in the hospital setting. This does not necessarily mean that all such patients should be referred for specialist palliative care advice. Not only would this overwhelm specialist palliative care teams, it would also be inappropriate. The most important part of the role of hospital palliative care services is education and this needs to be recognised, valued, and evaluated. Instead, the activities of most HPCTs is measured in terms of numbers of patients seen or patient contacts.

It is vital that the hospital palliative care team are as clear as possible to users about their role, the service that they offer and the system for accessing their service. In Southampton, referrals are accepted from any health care professional, but specifically with the permission of the patient's consultant and in collaboration with the patient and the key nurse. The notion of consultant permission may not sit easily with nurses reading this. Nurses may justifiably feel that doctors should not decide on the appropriateness of a nurse referring to another nurse, albeit a clinical nurse specialist, Macmillan nurse or similar. Our own experience has been that a large proportion of our referrals are for pain and symptom control advice (55%). Because management of symptoms often relies heavily on appropriate drug prescribing and use, the patient's own doctor's co-operation is vital. Medical members of the hospital palliative care team do not write on prescription charts. The reason for this is twofold: first, our aim is to encourage the referring team to understand the rationale behind our advice and to learn through that understanding; second, as patients often only see a nurse on the team it avoids confusion about who can prescribe and who cannot.

When is the right time?

Dying or not?

All those who work in palliative care will be familiar with the difficulty of identifying when patients are dying and when they are not. We have all been tripped up by the patient who we expect to live for months dying quite suddenly and, perhaps even more commonly, by the patient whom we expect to die, living for a considerable time. Although there are conflicting reports in the literature, most health professionals recognise that it is usually difficult to give a precise prognosis for patients with cancer. We get nice surprises and we get nasty surprises. Sometimes, and probably mostly, we simply don't know. Frequently, it is even harder to prognosticate in patients with non-malignant conditions. The operational policy of our HPCT states that we will accept referrals of patients with potentially life-threatening disease. What does this really mean? Is referral of a patient with severe peripheral vascular disease for pain control and psychosocial support to a specialist palliative care team appropriate? Our experience, to date, has suggested that many of these patients die within a few months of referral and some do not leave hospital. Is this because the staff on the vascular ward are adept at choosing those patients with a short prognosis? Could the interventions that we suggest shorten life, albeit through double effect? Should we be seeing them at all? If we don't who will? In some centres such patients would be referred to a chronic pain team rather than a palliative care team. Some of these questions may be unanswerable but we believe that it is vital to keep talking about them and in particular to engage staff working in the acute setting in these discussions. Everybody involved needs to be aware of the complexity of trying to determine when patients with severe non-malignant disease become terminally ill. This label is often avoided but can be useful not only to the patient and their family but also to providers of health and social care.

Diagnosis with a poor, but not definitely fatal prognosis

The group of patients for whom the prognosis is poor but not definitely fatal presents particular difficulties.

> Claire is an attractive young woman who has suffered from an unusual autonomic gut neuropathy since a teenager. Survival for Claire is dependent on intermittent supplemental parenteral nutrition via a central line. A long history of infected lines, haemorrhages and thromboses complicates her situation. Not surprisingly Claire has suffered from a number of complex psychological problems including anorexic behaviour, clearly a very undesirable trait in someone in whom nutrition is already severely compromised. Claire has an ileostomy and many scars from line insertions. A young lady who takes great pride in her appearance, she also has a lot of problems related to body image.
>
> Staff in the unit where she is frequently admitted asked us to see her to offer some psychological support. Claire obviously has a life threatening illness and many emotional problems related to a number of losses. From time to time she has symptom control needs; she is often very depressed. Should Claire receive specialist palliative care services? Arguably many of her problems are compatible with our skills and experience. She will probably die from this disease but maybe not for a number of years. Claire appreciated our intervention. For her we represented professionals who were interested in her emotional state rather than her central line or magnesium levels. The doctors and nurses looking after her were relieved that there were others to share the difficulties with this patient. 'You're so good with her …' was a common statement.

Those working in palliative care will be familiar with the rewards associated with patients and staff who tell us that we are the only ones who have been able to help them or that they would not have got through an episode without us. The acute hospital setting is particularly likely to throw up this situation because there is often such an emphasis on the disease and its treatment. To the patient priorities may often seem to focus around investigations, theatre lists, and admissions and discharges, rather than the patient's individual problems and anxieties. Working with other health care staff in the hospital setting, palliative care personnel must be alert to the seductiveness of this scenario and these types of patients. We must remember not only to avoid de-skilling staff caring for patients, but also to be alert to the serious danger of discrediting staff to one another or to patients and their families. In a hospital there will always be patients with such complex social and medical problems that health care professionals do not know what to do with them. There will always be services which are under-resourced or even completely absent. In Southampton, a cut in funding resulted in the temporary cessation of a chronic pain service for in-patients for about a year. This resulted in a significant number of patients being referred to our service who would otherwise have been referred to the chronic pain service. The HPCT must be aware of trying to fill gaps in other services. Just because there is a need does not mean that the HPCT has to fill it; we do so at the risk of diluting our own skills and experience. How long can a team that is seen as the cure for all ills maintain its credibility?

Acute care in the terminal phase

Patients who are truly in the terminal phase of their disease may be admitted to an acute unit inappropriately because it is so difficult to predict when a patient with advanced non-malignant disease is dying.

Manny was a fifty-eight year old accountant who had been HIV positive for 6 years. His partner Jerry had watched Manny go through many opportunistic infections and recover unexpectedly on a number of occasions. With a CD4 count of virtually zero, Manny was admitted with his fifth bout of pneumonia. Intravenous antibiotics were started but there was little initial response. Jerry was told that Manny would die this time. The HPCT were invited to offer support to Jerry and to offer advice on symptom management. Startlingly after a couple of days Manny started to respond and 10 days after admission was planning to go home. Jerry described his anger to us. He had tried to prepare for his partner's death on many occasions. He was emotionally spent. This time he was prepared and as ready as he felt he ever would be. He didn't feel able to either continue caring for Manny any longer or to go through the process of preparing to lose him again. One more time would be one time too often. The nurses on the ward knew the couple well. This unexpected reaction from such a devoted partner was confusing and unexpected. Inevitably judgements crept in and the palliative care team found themselves supporting the nurses and doctors as much as Jerry in balancing these complex and contradictory feelings. With support and encouragement Manny and Jerry were able to get home and remain there for what proved to be a short final period. He died six weeks later.

As this case illustrates, HIV disease can present particular difficulties in prognostic prediction and thus in deciding the appropriateness of different approaches to care. Since the advent of triple therapy we see fewer patients admitted to hospital and this has further confounded the picture. Patients with HIV disease are, in general an empowered, knowledgeable, and vocal group and tend to want to explore every possible treatment and keep fighting the disease until death. It might be argued that this philosophy closely matches that of the acute hospital team. Certainly such patients are often in-patients near the end of their lives. Because of these factors the patient and the acute team may be reluctant to refer to the HPCT. However, this is not always the case and referral trends may vary in different hospitals resulting in some patients with HIV disease being referred to the HPCT. Once a patient is referred, then the challenge for the hospital palliative care team may be to help the doctors and nurses balance the traditional palliative care approach with the determination of these patients to continue active, or even what might be seen as potentially curative, treatment. Notwithstanding this both the HPCT and ward team have to be wary of allowing their clinical decision making to be influenced by their own value judgements and the juxtaposition of differing values. Perhaps this is the greatest challenge for palliative care specialists involved in the care of patients with HIV disease in the acute hospital setting.

Are doctors reluctant to recognise patients as terminally ill?

There may also be differences in the perceptions of different members of the interdisciplinary team. For instance, nurses may recognise a patient as being terminally ill before a doctor does. In a survey of leading physicians and nurses in a 1000-bed Paris university hospital it was found that nurses are more influenced by the absence of curative possibilities than doctors (Vidal-Trecan 1997). This may illustrate a difference in nursing and medical training and culture. Medicine may be seen as having a more scientific basis whilst nursing may be thought of as a mixture of compassion and science. This cannot, however, be the only explanation since we have always collected data on which health professional initiated a referral to the HPCT and, in the early days of the team, nurses made the majority of referrals; however, over time, the trend reversed and far more doctors than nurses referred patients.

The reasons for this are probably complex and may include, at least in part, an unwillingness of medical staff to see the patient as incurable. Some doctors may feel a sense of failure in the face of the dying patient. Some may be unwilling to refer to other colleagues especially to a palliative care team, and particularly one in which most of the team are specialist nurses, whose role they regard as solely care of the imminently dying. It may be that such factors influence their decisions about referring patients with non-malignant disease. Regrettably, there are some patients with non-malignant disease who are referred because nobody knows what else to do with them. Whatever the reason or reasons, we have found that as these medical staff got to know and trust us, to realise that we were not harbingers of doom, and even told the occasional joke, they seemed more willing to refer patients. Until research sheds light on the decision-making process of whether or not to refer a patient to a hospital palliative care team, these explanations must remain speculative.

It is important that people in our position as providers of specialist palliative care have knowledge of the natural history of the diseases that we see or, at least, are not afraid to ask when we are unsure. An educated guess about whether or not a patient is dying sooner rather than later underpins everything that we do: approach, attitudes, clinical decision-making, and what we choose to say to the patient and relative. Everyone involved may have many different views about this:

'Shut the door' he said to his wife, 'I know I'm dying, you know I'm dying and I'm going to say good-bye to you and be done with it.'

He died three weeks later. Jo was a 63 year old man with severe, chronic obstructive pulmonary disease who had spent most of his last year in and out of an acute medical ward. Bronchodilators, antibiotics, corticosteroids, and respiratory stimulants were less and less helpful to him. At the suggestion of the nursing staff on the ward the doctors reluctantly referred him to us. A fiercely independent man, struggling to maintain control of his dwindling life and to breathe, Jo was very suspicious of us. We let him set the rules, which included taking things at his pace and following his agenda. Some days he was optimistic and planned for the future, other days he wanted us to help him prepare to die. We believed that he was dying, albeit slowly. Decisions about the use of opioids and benzodiazepines were carefully negotiated with the nursing and medical teams but were often questioned by different doctors especially those from other teams on call at night. At one point there was debate over whether the most appropriate course of action was a subcutaneous infusion of diamorphine and midazolam or an intravenous infusion of doxapram. He was referred to us five months before his final admission and was able to go home for a few months with moderately improved symptoms. His final admission to hospital lasted two months.

A year after his death his wife agreed to be interviewed for this chapter and said, 'The man I knew died two years before.' We learned a number of interesting and useful facts from her. Because her husband had MRSA and had been nursed in a side room it had never occurred to either of them that the HPCT were anything other than members of that ward's team. Similarly she was unable to identify the difference between the doctor and the nurse on the team (although this may have been about the fact that the doctor was a woman and the nurse a man!). However she was able to identify a number of ways in which the team had been helpful: 'I think he was more comfortable ... I know he had a lot of faith in you, I don't think he had any pain ... I just used to think of you as the man with the tie who used to see to Jo's pain. I don't think he was scared of dying at the end because of what you had done.'

Patients with cancer and non-malignant disease

The whole picture grows even more interesting when we consider the not insignificant group of patients who have diagnoses of both cancer and non-malignant diseases.

> Kathleen was a seventy-three year old lady with a three-year history of breast cancer. She was referred to the team, having been admitted to an acute medical ward, with a recent diagnosis of brain metastases confirmed on CT scan. Her problems were of short-term memory loss and confusion. Steroids had no effect on these symptoms. On close questioning of the family it became apparent that these symptoms had been gradually coming on over the last few years. It seemed that this lady's symptoms were more related to dementia than her malignant diagnosis. However, it might be argued that dementia is indeed a terminal illness and that this patient therefore had clear palliative care needs. Eventually it was agreed with the elderly care unit that they were better skilled to take over this lady's care.

Those working in palliative care will be familiar with the challenge of referrals of elderly men with prostate cancer. Often these patients' needs will be far more related to advancing age and all the medical problems that this may bring, than to the cancer. The initial knee jerk reaction may be to deflect these patients to an elderly care unit, social services, or a nursing home. However if we are to develop palliative care for patients with non-malignant disease should we include these patients? Where do we draw the line? The challenge is not only identifying which group of patients should be offered our service and expertise, but also those who are not appropriate for us to see. The need for careful consultation and discussion with the wider team and, where appropriate, those in other specialties cannot be overstated.

Furthermore, attention has been increasingly drawn to the palliative care needs of patients earlier in the course of their illness. For example we have met in-patients with recently-diagnosed motor neurone disease who require psychological support coping with the diagnosis, threat of loss of function, and fears of a distressing death, as well as symptom control interventions.

Conclusion

In writing this chapter we are aware that we have raised more questions than we have answered. But perhaps this reflects the real world. Palliative care is still a relatively young specialty and the application of this specialty to patients with non-malignant disease is even younger. It is therefore not surprising that we are still at the beginning of our knowledge trail. It has been stated that, 'maintaining high standards of care depends on advances in knowledge and in order to achieve this there is an obligation to contribute to these advances' (Calman and Hanks 1998). Only through identifying the issues for debate and then stimulating that debate can we advance such knowledge. Furthermore it is not good enough for us simply to continue to extrapolate our knowledge of patients with non-malignant disease from our knowledge of patients with cancer. We must develop a research base specific to the needs of patients with non-malignant disease and, in particular, to how these patients' needs relate to the treatment they receive in the acute setting. The current dearth of research and audit on this subject means that those palliative care specialists who are involved in the care of patients with non-malignant disease in the hospital setting would be hard pushed to claim that their clinical practice is evidence based.

The hospital setting is an excellent training and research environment for palliative care for patients with non-malignant disease. We have described what we believe to be the unique challenges of and opportunities for offering specialist palliative care to patients with non-malignant disease in the acute hospital setting. In particular we hope that we have convinced readers of the great value of working in partnership with the hospital doctors and nurses. This partnership must be nurtured and built on so that, together, we can identify the research agenda and collaboratively, embark on the appropriate research projects to develop specialist and generic palliative care for patients in hospital who do not have cancer, but, still have life threatening and terminal illnesses.

References

Addington-Hall, J.M., MacDonald, L.D., Anderson, H.R., and Freeling, P. (1991). Dying from cancer: the views of bereaved family and friends about the experiences of terminally ill patients. *Palliative Medicine* 5: 207–14.

Bates, T., Hoy, A., Clarke, D., and Laird, P. (1981). A new concept of hospice care: St Thomas' terminal support team. *Lancet* 1: 1201–3.

Brescia, F.J., Adler, D., Gray, G., *et al.* (1990). Hospitalised advanced cancer patients: a profile. *Journal of Pain and Symptom Management* 5: 221–7.

Calman, K. and Hanks, G. (1998). Clinical and health services research. In Doyle, D., Hanks, G.W.C., MacDonald, N. (eds), *Oxford Textbook of Palliative Medicine.* Oxford: Oxford Medical Publications, pp. 159–65.

Eve, A. and Smith, A.M. (1994). Palliative care services in Britain and Ireland—update 1991. *Palliative Medicine* 8: 19–27.

Gibbs, L.M.E., Addington-Hall, J.M., and Gibbs, J.S.R. (1998). Dying from heart failure: lessons from palliative care. *British Medical Journal* 317: 961–2.

Hinton, J. (1963). The physical and mental distress of the dying. *Quarterly Journal of Medicine* 32: 1–21.

Hinton, J. (1979). Comparison of places and policies for terminal care. *Lancet* 1: 29–32.

Hockley, J.M., Dunlop, R., and Davies, R.J. (1988). Survey of distressing symptoms in dying patients and their families in hospital and the response to a symptom control team. *British Medical Journal* 296: 1715–17.

Hospice Information Service (1996). *Hospice Facts and Figures. Fact sheet 7.* London: HIS.

Lynn, J., Teno, J.M., Phillips, R.S., Wu, A.W., Desbiens, N., Harrold, J., Claessens, M.T., Wenger, N., Kreling, B., and Connors, A.F. Jr (1997). Perceptions by family members of the dying experience of older and seriously ill patients. *Annals of Internal Medicine* 126: 97–106.

Lynn, J., Harrell, F., Cohn, F., Wagner, D., and Connors, A. (1997). Prognoses of seriously ill hospitalised patients on the days before death: implications for patient care and public policy. *New Horizons* 5: 56–61.

Mills, M., Davies, H.T.O., and Macrae, W.A. (1994). Care of dying patients in hospital. *British Medical Journal* 309: 583–6

Mount, B.M. (1976). The problem of caring for the dying in a general hospital; the palliative care unit as a possible solution. *Canadian Medical Association Journal* 115: 119–21.

Mount, B.M., Jones, A., and Patterson, A. (1974). Death and dying: attitudes in a teaching hospital. *Urology* 4(6): 741–8.

National Council for Hospice and Specialist Palliative Care Services (1996). *Palliative Care in the Hospital Setting.* Occasional Paper 10. London: NCHSPCS.

National Council for Hospice and Specialist Palliative Care Services and Scottish Partnership Agency for Palliative and Cancer Care (1998). *Reaching Out: Specialist Palliative Care for Adults with Non-malignant Diseases.* Occasional Paper 14. London: NCHSPCS.

O'Brien, T., Welsh, J., and Dunn, F.G. (1998). ABC of palliative care: non-malignant conditions. *British Medical Journal* **316**: 286–9.

Parkes, C.M. and Parkes, J. (1984). 'Hospice' versus 'hospital' care—re-evaluation after 10 years as seen by surviving spouses. *Postgraduate Medical Journal* **60**: 120–4.

Seale, C. (1991). A comparison of hospice and conventional care. *Social Science and Medicine* **32**: 147–52.

Simpson, K.H. (1991). The use of research to facilitate the creation of a hospital palliative care team. *Palliative Medicine* **5**:122–9.

Vidal-Trecan, G. (1997). The management of terminal illness: opinions of the medical and nursing staff in a Paris University hospital. *Journal of Palliative Care* **13**(1): 41–7.

Chapter 14

Palliative care for non-cancer patients: a UK perspective from primary care

Stephen Barclay

Introduction

The last century has seen an increasing institutionalisation and medicalisation of death (Field 1994). Death, like birth, is a family affair, but hospitals are increasingly the site of both: there is a growing feeling that hospital is frequently an inappropriate place for the beginning and ending of life (Bowling 1983). Table 14.1 summarises the place of death data for England and Wales in 1995. Deaths in the patient's own home, in residential, or nursing homes all occur under the care of the primary health care team. In 1995, 38% of cancer deaths and 40% of non-cancer deaths thus were within the remit of primary care. Compared with deaths from cancer, non-cancer deaths were more likely to occur in NHS

Table 14.1 Place of death in England and Wales in 1995

	Cancer (%)	Non-cancer (%)
NHS hospitals (1)	48.3	55.0
Voluntary hospices (2)	13.3	0.2
Psychiatric hospitals	0.3	1.0
Own home	25.8	19.9
Nursing home (3)	7.3	10.9
Residential home (4)	3.6	9.6
Other homes/places (5)	1.6	3.4

(1) All non-psychiatric NHS hospitals, including acute, community, long-stay stay elderly hospitals and NHS hospice units.

(2) Office for National Statistics currently only codes for non-NHS hospices.

(3) 'Non-NHS other hospitals and establishments for care of the sick'.

(4) 'Other community establishments'.

(5) Cancer: largely deaths while staying with relatives.

  Non-cancer: largely sudden deaths and accidents.

Source: Office for National Statistics Mortality Data (England and Wales, 1995).

hospitals, less likely to occur at home, very much less likely to occur in voluntary hospices, and more likely to occur in residential or nursing homes. Four-fifths (85%) of deaths in nursing homes and nine-tenths (93%) of those in residential homes were of people aged 75 and over. Approximately half were of deaths of women aged 85 or over (47% and 57%).

Most of the last year of life is spent at home, and many patients are admitted to hospital shortly before death. There is, therefore a paradox: 'most of the final year is spent at home, but most people are admitted to hospital to die' (Thorpe 1993). There is a trend towards more hospital care in the final year of life: two national studies of deaths from all causes in England (Cartwright 1991) revealed that 63% had spent 11 or more of their last 12 months at home in 1969: in 1987 this figure was 54%. Nevertheless, most people still spend most of their last year of life at home. Home is where most dying patients would prefer to be (Dunlop *et al.* 1989; Townsend *et al.* 1990), as well as being the place that their lay carers (Addington-Hall *et al.* 1991) and GPs (Haines and Booroof 1986) would prefer for them: although there is evidence that these preferences for home death decrease as illness progresses (Townsend *et al.* 1990; Hinton 1994). Maintaining a normal life for as long as possible, being in familiar surroundings cared for by a relative, and supported by health professionals well known to them, have all been found to be aspects of home care services valued by patients and carers (Grande *et al.* 1996; Grande *et al.* 1997b). Home is, therefore, both the place where most people spend most of their last months of life and the place where most would want to die, although many do not achieve this. The primary location of palliative care therefore remains in the community, under the care of the patient's GP and district nurse.

This chapter explores the quality of palliative care provided in the community in the UK, the relationship between primary care services and specialist palliative care services, and suggests a community view of the extension of specialist palliative care services to non-cancer patients. It begins, however, with an overview of the provision of health and social care in the community in the UK, with particular emphasis on recent changes which have impacted on palliative care.

Care in the community in the UK

The primary health care team

GPs

The cornerstone of primary care in the UK is a patient's registration with their general practitioner (GP), who is responsible for provision of personal medical services to their patients 24 hours per day, 365 days per year. They act as 'gate-keepers' for referrals to secondary and tertiary care. GPs are self-employed independent contractors. Continuity of care is a central feature of the work of a GP, who may serve a local population for a working lifetime of 30 years. By the time a practitioner comes to retire, the mothers in the antenatal clinic may well be women that (s)he remembers caring for before they were born. Continuity of care has, however, been eroded in recent years by the decline in the number of single-handed GPs (from 22% in 1969 to 10% in 1996) and the associated increase in group practices, especially large practices: 44% of GPs now practice in partnerships of five or more doctors (Department of Health 1997b). These group practices frequently operate a shared list system, with patients likely to receive care from more than one family doctor.

Home visiting by general practitioners has progressively declined over recent decades, with an increase in consultations on GP surgery premises. Between 1971 and 1995, the percentage of GP consultations at home has fallen from 22% to 9%, surgery consultations risen from 73% to 84%, and telephone consultations risen from 4% to 7% (General Household Survey data). A national survey of deaths from all causes (Cartwright 1990) identified that home visiting was the most frequent source of criticism of GPs, 14% of respondents indicating that they felt that the deceased's GP was reluctant to visit, and 21% that they would have liked the GP to visit more. Satisfaction with GP care was strongly related to the number of GP visits.

In 1995 there was a new agreement between the government and GPs concerning out-of-hours care. This has resulted in major changes in the delivery of care overnight and at weekends. GP co-operatives have developed in many areas, and are estimated to cover over half the UK population. Previously, out-of-hours care was based on a system of home visiting provided by a rota of doctors within a practice. This has now been replaced by a rota of local GPs, working 3- or 6-hour shifts, with an increase in telephone consultations, and an expectation that mobile patients will attend an emergency centre; home visits are largely restricted to the house bound. While co-operative care has been found to be satisfactory for most patients, concern has been expressed that the discontinuity of care that is now enshrined out of hours may disadvantage palliative care patients (Barclay et al. 1997b).

District nurses

Nursing care in the community is provided by district nurses. Although they are employees of community NHS Trusts, not general practioners, they are usually attached to a practice, delivering care to patients of the practice in their own homes and residential homes (but not nursing homes). Highly-skilled, qualified district nurses lead teams of staff nurses and nursing auxiliaries. Much of the work of these teams is with the elderly patients of the practice, many of whom are coming towards the end of their lives. Their work has changed fundamentally in the last decade as result of changes in community care legislation: they are providing less personal hygiene care, and undertaking more assessment and complex care, such as palliative care. Personal care traditionally provided within the NHS by district nurses is now undertaken by home care assistants (previously known as home helps), provided by social services or purchased by social services from private agencies.

Community care

The 1989 White Paper 'Caring for People' led on to the 1990 'National Health Service and Community Care Act', which saw a fundamental change in the provision of community care for the elderly in England and Wales. The central feature was a movement of costs for long-term care from publicly-funded health care to personally-funded social care. All those whose needs extend beyond health care are now assessed by the local authority Social Service Department to decide on what services to provide: such assessments apply both to people seeking domiciliary and day care services and to people seeking admission to residential and nursing homes. Currently, each local authority has its own eligibility criteria for such services, and its own charging structure (Audit Commission 1994): these are means of reconciling needs and resources by allowing through only a firmly limited amount of need.

While health care is seen as having a special legitimacy and is available free of charge, social care is now seen as an area of personal responsibility, for which the client must pay personally. The 'charging border' between health and social services remains a difficult issue.

A bath deemed to be necessary on health grounds is provided free by a member of the district nursing team: other baths are provided by a home care assistant employed by the social services and a charge is incurred. Clients must now also pay for residential care (subject to means testing), while they may pay very little for a package of domiciliary services, which in some cases can cost more than institutional care. There is evidence that rises in charges for local authority services are associated with reductions in service take-up (Association of Metropolitan Authorities 1994). In addition, from 1996, health authorities became obliged to define their eligibility criteria for NHS continuing care on health grounds. The small numbers of patients meeting these criteria make no financial contribution themselves, whatever their means, for NHS care is 'free at the point of use'. The criteria are locally decided, with no national guidelines for establishing who is eligible to be directly supported by the health authority in an NHS hospital, an NHS nursing home, or a purchased place in a private nursing home.

The 1990 Community Care Act clearly defined local authority social service departments as the lead agencies for community care. This signalled an opportunity for the NHS to relinquish its long-term care responsibilities, which has resulted in a national programme of institutional closures during the 1990s. There has been a consequent decline in NHS provision of general beds for the elderly and for the elderly mentally infirm, and in local authority residential accommodation. Associated with this decline in state provision of care places has been a marked rise in private sector provision of places in residential homes, and nursing homes, with a more modest rise in provision in voluntary sector residential homes. More recent years have seen a continuation of these trends, with a considerable rise in 'Dual Registered' homes that provide residential and nursing care under the same roof, thus permitting patients to stay with familiar friends and staff as they deteriorate physically or mentally, and move from residential to nursing wings of the same institution. While there is usually a range of local care homes to choose from, entry into such care often takes place at a time of crisis: in practice this may mean that there is little choice (Bradshaw and Gibbs 1998).

The impact of community care changes on primary care

The changes in community provision of residential and nursing homes represents an increasing challenge to the already stretched resources of primary care. Medical care for all people in residential and nursing homes is provided by local GPs: much of this care was previously provided by hospital medical staff, particularly for many nursing home residents who would previously have been in long-stay NHS care. The changing provision of long-term care for elderly people (together with the de-institutionalisation of psychiatric patients and demographic change) has significantly increased GP workload (Kavanagh et al. 1998). A GP working in a retirement area with a list of 1900 patients may have 30% of his patients aged over 65, around 90 of whom would be in residential or nursing home care (Bowman 1998). This represents a considerable workload for the GP, whose only compensation is an augmented capitation fee for over-65s. The General Medical Services Committee of the British Medical Association has proposed that patients in nursing homes should be excluded from GPs' core services, and are currently seeking to negotiate additional payment outside of General Medical Services for this additional workload.

GPs may welcome the facility to 'keep on' a patient with whom they have a relationship going back over many years, when they enter a residential or nursing home. They may feel very differently about the opening of a nursing home close to their practice, which is then filled with patients decanted from hospital wards with varying levels of physical and mental frailty, concerning whom there may be little information about past medical history, and with whom the GP has no previous relationship. An attitude of resignation and resentment may arise at this 'dumping' of work from secondary to primary care: care that is solely reactive to calls from staff may follow, rather than good quality pro-active care, building in a structure of planned care with regular reviews. The introduction of a system of pro-active and systematised care results in a reduction in emergency calls, and the development of good working relationships with care staff (Bowman 1998). The provision of palliative care in nursing homes is discussed in Chapter 12.

Palliative care in the community

As already outlined, the primary location of palliative care in the UK is in the community, under the care of the patient's GP and (if they live in their own home or a residential—but not nursing—home) the district nursing team. This is not always recognised, and greater acknowledgement needs to be given to the fact that most of the professional care received by people reaching the end of life is given by the primary health care team (Kurti and O'Dowd 1995). This central role of the primary health care team in palliative and terminal care was endorsed in an expert report for the UK government (Department of Health 1992) which stated that: 'The primary health care team … already provide, and will continue to provide, the mainstay of support to patients and families facing terminal illness, even when the final act of dying may take place in hospital.' This report went on to recommend that future developments of palliative care services should be focused around primary care, maintaining long-standing relationships between GPs and patients.

Of the 1881 patients on the list of an 'average' GP, 20 die each year (ONS mortality data 1995): 15 from non-cancer diagnoses, of whom 6 will die under the care of their GP (Table 14.1); 5 from cancer, of whom 2 will die in their GP's care. Although a small part of their work, GPs see palliative care as an important and integral part of their role, which contributes significantly to their job satisfaction (Haines and Boroof 1986; Field 1998). Palliative care is not thought to be of a very different nature from the rest of their work: the quality of their care of people who are dying encapsulates their ideals of patient care, and is seen as a marker of their general standards of patient care (Field 1998; Brooks 1995).

Why primary care is suited to palliative care

The primary care team has three qualities which makes it particularly suited to providing palliative care: continuity of care, a family perspective, and its multidisciplinary nature:

Continuity of care

In a study of attitudes to palliative care (Field 1998), GPs emphasised continuity of patient contact to be the main difference between the way they had previously cared for dying patients while working as hospital doctors, and now as general practitioners. They were likely to have built up relationships with the patient and family over some years prior to the final illness. Palliative care specialists rarely have the opportunity to develop such relationships that are so important to patients (Grande *et al.* 1996; Grande *et al.* 1997b). However, as outlined above, changes in general practice in the UK are reducing opportunities for continuity of care, and this may have important consequences for palliative care in the community.

Family perspective

Primary care is embedded in family and community relationships. In providing care for a dying patient, the family and wider community networks of friends are all recipients of care, both during the final illness, and then afterwards when bereavement care may be offered (Field 1998). It is not uncommon for the patient, their spouse, and children all to be registered with the same GP. Psychological and social support for the patient and their carers is an important aspect of palliative care, and one that the primary health care team is uniquely positioned to provide.

Multidisciplinary in nature

Caring for dying patients requires a team approach: such a team already exists for every patient across the country in the form of the primary health care team. GPs and district nurses identify a team approach as the most important aspect of their palliative care provision (Kurti et al. 1995), and guidelines for palliative care in primary care have emphasised the importance of such teamwork (Robinson and Sacey 1994; Rogers et al. 1998). Recent research (Grande et al. 1997a) has emphasised the complementary roles within the primary health care team in the provision of palliative care. A sample of 127 GPs and 73 district nurses rated how difficult they found symptoms to control: district nurses reported that it was easier to control loss of bowel control, loss of bladder control, bad smell, and bedsores than did their GP colleagues. In contrast, GPs found it easier to control depression, anxiety, nausea/vomiting, constipation, sleeplessness, and pain than did their district nurse colleagues. This would suggest that the two professions working together would provide better patient assessment and care than either working alone.

GPs' knowledge and skills in palliative care

How well prepared are GPs for this task of providing palliative and terminal care at home? The Cambridge University Health Services Research Group undertook a postal questionnaire study of a random sample of 450 East Anglian GPs concerning their training and knowledge in Palliative Care (Barclay et al. 1997a). Training was frequently absent during the years as medical students and junior doctors, although there was evidence that training has become more common in recent years. During the GP registrar (trainee) year, or as GP principals, the majority of respondents reported receiving training in all areas (apart from those who were trained prior to the introduction of syringe drivers).

In a subsequent questionnaire, the East Anglian GPs were asked what drugs they would prescribe when starting a patient on a strong opioid. One would expect them to prescribe a laxative, and also an anti-emetic for the first week or two in a community setting: 51% of respondents suggested a laxative and 54% an anti-emetic. These figures are strikingly similar to a study of hospice admissions from the community (Seamark et al. 1996), which found that of patients receiving morphine 49% were also receiving a laxative and 61% an anti-emetic.

The GPs were also asked the following question concerning the conversion of oral morphine to subcutaneous diamorphine: 'What dose of diamorphine given over 24 hours would you regard as equivalent to MST 60 mg bd?' Nineteen per cent gave the strict pharmacological equivalent of 40 mg of diamorphine, and 27% indicated a dose of up to 60 mg, which is possibly appropriate; 16% suggested less than 40 mg (significantly under-dosing the patient); and 16% suggested over 60 mg (significantly over-dosing the patient). Why does this conversion pose such difficulty to GPs? While specialists in palliative medicine prescribe for syringe drivers daily, a GP will perhaps only have one or two patients a year needing a syringe driver. The question is thus small print to a GP, who cannot be expected to retain such detailed information over the wide spectrum of knowledge needed for general practice. Advice in printed form (as now available in the British National Formulary), and the ready availability of a specialist for advice is essential in such an uncommon situation in primary care.

Quality of palliative care in the community

Research continues to reveal variable quality of palliative care in the primary care setting: 'home is either the best or the worst place to die' (Parkes 1978). As mentioned above, one of the reasons may be a lack of training in palliative care. In addition, a GP may not necessarily know about all of a patient's symptoms, and would thus be unable to treat them. Patients in the last year of life have been found to consult their GP about only two-thirds of their symptoms: some of the symptoms of which the GP is unaware may cause considerable distress (Cartwright et al. 1973). A better understanding of which symptoms GPs are not informed, and why, is needed.

Symptom control

Many patients still do not receive optimal control of pain (Parkes 1978; Addington-Hall et al. 1991; Addington-Hall and McCarthy 1995; Herd 1990; Sykes et al. 1992), although there is some evidence that pain control in primary care may be improving (Jones et al. 1993). A study of a few years ago (Haines and Boroof 1986) found that 32% of GPs reported difficulty with controlling patients' pain, and another (Herd 1990) found that symptom control was the most common medical reason for admission. Two more recent studies (Seamark et al. 1996; Grande et al. 1997a) have both found that only 8% of GPs report pain as difficult to control. It may be that a more confident approach to the management of pain has entered general practice over recent years (Seamark et al. 1996): or perhaps a degree of complacency, given the continuing reports of problems with pain control in the community. Some GPs see symptom control as the basic aspect of care that could be taken for granted, with the provision of psychosocial support to patients and relatives as being more important (Field 1998).

Vomiting and constipation, dyspnoea, anxiety, and depression remain sources of considerable patient distress (Addington-Hall et al. 1991; Addington-Hall and McCarthy 1995; Higginson and McCarthy 1989; Hinton 1994).

Satisfaction with GP care

Many GPs report difficulty in coping with the emotional distress of dying patients and their relatives (Haines and Boroof 1986; Wakefield et al. 1993). Those GPs who have difficulty with their own emotional responses are more likely to have difficulty communicating with dying patients and their relatives, and responding to their needs (Cartwright 1990). A national study of deaths from all causes, which included interviews with GPs as well as bereaved carers (Cartwright 1990) found that 87% of bereaved carers felt that the GP was an easy person to talk to, 82% that the GP had time to discuss things, 83% that the GP looked after the dying patient in an understanding way, and 74% felt that the GP care was excellent or good. However, half of the GP respondents felt they were able to give enough time to dying patients, and 43% of GP respondents would have liked to have given more time. Informal carer satisfaction with GP palliative care has been found to be positively associated with larger numbers of GP visits, and the GP giving the carer information concerning diagnosis and management (Fakhoury *et al.* 1996).

Supporting informal carers

The vast majority of care in the last year of life is not provided by professionals, but by relatives and friends (Seale and Cartwright 1994), especially wives and daughters. The support provided by a family caregiver may make all the difference for the dying person in their place of death: some have reported that up to 90% of terminal admissions to hospice are due to the stress of caring on the relatives, or lack of resources available to support the patient at home (Doyle 1980; Draper *et al.* 1992). The physical demands of caring are commonly the most difficult for carers, who find they become very tired (Kurti and O'Dowd 1995). A 1992 survey of nearly 3000 carers (Carers' National Association 1992) revealed that 65% felt that caring had affected their health. The relationship between carers and professionals is often an ambiguous one (Twigg and Aiken 1991). For over half of carers, the only supportive service that they are in touch with is the GP (Allott and Robb 1998) .

Meeting the support and equipment needs of patients and their carers in the community presents difficulties: relatives have reported insufficient levels of nursing care, particularly practical help with daily care needs and support during the night (Sykes *et al.* 1992; Addington-Hall *et al.* 1995). Lay carers often experience considerable strain as a consequence (Herd 1990; Hinton 1994): one-third of families describe severe anxiety, fears, or worries (Higginson 1995).

District nurse care

District nurses have a central role in palliative and terminal care, providing the great majority of nursing care for the terminally ill (Seale 1992). They have a major role in both providing and arranging care, together with an increasing role in giving information and psychosocial support (Seale 1992). Due to the protracted nature of many non-malignant illnesses, and the associated major nursing needs, district nurses may have contact with these patients several times a week over many months or years. The district nurse is often the most useful point of contact for carers of patients with end-stage non-malignant disease, as there may be relatively little contact with the GP (Kurti and O'Dowd 1996).

District nurses have to cope with substantial amounts of stress arising from their close and long-term patient contact, and emotional involvement with families where a person is dying. They may feel a lack of control over important determinants of distress such as drug doses, telling the prognosis, or arriving early enough in the course of disease (Seale 1992). This may give rise to tensions in relationships with GPs who have more control over these matters, but less daily involvement.

In a national survey of deaths from all causes, 1 in 5 (22%) of bereaved informal carers felt that their loved one needed more district nurse care than was received, and 12% of those who did not receive any district nurse help were said by their carers to have needed such help (Seale 1992). However, of all the people saying more nursing help was needed, only a quarter had asked for it. Most referrals of terminally ill patients to district nurses come from GPs: 48% of district nurses in this study felt that terminally ill patients were referred to their teams by the GPs too late to develop a good relationship. In addition, 59% felt that the initial GP referral had provided inadequate information, particularly with regard to medical information, information concerning the family, and what the patient and carers knew about the diagnosis and prognosis. Multidisciplinary guidelines for palliative care in primary care (Robinson and Sacey 1994) have emphasised the importance of involving district nurses at an early stage, and the value of effective teamwork.

Many district nurses feel that they could do more for their dying patients, especially spending more time talking or being with patients, and that they would like to do so were it not for time constraints (Seale 1992). Caregiver satisfaction with district nurse care is positively associated with the district nurse visiting frequently and on many occasions, ensuring the provision of night help, contacting other services on the patient's behalf, and visiting after the death (Fakhoury et al. 1996).

The provision of community nursing care at night is a major area of concern to district nurses and GPs (Boyd 1993; Barclay et al. 1999). In some areas of the UK, district nurse care is not available after 5 pm, although twilight or evening district nurse care may be available up to 10 pm. In many areas, overnight district nurse care is insufficient or unavailable. District nurses work on the basis of visiting patients at home: they are not available to stay for prolonged periods of several hours, as may be needed for patients with advanced diseases. The charity, Marie Curie Cancer Care, partly funds overnight nursing care, but the care available from Marie Curie nurses is limited in many areas to 2 or 3 nights per week, and is largely available only for patients with malignant disease. Home hospice or hospital at home services providing intensive 24-hour nursing care are welcome recent developments, whose cost-effectiveness requires more evaluation (Grande et al. 1999).

Community commissioning of palliative care

The prioritisation of health care is an important national debate (Smith 1996; Light 1997) . Over recent years, despite mixed feelings (Ayres 1996), GPs have become responsible for allocating an increasingly large proportion of the health service budget through fundholding, total purchasing, or GP commissioning groups (Yule et al. 1994; Mays et al. 1997; Graffy and Williams 1994).

A 1997 White Paper 'The New NHS' (Department of Health 1997a) signalled major changes in GPs' roles in commissioning, with the abolition of the internal market. Primary care groups (PCGs) and primary care trusts (PCTs) have been formed: typically serving around 100 000 patients, they are expected to progress up a four-stepped hierarchy of responsibility, from an advisory role in health authority commissioning, to the full allocation of a budget, commissioning care for their population on the basis of a public health function for their locality. PCG/Ts comprise, among others, all local GPs with their community nursing colleagues in 'a coming together of equals' (section 5:27). For the first time, community nurses are to take on a key role in the planning and commissioning of services.

In a study (Bowling 1996) of a large nationally representative sample of adults, 'special care and pain relief for people who are dying' was ranked as second in priority of 12 health services. A similar study of the public, GPs and consultants in inner London (Bowling et al. 1993) also found a high priority given to palliative care: such services might therefore be expected to be early candidates for PCG/T commissioning, as most referrals to specialist inpatient care or home care teams come from primary care (Eve et al. 1997).

A recent questionnaire study (Barclay et al. 1999) of GPs and district nurses working in the area served by the Cambridge hospice investigated their development priorities for palliative care services. Both GPs and district nurses ranked the urgent admission of cancer patients to hospice for symptom control as the service of highest priority for future development, as found in other studies (Finlay et al. 1992). The GPs and district nurses both ranked the Marie Curie nursing service to be of high priority for future development, as found in other studies (Boyd 1993; Pugh 1996). Hospital at Home for Palliative Care (a non-specialist nursing service providing 24-hour nursing care at home for patients of all diagnoses in the last two weeks of life) was viewed by district nurses as a high priority for service extension, and obtained the largest inter-professional difference in priority ranking: this may reflect the greater awareness of district nurses concerning the nursing and night-sitting needs of patients, and the stresses and needs of their lay carers (Grande et al. 1997b). The admission of patients with non-malignant diagnoses to hospice for respite care came low down the list of development priorities for both GPs and district nurses: district nurses were significantly more likely to rank terminal care admissions for these patients to be a high development priority than GPs.

GPs and district nurses gave the highest priority to the further development of services providing immediate clinical care, particularly in the final stages of illness: such an emphasis on individual care is the hallmark of primary care, and has been found in previous studies of needs assessment in primary care (Jordan et al. 1996; Audit Commission 1996) . To prevent an unduly short-term view becoming predominant in PCG/Ts, strong partnerships with public health medicine will be needed to ensure a more systematic and pro-active needs assessment, which may include the need for professional education. The inclusion of district nurses in PCG/Ts marks a significant change from the previous GP-led models. The greater contact district nurses have with dying patients and their families enables them to become their advocates in a special way. It is not clear how the differing professional priorities will be managed within PCG/Ts, and a consensus reached: given the tendency of doctors to take the lead, and of nurses to defer to doctors, some mechanism of achieving consensus may need to be developed.

The relationship between primary care and palliative care specialists

The major part of continuing care for palliative patients is provided by the primary health care team (Boyd 1995), whether with malignant or non-malignant diagnoses: such continuing care cannot realistically be the responsibility of specialist palliative care (NCHSPCS 1998). Both generalists and specialists have a role in palliative care, working together, recognising, and respecting, each others' skills (Boyd 1993; Charlton 1995).

There is a need for specialists to involve GPs and district nurses as full partners, and to agree an appropriate modus operandi, which is not simply dictated on the specialists' terms (Field 1998). Flexible specialist working patterns are needed, which involve several levels of involvement (NCHSPCS 1998), and which build in regular reviews to agree the working relationship for individual patients. Such a relationship, with clearly defined levels of involvement, will clarify the objective of each referral, facilitate the provision of more focused care, and enable a larger number of patients with a wider range of diagnoses to benefit from specialist advice (Boyd 1995).

One controversial issue is whether specialist palliative care providers should 'take over' patient care. It has been noted that: 'there is a danger that specialists may imply that good quality care can only be provided by their experienced team: such a conclusion would progressively undermine the skills of primary and secondary health care colleagues in this area of work. It is never necessary for the specialist team to take over the care of a patient unless that is what the patient and his practitioner want' (Pugsley and Pardoe 1986). While in the short term it may be difficult for specialist providers to limit their involvement with individual patients, it does allow for the development of mutual trust and respect, and the sharing of specialist skills and knowledge over time. One of the most important attributes of a good GP is the wisdom to know when to refer to specialist services. Calling in specialist help may carry a price for the GP and district nurse, in the loss of control of the patient (Wakefield *et al.* 1993; Brooks 1995), and de-skilling if the care is taken over (Field 1998). Specialist teams perceived by local GPs to 'take over' patients referred may receive fewer referrals, thus denying patients the potential benefits of specialist input and advice. 'It is better to help a colleague with a difficult case than to tell him he is wrong, and that he should make way for the expert' (Pugsley and Pardoe 1986).

District nurses may feel ambivalent towards clinical nurse specialists in palliative care (Nash 1990; Nash 1992; Barclay *et al.* 1999). District nurses provide the great majority of community nursing for the dying (Seale 1992), so they may feel unsure who has overall responsibility for the patient care, and even that their own contribution is underrated (Seamark *et al.* 1993). This may in part reflect an ambivalence of generalist district nurses towards the growing number of specialist nurses in many areas of care, who may be insufficiently integrated into the primary health care team (Hatcliffe *et al.* 1996), and who may leave them feeling de-skilled (Nash 1990). A further factor may be unease with the evolving role of the clinical nurse specialist in palliative care (Webber 1993), from one of psychosocial support (Grande *et al.* 1996; Cox *et al.* 1993; Nash 1993), to an educational and advisory role, only visiting the patient once or twice (Nash 1990). A recent study of specialist nursing care in patients with chronic obstructive airways disease questioned the value of input from specialist nurses if it is limited to a few patient contacts (Ketelaars *et al.* 1998).

It has been estimated that approximately 50% of cancer patients receive specialist care from some kind of palliative care team or nurse (Eve *et al.* 1997). For many this represents a brief period of care, or a single contact with a service: the majority of the care remains, appropriately, with the general services in community or hospital. A recent report (NCHSPCS 1998) commented that:

> specialist palliative care is not unique in its stated emphasis on the quality of life and holistic care. The language of general practice, geriatric medicine and nursing also emphasises the need to see patients as more than physical bodies and to recognise their holistic needs. Although evidence suggests a gap between rhetoric and reality, there are of course examples of excellent care of patients with chronic diseases from services and practitioners outside palliative care who provide excellent multi-professional care.

A similar gap may exist between the rhetoric and the reality of specialist palliative care. Some specialists give the impression of being the major providers of palliative care in their areas: this is not true of cancer palliative care (Eve *et al.* 1997), and most certainly not true of non-cancer palliative care. The reality is that primary care and the generic hospital services currently provide, and will continue to provide, the great majority of palliative care.

While undoubtedly having skills and approaches in symptom control, specialists and generalists need an open admission that some symptoms may have to be borne, or at best only partially relieved. It has been suggested that the medicalisation of death (Field 1994), and the advent of the specialty of palliative medicine, may be causing the hospice movement to lose its early vision of the team sharing the burdens of the patient and family as fellow travellers. Fatigue and weakness, with the consequent dependence on others for care needs, are among the most common and distressing symptoms of advanced disease, and an integral part of dying. Such symptoms cannot be removed: they can at times be relieved somewhat, by good holistic medical and nursing care, with a loving sharing of the awfulness of what is happening to patient and family.

A primary care perspective on specialist palliative care for patients with non-malignant diseases

Every GP has several hundred patients with incurable chronic disease at any one time: a holistic approach to the care of these patients is an integral aspect of the GP's role, which includes the combining of disease modifying active treatment and symptom controlling palliative treatment. For patients with chronic lung disease, cardiovascular disease, neurological disease, or stroke, the interval between diagnosis and death may be many years, during which the relative importance of active and palliative treatments change continuously (Fordham et al. 1998). Patients with rheumatoid arthritis, osteoarthritis, or degenerative arthritis of the vertebral column may suffer many years of severe pain and disability. Diabetes often carries major physical and psychosocial consequences. The GP, as the clinician with long-term responsibility for these patients, should incorporate the palliative care approach from the time of initial investigation and diagnosis, intercurrent disease exacerbations, and on into the more advanced stages, considering and addressing the psychosocial issues throughout. This approach is the bedrock of general practice: such care of chronic disease forms a major part of the workload of every GP across the land.

There is, however, an issue of equity of access to specialist palliative care services, 96–97% of whose current activity is currently focused on cancer patients (Eve et al. 1997). Since patients with malignant and non-malignant conditions have similar experiences of symptoms (Addington-Hall and McCarthy 1995; McCarthy et al. 1996; McCarthy et al. 1997), it is inequitable that they should be excluded from specialist palliative care services (NCH-SPCS 1998). This is certainly valid, but the question must then be asked: 'When does palliative care start?' 'The point at which illness becomes progressive or terminal rather than chronic' (Higginson 1998) or 'proximity to death' (NCHSPCS 1998) appears to be the common view among specialists. The implied agenda here is one of clinician focus (the end of life), rather than patient focus (the need for symptom control and psychosocial support at any point of the illness trajectory).

The present author is a general practitioner, and responsible for the care of all the patients on his list, whatever their diagnosis or prognosis. I would like to broaden the issue of equity further still. By all means include patients with non-malignant disease, but why limit the focus to the end of life? Patients with widespread joint disease who suffer severe pain over many years, or those with personality disorders and frequent emotional crises, may need an intensity of symptom control and support over many years that is comparable with (or greater than) that needed by patients in the palliative and terminal stages of illness. The latter are seen as candidates for specialist palliative care, and are given the GP's home phone number, not the former. It may be that the time-limited nature of the intensive professional commitment to the dying, and its emotional appeal to clinicians fosters the inequality of approach from GPs and specialists alike. One study of GPs (Field 1998) found that they do not see caring for their terminally ill patients as particularly different from the rest of their work: rather, the quality of their care for people who were dying encapsulated their ideals of patient care, and was seen by themselves and their patients as a marker of their general standards of care.

There are concerns for the long-term future of specialist palliative care, should a major move to incorporate non-malignant disease be made. Specialist palliative care services in many areas face the difficulty of striking a balance between maintaining a distinctive specialist role, and responding to local needs, some of which may be due to shortage of community services. For specialist teams to provide the complete package of care is inappropriate for most areas in the UK where primary care is already well developed, albeit imperfect (Boyd 1993). The great majority of the palliative care needs remain the responsibility of GPs and generalist hospital services, while specialist palliative care maintain a specialist advisory role for the majority of patients referred, and provide long-term continuity of care for only a small number of patients. This is an appropriate arrangement, and consistent with the generalist–specialist interface on which the NHS is founded. To suggest greater continuity of care for more patients from specialists is a service model that cannot be sustained: it has been suggested that the clinician that emerged would be little different from a GP with access to in-patient beds (Fordham *et al.* 1998).

There is a further vital role for specialists. By paying particular attention to undergraduate and pre-registration training for doctors, nurses, and other health professionals, and enhancing the skills of GPs and consultants (NCHSPCS 1998), there is the opportunity to influence the care of patients in a disproportionate way to the numbers of specialists. The hospice and palliative care movement has already deeply influenced the health care culture in the UK: but there is much more work to be done.

References

Addington-Hall, J.M., MacDonald, L.D., Anderson H.R., and Freeling, P. (1991). Dying from cancer: the views of bereaved family and friends about the experiences of terminally ill patients. *Palliative Medicine* 5: 207–14.

Addington-Hall, J.M. and McCarthy, M. (1995). Dying from cancer: results from a national population-based investigation. *Palliative Medicine* 9: 295–305.

Addington-Hall, J.M., Lay, M., Altmann, D., and McCarthy, M. (1995). Symptom control, communication with health professionals, and hospital care of stroke patients in the last year of life as reported by surviving family, friends and officials. *Stroke* 26(12): 2242–8.

Allott, M. and Robb, M. (eds), (1998). Understanding health and social care: an introductory reader. London: Sage.

Association of Metropolitan Authorities (1994). *A Survey of Social Services Charging Policies 1992–4.* London: AMA.

Audit Commission (1994). *Taking Stock: Progress with Community Care.* London: Audit Commission.

Audit Commission (1996). *What the Doctor Ordered. Fundholding: The Main Report.* London: HMSO.

Ayres, P. (1996). Rationing health care: views from general practice. *Social Science and Medicine* **42**(7): 1021–5.

Barclay, S., Grande, G., Todd, C., and Lipscombe, J. (1997a). How common is medical training in palliative care? A postal survey of general practitioners. *British Journal of General Practice* **47**: 800–5.

Barclay, S., Rogers, M., and Todd, C. (1997b). Communication between GPs and co-operatives is poor for terminally ill patients. *British Medical Journal* **315**:1235–6.

Barclay, S., Todd, C., McCabe, J., and Hunt, T. (1999). The differing priorities of general practitioners and district nurses for palliative care services: implications for commissioning by primary care groups. *British Journal of General Practice* **49**: 181–6.

Bowling, A. (1983). The hospitalisation of death: should more people die at home? *Journal of Medical Ethics* **9**: 158–61.

Bowling, A. (1996). Health care rationing: the public's debate. *British Medical Journal* **312**: 670–4.

Bowling, A., Jacobson, B., and Southgate, L. (1993). Health service priorities. Explorations in consultation of the public and health professionals on priority setting in an Inner London Health District. *Social Science and Medicine* **37**(7): 851–7.

Bowman, C. (1998). Institutional Care for Older People in the Community. In Beales, D., Denham, H., and Tulloch, A. (eds), *Community Care of Older People.* Oxford: Radcliffe Medical Press.

Boyd, K. (1993). Palliative care in the community: views of general practitioners and district nurses in East London. *Journal of Palliative Care* **9**(2): 33–7.

Boyd, K. (1995). The role of specialist home care teams: views of general practitioners in South London. *Palliative Medicine* **9**: 138–44.

Bradshaw, J. and Gibbs, I. (1988). *Public Support for Private Residential Care.* Aldershot: Avebury Press.

Brooks, D. (1995). Palliative care in general practice: should GPs do it at the expense of commoner problems? *British Medical Journal* **311**: 1502–3.

Carers' National Association (1992). *Speak Up: Speak Out,* London: Carers' National Association.

Cartwright, A. (1990). *The Role of the General Practitioner in Caring for People in the Last Year of Their Lives.* London: King Edward's Hospital Fund for London.

Cartwright, A. (1991). Changes in life and care in the year before death 1969–1987. *Journal of Public Health Medicine* **13**(2): 81–7.

Cartwright, A., Hockey, A., and Anderson, J. (1973). *Life Before Death.* London: Routledge and Kegan Paul.

Charlton, R. (1995). Palliative care in general practice: palliative care is integral to practice. *British Medical Journal* **311**: 1503.

Cox, K., Bergen, A., and Norman, I. (1993). Exploring consumer views of care provided by the Macmillan nurse using the critical incident technique. *Journal of Advanced Nursing* **18**: 408–15.

Department of Health (1992). Joint Report of the Standing Medical Advisory Committee and Standing Nursing and Midwifery Committee. *The Principles and Provision of Palliative Care.* London: Department of Health.

Department of Health (1997a). *The New NHS.* London: Department of Health.

Department of Health (1997b). *Statistics for General Medical Practitioners in England.* London: Department of Health.

Doyle, D. (1980). Domiciliary terminal care. *The Practitioner* **224**: 575–82.

Draper, B., Poulos, C., Cole, A., and Ehrlich, F. (1992). A comparison of caregivers for elderly stroke and dementia victims. *Journal of American Geriatric Society* **40**: 896–901.

Dunlop, R., Davies, R., and Hockley, J. (1989). Preferred versus actual place of death: a hospital palliative care support team experience. *Palliative Medicine* **3**: 197–201.

Eve, A., Smith, A., and Tebbit, P. (1997). Hospice and palliative care in the UK 1994–5, including a summary of trends 1990–5. *Palliative Medicine* **11**: 31–43.

Fakhoury, W., McCarthy, M., and Addington-Hall, J. (1996). Determinants of informal caregivers' satisfaction with services for dying cancer patients. *Social Science and Medicine* **42**: 721–31.

Field, D. (1994). Palliative medicine and the medicalisation of death. *European Journal of Cancer Care* **3**: 58–62.

Field, D. (1998). Special, not different: general practitioners' accounts of their care of dying people. *Social Science and Medicine* **46**(9): 1111–20.

Finlay, I., Wilkinson, C., and Gibbs, C. (1992). Planning palliative care services. *Health Trends* **21**(2): 139–41.

Fordham, S., Dowrick, C., and May, C. (1998). Palliative medicine: is it really specialist territory? *Journal of the Royal Society of Medicine* **91**: 568–72.

Graffy, J. and Williams, J. (1994). Purchasing for all: an alternative to fundholding. *British Medical Journal* **308**: 391–4.

Grande, G.E., Todd, C.J., Barclay, S.I.G., and Doyle, J.H. (1996). What terminally ill patients value in the support provided GPs, district nurses and Macmillan nurses. *International Journal of Palliative Nursing* **2**(3): 138–43.

Grande, G.E., Barclay, S.I.G., and Todd, C.J. (1997a). Difficulty of symptom control and general practitioners' knowledge of patients' symptoms. *Palliative Medicine* **11**: 399–406.

Grande, G.E., Todd, C.J., and Barclay, S.I.G. (1997b). Support needs in the last year of life: patient and carer dilemmas. *Palliative Medicine* **11**: 202–8.

Grande, G., Todd, C., Barclay, S. and Farquhar, M. (1999). Does hospital at home for palliative care facilitate death at home? A randomised controlled trial. *British Medical Journal* **319**: 1472–5.

Haines, A. and Boroof, A. (1986). Terminal care at home: Perspective from general practice. *British Medical Journal* **292**: 1051–3.

Hatcliffe, S., Smith, P., and Daw, R. (1996). District nurses' perceptions of palliative care at home. *Nursing Times* **92**(41): 36–7.

Herd, E.B. (1990). Terminal care in a semi-rural area. *British Journal of General Practice* **40**: 248–51.

Higginson, I. (1995). *Palliative and Terminal Care: Health Care Needs Assessment. The epidemiologically based needs assessment reviews,* 2nd series. Oxford: Radcliffe Medical Press.

Higginson, I. (1998). Who needs specialist palliative care? *Journal of the Royal Society of Medicine* **91**(11): 563–4.

Higginson, I. and McCarthy, M. (1989). Measuring symptoms in terminal care: are pain and dyspnoea controlled? *Journal of the Royal Society of Medicine* **82**: 264–7.

Hinton, J. (1994). Can home care maintain an acceptable quality of life for patients with terminal cancer and their relatives? *Palliative Medicine* **8**: 183–96.

Jones, R.V.H., Hansford, J., and Fiske, J. (1993). Death from cancer at home: the carers' perspective. *British Medical Journal* **306**: 249–51.

Jordan, J., Wright, J., Wilkinson, J., and Williams, D.D.R. (1996). *Health Needs Assessment in Primary Care: a study of understamding and experience in three districts.* Leeds: Nuffield Institute for Health.

Kavanagh, S. and Knapp, M. (1998). The impact on general practitioners of the changing balance of care for elderly people living in institutions. *British Medical Journal* **317**: 322–7.

Ketelaars, C., Huyer Abu-Saad, H., Halfen, R.J., Schlosser, M.A., Mostert, R., and Wouters, E.F. (1998).

Effects of specialised community nursing care in patients with chronic obstructive pulmonary disease. *Heart and Lung* **27**(2): 109–20.

Kurti, I. and O'Dowd, T. (1995). Dying of non-malignant diseases in general practice. *Journal of Palliative Care* **11**(3): 25–31.

Light, D.L. (1997). The real ethics of rationing. *British Medical Journal* **315**: 112–15.

McCarthy, M., Addington-Hall, J.M., and Altmann, D. (1997) . The experience of dying with dementia: a retrospective study. *International Journal of Geriatric Psychiatry* **12**: 404–9.

McCarthy, M., Lay, M., and Addington-Hall, J.M. (1996). Dying from heart disease. *Journal of the Royal College of Physicians* **30**(4): 325–8.

Mays, N., Goodwin, N., Bevan, G., and Wyke, S. (1997). What is total purchasing? *British Medical Journal* **315**: 652–5.

National Health Services Management Executive Value for Money Unit (1992). *The Nursing Skill Mix in the District Nursing Service*. London: HMSO.

Nash, A. (1990). The role of the Macmillan nurse. *Nursing Standard* **5**: 33–37.

Nash, A. (1992). Patterns and trends in referrals to a palliative missing service. *Journal of Advanced Nursing* **17**: 432–40.

Nash, A. (1993). Reasons for referral to a palliative nursing team. *Journal of Advanced Nursing* **18**: 707–13.

National Council of Hospices and Specialist Palliative Care Services. (1998). *Reaching Out: Specialist Palliative Care for Adults with Non-malignant Diseases*. Occasional Paper 14. London: NCHSPCS.

Parkes, C.M. (1978). Home or hospital? Terminal care as seen by surviving spouses. *Journal of the Royal College of General Practitioners* **28**: 19–30.

Pugh, E. (1996). An investigation of general practitioner referrals to palliative care services. *Palliative Medicine* **10**: 251 7.

Pugsley, R. and Pardoe, J. (1986). The specialist contribution to the care of the terminally ill patient: support or substitution? *Journal of the College of General Practitoners* **36**: 347–8.

Robinson, L. and Sacey, R. (1994). Palliative care in the community: setting: practice guidelines for primary care teams. *British Journal of General Practice* **44**: 461–4.

Rogers, M.S., Barclay, S.I.G., and Todd, C.J. (1998). Developing CAMPAS: a palliative care audit for primary health care teams. *British Journal of General Practice* **48**: 1224–7.

Seale, C (1992). Community nurses and the care of the dying. *Social Science and Medicine* **34**(4): 375–82.

Seale, C. and Cartwright, A. (1994). *The Year before Death*. Aldershot: Avebury Press.

Seamark, D.A., Lawrence, C., and Gilbert, J. (1996). Characteristics of referrals to an in-patient hospice and a survey of general practitioners' perceptions of palliative care. *Journal of the Royal Society of Medicine* **89**(2): 79–84.

Smith, R. (1996). Rationing health care: moving the debate forward. *British Medical Journal* **312**: 1553–4.

Sykes, N.P., Pearson, S., and Chell, S. (1992). Quality of care of the terminally ill: the carer's perspective. *Palliative Medicine* **6**: 227–36.

Thorpe, G. (1993). Enabling more dying people to remain at home. *British Medical Journal* **307**: 915–8.

Townsend, J., Frank, D., Fermont, D., Dyer, S. *et al.* (1990). Terminal cancer care and patients' preference for place of death: a prospective study, *British Medical Journal* **301**: 415–17.

Twigg, J. and Aitken, K. (1991). *Evaluating Support to Informal Carers*. York: Social Policy Research Unit, University of York.

Wakefield, M., Belby, J., and Ashby, M. (1993). General practitioners and palliative care. *Palliative Medicine* 7:117–26.

Webber, J. (1993). *The Evolving Role of the Macmillan Nurse.* London: Cancer Relief Macmillan Fund.

Yule, B., Healey, A., and Grimshaw, J. (1994). Fundholding: the next five years. *Journal of Public Health Medicine* 16(1): 36–40.

Chapter 15

Specialist palliative care and non-malignant diseases

Robert Dunlop

Introduction

The modern hospice movement was founded in 1967 by Dame Cicely Saunders. However, hospices for the care of the dying pre-dated the opening of St Christopher's Hospice. The earliest examples were opened in the mid-nineteenth century. Most were associated with religious orders which had a mission to serve the dying poor. For example, Mary Potter, a Catholic nun who founded the Little Company of Mary, was moved to establish institutions for the care of the dying by a 'certain solicitude for the eternal salvation of the dying and a conviction that great spiritual fruit might be gained from physical presence at the death-bed'. She was, at the time, convalescing after an illness from which some had thought she would never recover. The vivid memory of the solicitude, fear, weakness, and inability to pray, which she had experienced during the days of crisis, caused her to think how useful it would be if there were 'a group of religious Sisters dedicated to the spiritual and, where possible, the physical assistance of those in danger of death' (Dougherty 1961). The early hospices made no distinction between the needs of patients dying from cancer and patients dying from non-malignant conditions.

At the turn of the century, the most feared 'killer' disease was tuberculosis (Kastenbaum 1988; Rothman 1994). St Joseph's Hospice, which was opened in 1905 by the Irish Sisters of Charity, initially cared for patients with tuberculosis from the East End of London. In the ensuing decades, the prevalence of tuberculosis declined, partly due to improvements in living standards and chemotherapy. When Cicely Saunders began working at St Joseph's Hospice, tuberculosis was 'curable' and cancer had become the most common diagnosis of hospice patients. It was with this group of patients that the routine administration of morphine had such a dramatic effect on the most feared symptom—pain.

When St Christopher's was first opened, it was envisaged that the in-patient service would be available to patients with non-malignant diseases. This decision was informed, in part, by the evidence from John Hinton's work published in 1963. He found that patients dying from non-malignant diseases were just as likely to experience distressing symptoms but were less likely to have these symptoms relieved. In practice, cancer remained the dominant diagnosis group. Within a few years, the range of non-malignant diseases had been narrowed to motor neurone disease (amytrophic lateral sclerosis) (O'Brien et al. 1992). Early experiences exposed the problems of indeterminate prognosis (for example, chronic liver disease) and behaviour management in a hospice in-patient unit (for example, Alzheimer's disease). Although some palliative care literature addressed the specific needs of patients with non-malignant diseases (Wilkes 1982), it was not until the emergence of AIDS in the mid-1980s that the hospice movement was systematically faced with the challenge of non-malignant conditions. Several recent studies (Addington-Hall *et al.* 1998; Hockley *et al.* 1988; Seale and Cartwright 1994) and reports (SMAC, SNMAC 1992; Addington-Hall 1997) have maintained this challenge by emphasising the un-met needs of patients with conditions other than cancer.

This chapter reviews the current role of specialist palliative care services in caring for patients with non-malignant diseases. These services are described and defined in the Introduction. Challenges for the future are outlined, particularly in the light of the differences in practice between the UK and the US.

The involvement of specialist palliative care services in the care of patients with non-malignant diseases

There are significant differences in the proportions and numbers of patients with non-malignant diseases that are served by specialist palliative care programmes in the UK and the US. According to the Minimum Data Set held by the NCHSPCS and St Christopher's Hospice, more that 96% of all patients receiving in-patient care, home care, or day hospice care had a diagnosis of cancer in 1994–95 (Addington-Hall 1997). The most recent figures (personal communication, Hospice Information Service) show little increase in the proportion of new patients with a non-cancer diagnosis (in-patient units 4.7%, day hospices 6.3%, home care services 3.8%, hospital support services 5.1%). Although the overall figures demonstrate that specialist palliative care services have minimal direct impact on this group of patients, it is interesting to note that some services do have greater involvement. The maximum proportion of new patients with a non-cancer diagnosis reported to the Minimum Data Set was 31.8% for an in-patient unit, 57.1% for a day hospice, 30.7% for a home care service, and 24.1% for a hospital support team.

Comparable figures are not available for the US. Banaszak-Holl and Mor (1994) reported that the proportion of hospice beneficiaries with non-cancer had increased from 12% in 1987 to 16% in 1989. Christakis and Escarce (1996) reviewed the diagnosis of Medicare hospice beneficiaries who received specialist palliative care in five major states in 1990. Of the 6451 patients enrolled in hospice programmes, 19.8% had a non-cancer diagnosis. Congestive cardiac failure was the most common diagnosis, followed by chronic obstructive pulmonary disease, stroke, dementia, and renal failure in order of frequency. In that study, the median survival for dementia and chronic obstructive pulmonary disease patients was significantly longer than that overall (74 and 76.5 days respectively versus 36 days). Also, the percentage of patients living longer than 180 days was greater in the non-cancer group. In all but the renal failure group, more than 20% of patients with non-cancer survived longer than 180 days, compared with 14.9% overall. According to the National Hospice Organisation, the proportion of hospice admissions for non-cancer diagnoses has continued to rise (Stuart *et al.* 1996). For example, in one large hospice programme, which currently serves more than 5000 patients at any one time, almost 50% of the patients have a non-cancer diagnosis.

A particularly interesting development in the US has been the involvement of hospice programmes in long-term care facilities (Kinzbrunner 1998). As hospices began caring for more patients with non-cancer diagnoses, some of these patients were transferred into nursing homes. The hospices perceived that this led to a decrease in the quality of care. Proponents of hospice care successfully argued for a change in eligibility for the Medicare hospice benefit. Patients who were living in a long-term care facility could receive the benefit because they were in their 'home'. Staffing levels in nursing homes are often inadequate to care for terminally ill patients. Hospice programmes have developed strategies for collaborating with nursing home staff to supplement patient care. For example, hospice staff, including physicians, registered nurses, chaplains, and social workers visit patients who have been transferred to nursing homes on a regular basis, advising and supporting the nursing home staff. In addition, hospices will provide additional hands-on care from nursing aides in their employ. These aides co-ordinate care with the nursing home staff, for example bathing the patient on alternate days. Bereavement support is provided by the hospice programmes. While some may question this new direction in palliative care, evidence is emerging that pain relief for cancer patients dying in nursing homes is significantly better when hospices are involved (personal communication—Mor, V.).

Why do specialist palliative care services only have limited involvement with non-cancer patients?

In the US, where palliative care is reaching more non-cancer patients, only 17% of all people who die access specialist palliative care services (Cassell and Vladek 1996). Even after 30 years of palliative care in the UK, the direct involvement of hospice services in the care of these patients is virtually negligible. Although specialist palliative care will not be appropriate for all deaths (sudden deaths, for example), it is clear that a large number of non-cancer patients have problems which are just as distressing as those of cancer patients. Addington-Hall et al. (1998) reported that a third of cancer patients who received specialist palliative care scored at or above the median on three measures of symptom experience in the last year of life: they had had 8 or more symptoms, 3 or more distressing symptoms, and three or more which had lasted more than 6 months. Nearly 1 in 5 (16.8%) of non-cancer deaths had had a similar symptom experience. They estimated that if palliative care services were to meet this un-met need, there would be a 79% increase in case load. This figure does not take into account those patients with non-malignant diseases who have less severe symptoms but who would also benefit from specialist palliative care.

Why is there a discrepancy between un-met need and actual service provision? The reasons for this discrepancy are complex and multi-factorial. The difference in coverage between the UK and the US points to a major factor—the availability of funding. The modern hospice movement in the UK developed on the back of charitable funding. Although many palliative care services are totally funded by the National Health Service, a substantial proportion of the funding is from community sources. In 1997–98, it is estimated that specialist palliative care services received £56.4 million from the National Health Service, compared with £171 million from donations, legacies, fund-raising, etc. Currently, there are 63 hospices represented in the top 500 charities in the UK; their combined income exceeds that of the largest medical or health charity. This reliance on charitable funding contrasts with the situation in the US. Very early in the history of the hospice movement, the Health Care Financing Administration approved the Medicare hospice benefit. The availability of a *per diem* patient benefit enabled hospice programmes to grow on the basis of a predictable income stream. When the benefit became available for patients with non-cancer, hospice programmes responded accordingly. It is of interest to note that recent attention by the Office of the Inspector General on the possibility of benefit fraud (based on higher length of survival for some non-cancer patients) may have made some hospices more cautious about admitting these patients.

The reliance of many UK hospices on charitable money has understandably made them feel very cautious, even frightened, of the prospect of a significant growth in service, whether for cancer or non-cancer patients. The National Health Service is very slow to shift resources into a new area of care such as specialist palliative care for non-malignant conditions. Therefore, any short-term growth in services has to be wholly funded from charitable donations, without the prospect of a secure longer-term income. In an effort to cope with the realisation of the enormous un-met need and the fear of having to expand without a guaranteed income, the palliative care movement in the UK has held on to the aim that the 'experience and teaching should be so accepted that the medical field as a whole will effectively carry out the care needed by dying patients, the majority of whom will die in their homes or in general hospitals and not in special centres' (Saunders 1980). In other words, hospice services should only care for a minority of patients and thence act as centres of excellence to indirectly improve the care of the majority. While this may be a pragmatic approach, it has become a major philosophical cornerstone which underpins the thinking of many in the specialty. However, the danger is that the philosophy per se drives strategic thinking and future developments, rather than the more fundamental issue which is lack of funding. Therefore, services do not seek to increase funding for expansion, which would require a medium-term effort, because this is contrary to the philosophy. This means that need remains un-met in the long-term. It is interesting to speculate about how specialist palliative care services in the UK would respond to an initiative such as the Medicare hospice benefit.

Even if funding were more available, there are several clinical issues which will hinder the development of palliative care services for non-cancer patients (Dunlop 1993):

* *Difficulty for physicians in coping with progressive incurable illnesses*—because of the medical emphasis on cure. The training of doctors perpetuates this emphasis. Although many medical schools have some teaching on palliative care in undergraduate curricula, the amount of time devoted to this specialty is minimal. The practice of 'saving' patients is reinforced by audit systems that focus on the negative impact of mortality statistics. The failure of the SUPPORT intervention (Lynn et al. 1997), which used nurse specialists to provide written advice to improve the care of terminally ill patients, has been attributed, in part, to the pressure on physicians to continue 'active' measures because of the risk of censure in post-death clinical audit meetings (personal communication—Williams JR).

* *Difficulty recognising when non-cancer patients are terminally ill.* Although this is a particular problem in non-cancer, it is not uncommon for patients with advanced cancer to be referred too late in the illness to benefit from specialist palliative care or not be referred at all. Although this relates in part to the focus on cure, there are other factors involved including a lack of awareness of the pathophysiology of advanced disease. This can result in a failure to recognise that patients are terminally ill and require different treatment to other patients. This lack of awareness of the pathophysiology is similar to the situation in

paediatrics, whereby children used to be treated with scaled down adult doses of medications before paediatrics emerged as a specialty.

- *Limitations of the medical description of diseases.* Doctors are taught that certain symptoms and signs are associated with specific diagnoses. For example, heart failure causes breathlessness on lying flat (orthopnoea), breathlessness at night (paroxysmal nocturnal dyspnoea), breathlessness on exertion, and peripheral oedema. Doctors focus on these symptoms and do not ask about other distressing symptoms like fatigue, pain from liver engorgement, constipation, and nausea.

- *The availability of 'active' treatments.* With many non-cancer diagnoses, there is a broad array of therapies, such as diuretics and angiotensin-converting enzyme inhibitors for congestive cardiac failure. The availability of these treatments protects physicians from a sense of therapeutic nihilism. For example, a patient with cardiac failure may be admitted with a recurrence of severe congestion. The diuretic dose may be increased, producing appropriate weight loss. When the doctors review the weight chart, they will encourage the patient that his condition is improving. However, this optimism will prevent the doctors from recognising that the patient may still be extremely limited by severe fatigue, worried about the future, and deeply concerned about the effect of his dependency on his wife.

- *Feelings of therapeutic ennui when 'active' treatments are not available.* There are some conditions for which no 'medical' therapies exist. Motor neurone disease was an example before the recent introduction of neuroprotective agents. These patients will be told that 'nothing more can be done', which response characterised the care of cancer patients 30 years ago when the modern hospice movement began. The emergence of community based support groups for these conditions testifies to the lack of satisfaction with this response.

- *Non-malignant diagnoses cause less distress to patients and families.* The diagnosis of cancer always upsets people. They automatically assume a limited prognosis and future pain. By contrast, patients with severe congestive cardiac failure may have a worse prognosis than cancer but they will usually not be aware of this.

- *Patients and families accept symptoms as inevitable.* This means that they do not complain and so fail to get attention. Sometimes, they do not want to bother the 'busy' health professionals. Often, there is a passive acceptance which is more common in older people.

Overcoming these issues will be a long and slow process. It will require education of patients and families as well as health care professionals. Public expectations of care are rising. However, the media often focuses on the spectacular new treatments and potential 'cures'. Specialist palliative care services have played a significant role in raising awareness about care at the end of life. In the UK, the needs of cancer patients have been foremost. Recent debates about euthanasia have highlighted the plight of some patients with non-malignant conditions, especially motor neurone disease. In the US, the results of the SUPPORT have been used to heighten awareness (Lynn *et al.* 1997). Education of the public will only work if health care professionals are also given more training and support to recognise these wider problems and involve palliative care services appropriately. However, palliative care is having to compete for space in the already overcrowded curricula of medical schools and other educational institutions. Future progress is likely to be slow. In the UK, this will give specialist palliative care services more time to prepare for the rising demand.

Challenges for specialist palliative care services in the future

The first major challenge is to get specialist palliative care services to recognise that they have a role in managing patients with progressive non-malignant conditions. Some services may feel that this is not appropriate, no matter if funding became available. While such a position may be reasonable if these services are wholly community funded, it would be harder to sustain if government funding were attached to a requirement to deliver services to patients with non-malignant conditions as well as cancer. It is important that the national representatives of palliative care in the UK, for example the NCHSPCS, should continue to affirm the responsibility of palliative care to address this group of patients. The consultation document (Addington-Hall 1997) is a valuable start.

The second major challenge is funding. In the UK, the NHS is unlikely to release sufficient amounts of new monies to fund significant expansion of specialist palliative care services. However, continuing dialogue is needed between the NHS and representatives of the voluntary hospice movement. Charitably funded services can begin the process of raising additional money but this will need a medium-term time frame. It is not clear how much additional money could be raised in this way but partnership schemes with the government may be feasible.

In the US, the Medicare hospice benefit is unlikely to be withdrawn from the care of non-cancer patients. However, as the services for non-cancer patients increase, the expenditure will rise. This is likely to increase the efforts by Federal and other funding agencies to cap expenditure. This could be done directly but more aggressive audits of services, for example withholding payments for patients who do not meet the guidelines outlined by the National Hospice Organisation (Stuart *et al.* 1996), could achieve the same effect. Another funding issue is the narrow focus of the Medicare hospice benefit. Patients who would benefit from a mix of palliative care and other services are currently required to make a choice between the two. The reimbursement system also makes it difficult for this group of patients to receive continuity of specialist palliative care support in the hospital and in the community environments. These issues argue for a closer collaboration between health care planners, funders, and representatives of specialist palliative care providers.

Even if the commitment and funding were available in the UK, there is a major issue about what would constitute best practice for non-cancer patients. Palliative care specialists are often uncertain about the clinical expertise that is needed, given that most, if not all, of their experience is with cancer patients. One area of concern is the use of opioids for pain. Patients with chronic non-malignant pain will be referred to specialist palliative care services because of the distress which they manifest over a long period of time (Hitchcock, Ferrell and McCaffery 1994). What if opioids could cause addiction in someone who turned out to have a long prognosis? Opioids can be used for prolonged periods in patients with non-malignant pain with reasonable effectiveness (Portenoy and Foley 1986). However, some of these patients have psychologically maintained pain, particularly if there is a past history of major depression, childhood abuse, alcohol abuse, family psychiatric history, or sexual abuse in childhood (Gamsa 1994). Their management requires an interdisciplinary approach, including skills which are not available to palliative care services. A combination of 'active' and palliative treatments will be needed for many other diseases. An evidence base needs to be collated, and clinical trials need to be conducted to provide more certainty and consistency of management. Studies should examine the cost-effectiveness of different models of service provision, for example in acute hospitals and nursing homes.

While many treatments and strategies for managing advanced cancer will be applicable to non-cancer patients, innovative methods will also be needed. For example, the uncertain prognosis of many non-malignant diseases potentially makes discussions about the future more difficult. With congestive cardiac failure, the patient could die suddenly tomorrow, next month or in six months time. When any patient asks 'How long have I got?', it is inappropriate to respond initially with some estimate of time, no matter how certain the prognosis. Like so many questions of this nature, the purpose of the question will not be as straightforward as it seems. Some effort should be spent understanding what the patient is actually asking. However, when information about time is needed, for example the patient wants to plan for an important event, an uncertain prognosis makes this very difficult.

Scenario planning, as used in business, offers a useful paradigm for this situation (Van Der Heijden 1997). Typically, business plans use forward projections based on past performance. If there has been a steady increase in income over the previous five years, future increases will be predicted using linear regression analysis. However, projections do not reflect the uncertainty of the future. Dramatic changes in economic environment can occur quickly, for example the Asian crisis. To prepare a business for contingencies, it is important to consider three or four scenarios which are equally likely. By examining the consequences of each scenario, staff become aware of the early signs of whichever scenario unfolds (De Geus 1998). The business can then respond accordingly. The scenario planning approach can be used in the clinical setting as well. Rather than guess at an uncertain prognosis, a patient and family can be encouraged to consider three possible outcomes: short-term, medium-term and longer-term time scenarios.

As the evidence base accumulates and as innovative treatment strategies evolve, the challenge will be to educate palliative care specialists and others. Didactic and other presentational methods will be insufficient to promote clinical competence and confidence. Staff will need to supplement teaching with clinical experience. This will be particularly important for physicians who are training to become palliative care consultants. Currently, most training at this level occurs in specialist palliative care units. Given the low proportions of non-cancer patients who are managed in hospices in the UK, this is unlikely to give sufficient clinical exposure. Hospital based advisory teams are better placed to provide more extensive clinical experience, provided the team accepts referrals and develops strong links with acute services that care for these patients, for example care of the elderly, cardiology, respiratory medicine, and neurology. Trainers will need to develop their own confidence in this field or liaise with other trainers to provide specific supervision and training.

Summary

The needs of patients with progressive incurable non-malignant disease and the needs of their families are similar to the problems of patients with advanced cancer. However, 30 years after the founding of the modern hospice movement, only a small minority of patients access specialist palliative care services. There is a significant difference in the depth of coverage between the UK and the US. This reflects, in large part, the availability of government money for the care of terminally ill non-cancer patients. There are several challenges to be overcome if the inequalities of service provision are to be addressed: more funding, greater commitment, better education, and further research are some of the most important. Greater political awareness and lobbying will also be needed. New paradigms of care will need to evolve. New models of care will also be needed, such as consultancy services and provision of hospice based health care aides for nursing homes, along with thorough evaluation. Hopefully, the next 30 years of the hospice movement will see similar improvements in care for non-cancer patients as have occurred for cancer patients.

References

Addington-Hall, J.M. (1997). *Reaching Out.* Report of the Joint NCHSPCS and Scottish Partnership Agency Working Party on Palliative Care for Patients with Non-malignant Disease. London: National Council for Hospice and Specialist Palliative Care Services.

Addington-Hall, J., Fakhoury, W., McCarthy, M. (1998). Specialist palliative care in nonmalignant disease. *Palliative Medicine* 12: 417–27.

Banaszak-Holl, J. and Mor, V. (1994). *Hospice Report: The Impact of Changing Medicare Coverage on Hospice Beneficiaries.* Providence, RI: Center for Gerontology and Health Care Research.

Cassell, C.K. and Vladek, B.C. (1996). Sounding board. ICD-9 code for palliative or terminal care. *New England Journal of Medicine* 335: 1232.

Christakis, N.A. and Escarce, J.J. (1996). Survival of Medicare patients after enrollment in hospice programs. *New England Journal of Medicine* 335: 172–8.

De Geus, A. (1998). *The Living Company: Growth, Learning and Longevity in Business.* London: Nicholas Brealey.

Dougherty, P. (1961). *Mother Mary Potter: Foundress of the Little Company of Mary.* London: Sands, p. 40.

Dunlop, R.J. (1993). Wider applications of palliative care. In Saunders, C. and Sykes, N. (eds), *The Management of Terminal Malignant Disease.* London: Edward Arnold, pp. 287–96.

Gamsa, A. (1994). The role of psychological factors in chronic pain. II. A critical appraisal. *Pain* 57: 17–29.

Hinton, J. (1963). The physical and mental distress of the dying. *Quarterly Journal of Medicine* 32: 1–21.

Hitchcock, L.S., Ferrell, B.R., and McCaffery, M. (1994). The experience of chronic non-malignant pain. *Journal of Pain and Symptom Management* 9: 312–18.

Hockley, J.M., Dunlop, R.J., and Davies, R.J. (1988). Survey of distressing symptoms in dying patients and their families in hospital and the response to a symptom control team. *British Medical Journal* 296: 1715–17.

Kastenbaum, R. (1988). Problems of death and dying. In Gilmore, A. and Gilmore, S. (eds), *Safe Death.* New York: Plenum Press, pp. 3–14.

Kinzbrunner, B.M. (1998). Hospice: 15 years and beyond in the care of the dying. *Journal of Palliative Medicine* 1: 127–37.

Lynn, J., Harrell, F. Jr, Cohn, F., *et al.* (1997). Prognoses of seriously ill hospitalised patients on the days before death: Implications for patient care and public policy. *New Horizons* 5: 56–61.

O'Brien, T., Kelly, M., Saunders, C. (1992). Motor neurone disease: a hospice perspective. *British Medical Journal* 304: 471–3.

Portenoy, R.K. and Foley, K.M. (1986). Chronic use of opioid analgesics in non-malignant pain: report of 38 cases. *Pain* 25: 171–86.

Rothman, S.M. (1994). *Living in the Shadow of Death: Tuberculosis and the Social Experience of Illness in American History.* Baltimore, MD: Johns Hopkins Press.

Saunders, C. (1980). *Hospice Care*. In Ajemian, I. and Mount, B.M. (eds), *The RVH Manual on Palliative/Hospice Care: A Resource Book*. New York: Arno, p. 22.

Seale, C., Cartwright, A. (1994). *The Year before Death*. Aldershot: Avebury Press.

Standing Medical Advisory Committee, Standing Nursing and Midwifery Advisory Committee (1992). *The Principles and Provision of Palliative Care*. London: SMAC, SNMAC.

Stuart, B., Connor, S., Kinzbrunner, B.M., *et al.* (1996). Medical guidelines for determining prognosis in selected non-cancer diseases (2nd edn). Arlington: National Hospice Organisation.

Van Der Heijden, K. (1997). *Scenarios: The Art of Strategic Conversation*. Chichester: Wiley.

Wilkes, E. (ed.) (1982). *The Dying Patient: The medical management of incurable and terminal illness*. Lancaster: MTP Press.

Chapter 16

Patients' perspectives

Cynthia Benz

Introduction

To dare to speak of patients' perspectives is risky. The very title seems to buy into a traditional division. Some are 'doers' in a professional capacity to others who receive the care deemed needful. And the recipients are allowed perspectives.

I both shrink from and am challenged by the invitation to share *patients'* perspectives of palliative care. I find myself uncomfortable with the label of patient, despite its pragmatism. Rather I would seek to explore the mutuality of care. My concern is how one fellow human being cares for another in need. My perspectives are still in their formative stage. What suffering I have so far escaped myself is powerfully obvious in the living and dying of others and expressed through their testimonies.

My personal experience is limited to my own capricious dance, mostly clumsy, rarely supple, and ever variable in speed, with the neurological condition labelled multiple sclerosis (MS). In addition, in professional and volunteer capacities, I have sat alongside others with a myriad of other diagnoses. In the home, counselling room, or hospital ward we have engaged together, struggling to identify for ourselves our need of care for body, soul, and spirit. 'Each of us is unique, yet the story of any one of us is in some measure the story of us all' (Mayne 1995: 8).

I hope that a primary focus on multiple sclerosis will prove sufficiently inclusive of other conditions. A common disease of the central nervous system, MS interrupts and threatens to devastate the lives of (in the main) young people. MS can build up slowly and unannounced or explode like a bombshell that knocks you to the ground. Its impact is felt most keenly in relapses, and hope returns in remissions. However, relapses can blur together, inexorably invading and incapacitating. Living with MS often calls for care that is palliative; and dying of or with MS certainly does.

I am torn between wanting to whisper—for these matters are personal and sensitive—and needing to proclaim. Suffering that is protracted, overlooked, minimised, and inadequately attended to demands a response. Hopefully the range of perspectives that emerge will be recognisable to other patients represented in this book and critically reflect on our collective dilemmas. This is my embryo of becoming 'fulfilled by a gradual build-up of private discoveries' (Blythe, Foreword in Mayne 1995).

What is palliative care? Beginning the search

To the non-user, palliative care is something done for the needy, on offer to those being eased towards and into death. It is hard to grasp what palliative care really is although we are all only 'temporarily able-bodied', prone to cyclic experiences of well-being and liable to flirt with death at any time (Frank 1995). Generally palliative care comes into its own once investigations and treatments have reached an end, and that end is presumed final. When distress becomes visible, support is all. I welcome an initial definition of palliative care as an appropriate response and right of all human beings facing any threatening, degenerative, destructive, or life-taking condition. It must be available at every stage of loss of health, temporary or terminal. It is vital '*the active total care* of patients whose disease is not responsive to curative treatment' may also be 'applicable earlier in the course of the illness' (WHO 1990). Such systems of support for patients, their families and friends need to be practical expressions of an integrative philosophy that 'affirms life and regards dying as a normal process.'

This chapter will seek to explore the palliative care we wish for as we undergo our journey. Good palliative care never negates that strong desire we have to be ourselves and for continuity. 'My old clothes could easily bring back poignant, painful memories. But I see in the clothes a symbol of continuing life. And proof that I still want to be myself. If I must drool, I may as well drool on cashmere' (Bauby 1997: 24). I firmly believe that the 'indivisible nature of human life—the physical, emotional, social, and spiritual'—demands that we learn to incorporate care as a life skill that enhances the quality of living, not simply as a necessity on offer at the end. If we are indeed 'a people who inhabit a broken land between life and death, joy and pain; a people who live from the heart' (Hall 1998: 32), palliative care must focus on the quality and mystery of life, or we will find ourselves 'parching the essence of life of one of its wellsprings' (Mitterand, Foreword in de Hennezel 1997: vii). Sensitivity is needed to balance increasing loss of function with awareness and discovery—perhaps for the first time—of those 'unsuspected resources' within. 'The treasure one has never mined' lies buried in 'the deep neglected registers of our deepest selves' (de Hennezel 1997: 159, 160). Although such resources sound almost ethereal, they are palpably present, simple, natural, gutsy, and real to those in tune with the person being cared for.

Routes

It matters to us how we got to this point of needing care. Our story defines us more than the current decay of our body. We all try to make sense of how we have arrived here. Some are catapulted into the need for palliative care by sudden illness, taken brutally unawares by malfunction of heart, kidneys, or liver. Others have skirted the possibility for a lifetime, hoping to be one of the lucky ones whose remission, careful management, or slow progression of our disease would keep us one degree under, yes, but not that far under. I write this chapter on behalf of all who fall between the categories of 'tourist', the patient who *will recover*, and the 'comatose . . . plunged into endless night' (Bauby 1997: 40)

As in any cross-section of humankind, patients are unique in character, life experience, specific hopes, and fears. Add our particular illness (or cocktail of illnesses), together with the routes negotiated before arriving in need of palliative care, and the countless variables make for a heady mix indeed. Yet right now, not over the threshold of death's door, we are highly aware of our separateness. Differences of culture, education, psychological make-up, and belief systems mean that, despite the labels—'patient in need of care' or 'patient facing imminent decease', we do have differing perspectives.

Lumping patients together as 'a single monolithic entity' neglects the routes by which we have come (Pattison 1989: 11). Even within a single illness experiences and reactions range so widely and wildly that only at the bedrock of human existence do we feel the pulse of commonality in the struggle between life and death. Given that 'there is probably an element of ambiguity in all ways of perceiving and of healing illness', it seems inevitable that those who suffer will not share the same perspectives and neither will those who care for them (Pattison 1989: 17). In addition, if 'not all disorders are best seen within the paradigm of the medical model', this raises the question as to whether the problems of palliative care and dying are not essentially medical either (Pattison 1989: 24).

Expectations and dilemmas

In need of palliative care?

Disease stubbornly disregards society's cry for immediate answers. We expect the medical profession to deliver what we hope for. However, cure is rarely on offer. Honesty and care may be—a discomforting fact possibly more readily accepted by patients than by many in the medical professions.

Few wish to anticipate the need to be looked after—either in old age or illness. Should we land in hospital weak, ill, or in a coma, we reckon we will be glad for the care on offer but somehow picture ourselves too sick to be much bothered—survival will be all that counts. Care is envisioned as a temporary measure, a perspective nursing staff are ready to encourage. No accolades are given to whoever accommodates too readily to being cared for. Independence is fostered by both patient and carer. We are challenged to fight disease by maintaining a positive attitude and mostly do so, cutting more and more corners en route until we find ourselves eroded. There are no more corners to cut.

Sometimes we rationalise that if we must be ill, something clear-cut in its impact and prognosis is preferable. Devastating though any illness is, there is a general consensus that malfunction of heart, kidneys, or blood is somehow explicable. At best it is curable, swiftly fatal, or may be patched up enough to get by for a while. On the other hand, mystery surrounds patients who have had a stroke, or live with neurological conditions like Parkinson's disease, or the results of head injuries. Their varying and variable symptoms, particularly impaired cognition and communication, are discomforting and alienating, improvement unlikely, treatment uncertain, and the knock-on effects unknown. Exhortations to 'hang on in there' and summon more courage to fight on is considered fair enough practice. We learn to live by managing our lives, usually bereft of palliative care. And we can run out of resources and fighting spirit. People do indeed die from multiple sclerosis, Parkinson's, and other chronic diseases. The gradual but relentless build-up to incapacity long-term may lull patient as well as professional and carer into a sense of false security. Sometimes the end is suddenly terminal within days, during which time true palliation is rarely available. It feels as if the non-cancer patient outside of a medical setting is not expected to deteriorate and die. But die we do.

To be excluded in time of need and dire distress is a cruel anomaly in the arena of health care, no matter whether it results from paucity of provision, thoughtlessness, disbelief at to the severity of our ailments, or misconceptions about what conditions are life-threatening.[1] How many suffer agonising slow deaths, their carers at home similarly worn to breaking point, because no one recognises their plight? When even the articulate voice is ignored, what chance do the mumbling majority stand? Too often it takes the intervention of an authority figure, willing to pull strings and rank, to shame the system into providing care. Tragically there are too few saviours to champion wider provision of palliative care and too many in need.

> I believe now is the time to grasp the nettle and try and work out what signs, symptoms and investigation results point towards the need for early palliation. We need hard facts so that we can actually know rather than just hope we are doing what is best for our patients. Without more research in this area we are in danger of failing to meet the palliative care needs of a large number of dying patients.

> (Jarrett 1997)

Tailoring care

Any illness 'catapults us into an undiscovered world of limitations. We live in bodies that restrict our choices. We perceive strong links between our symptoms and our reactions. We reason that care packages need to address these' (Benz 1997). Most get on with making the best of each day, forgetting any bad experiences of the past. Our approach is pragmatic and realistic, without dismissing hope. We have experience of pushing back the limits of endurance. Beyond lies a sensitive zone of transition where we still expect the right to 'quantify the quality of life'.[2] We set personal criteria as to what constitutes such quality, inevitably changing the goalposts as illnesses progress and tolerance increases out of necessity. We develop expertise in managing our condition, learning to accommodate deterioration and renegotiate control of our lives. We look for care that reflects our inner and social worlds. Too often care is perfunctory, and practical, an informed nursing response to the clearly visible need for physical care. We long for someone who cares for the totality that is us. When plummeted into needing palliative care, J was surprised to experience a totally new concept of care, in which the 'whole problem of J' was addressed. 'Enveloped in love within a peaceful setting, after being abandoned, stranded and without help', she emerged confident, enabled to clarify her needs for the first time and also face her dying.[2] There is 'a way of taking care of a body that makes one forget all physical damage, because it is the whole person that is being enveloped in tenderness. It is a way of taking care of a dying man (or woman or child) that allows him (or her) to feel that his soul is alive until the very end' (de Hennezel 1997: 4).

How those receiving palliative care feel about it is largely anecdotal. It is intrusive to question someone who is dying. If you are intimately and sensitively attuned with that person

---

[1] In such circumstances sadly we might even wish we had cancer instead—only because then our condition might be deemed more worthy of attention and care.

[2] I wish to express warm appreciation to all who agreed to talk to me about this experiences and perspectives as receivers or givers of care. In particular I acknowledge with gratitude: P. Ashmore, C. Bar-Isaac, G. Burton, F. Campling, R-A. Canning, C. Dann, M. Dickson, J. Glennon, C. Gould, J. Henderson, V. Lewis, J. MacDonald, D. Rook, S. Tomlinson & R. Wigmore.

you may glimpse and share what it is like to be moving towards death. A privilege indeed. Further appreciation of what issues are crucial may come from those whose illnesses relapse and remit or from those suspended at a point of suffering, who find a way of sharing the experience. Most of us are very willing to discuss our success in managing our care thus far but hesitate to speculate further.[3]

Or we can shut our minds completely to the realities through fear. This may result in our refusing care or demanding it ahead of need. The label of saint or sinner is self-imposed as often as not. How people deal with losses, including loss of health and life, helps explain our differing reactions. Once we accept responsibility for our reactions, we may invest in removing some of the barriers we raise unwittingly against care.

Fears

Facing the unknown is frightening. Of all emotions that colour our living and dying, fear lurks longest: general fears for the future and how we'll cope, and fears for those we love and must leave. We fear those early visible margins to be negotiated, not being able to walk or drive. We fear not being able to address our own personal needs. We can hardly contemplate being unable to communicate. We fear how we might get round the encroachments of cognitive malfunction. We do not want to be sidelined before our time comes for the final off-line. We experience panic as, in our deterioration, we maintain fewer links with the outside world and find ourselves severed from ways of expressing ourselves previously taken for granted. 'My mind teems with new ideas, fresh projects: can I acquire the technology to communicate them? Can I acquire the time? Sometimes I feel as if I am trapped in a runaway train that will inevitably crash into the terminus' (Richards 1990: 104). We fear being left alone, without a voice, and unattended, particularly in a hospital setting.

We fear the loss of dignity. Of all single words, dignity is mentioned most often. It matters that we retain our identity and self-worth. Vaughan resolved his dilemma over taking drugs or letting Parkinson's disease show by choosing 'the moderately "off" state in which I am coping by drawing on stored resources. . . . These magic moments are the only times when I am whole again and unpossessed' (Vaughan 1986: 200). Perhaps 'having the disease is just another way of *being* in the know' about life.[4] We fear being taken over by seductive potions of drugs and therapies that will extend life, hopefully free of physical pain, but at what cost to our emotional, mental, and spiritual selves? 'I will never beat MS and it won't beat me. I don't want to say we co-habit although we do. We do more than co-exist. It's like having a ringside seat at my own disintegration.'[3] Some of us will put up with a lot to stay real.

We have contradictory fears about the provision of care. We erect barriers against being seen in need of support. Sometimes we even resist carers who desperately want to make it better for all the right reasons. And we would certainly want to push away those who in their caring do so more for themselves than for us. We fear no system of care will support and contain us, and that care will be too long coming. We also fear the system will swallow us up

---

3 Notable exceptions are courageous people like Annie Lindsell and Jane MacDonald, bonded by their belief that voluntary euthanasia should be made a safeguarded option.

4 Jonathan Miller ponders whether 'there is a sense in which he [Vaughan] is more "himself" when off the drug than when he is relieved of symptoms and on it' (Vaughan 1986, Introduction: xiv).

without escape, bar death. We are unsure if palliative care is on general offer or by prescription only.[5] We desperately want reassurance that, at our dying especially, care will include support and encouragement for us as well as for those close to us. They deserve it in bountiful supply, full measure and running over. And so do we.[6]

Quality of life

Care is something of a dilemma. We are ambivalent about care. Even when we need care, we fear being taken over, to the point that a significantly high proportion of us contemplates the provision of voluntary euthanasia as a desirable future option. We worry about the sacrifices those close to us have to make. We dread the non-availability of services. We fear witnessing our personhood slipping away as a result of a disease-ravaged body and the sheer necessity of being cared for in order to survive—rather like being present at our own long drawn-out wake.

(Benz 1997: 8)

Today's multidisciplinary care teams do more than comfort the afflicted. They combine caring with testing, measuring, and monitoring, most of which reassures us that treatments can be effective and even cures hover on the horizon. This spells hope to any newly initiated to illness and disease. But patients are concerned with quality as well as quantity, and judging what constitutes the quality of another person's existence is not easy. Maintaining quality of life may be the right of every individual but patients soon realise that we are in no strong position to insist on our choices. Each has only one voice in the chorus of all who jostle to contribute to the 'quality of life package' deemed reasonable. So who does determine quality of life in theory *and* practice?

Traditional questionnaires focus on how far function and pain affect the patient, but are only indicative of health status. Quality of life is determined by what a person says it is. Hence, the individual variations.[7] There is often a mismatch between what is important to the patient and the assumptions of others. Patients target and seek compensation for areas of life affected by their long-standing illnesses (Bowling 1996). For example, those with arthritis most value getting out and going shopping. Patients with gastrointestinal disorders are most concerned about dietary restrictions while those with mental health problems prioritise securing a job.

....

[5] The section on severe disability in 'The 1997 Standards of Health care for People with MS' states the key issues are providing appropriate, long-term care facilities, adequate community care and community mobility, access to information, expertise, communication, co-ordination and respite care. However, little choice is available, especially for young severely disabled people, who discover a dearth of palliative care.

[6] I am struck by the way patients are assumed passive and unresponsive when dying. I trust continuing support and encouragement are implicit in the management aims but Aim 3 specifies it for carers only. (*Changing Gear—Guidelines for Managing the Last Days of Life in Adults*, Working Party on Clinical Guidelines in Palliative Care, December 1997).

[7] First-hand evidence comes from research commissioned by The MS Society into the attitudes of people with MS to living with the disease compared with those of their carers at home and professionals. The range of individual preference recorded by those with MS was frequently judged too wide of the mark, as if those giving care considered themselves more in the know than those in need of it.

Tailoring treatment or care plans to the individual's own priorities makes sense. Health may not be our first choice, nor even figure in our top five. Health often comes further down in the list. Even pain relief may not be most important. Many express more concern about social interaction with family and friends, and staying alert and aware. This demands a reformulation of care, based less on treating diseases and more on treating people. It takes time and skill to encourage patients to pinpoint the most important areas of life for them and also how important they are in relation to each other. Patient participation in such reviews is not only beneficial in practice but invites personal investment too. It encourages contributing 'an opinion as opposed to just answering a question'. Unless the patient can state a preference, even a close relative may not be relied upon to know what the patient's own perception of quality of life is. It is high time that patients' own assessments were built into health care provision. Combining patients' priorities with good basic care would result in the quality of life patients want for themselves, and perhaps even an underspend in budgets. Presumably improved rapport all round would also have a positive effect.

Independence versus dependence

'Yet again I gave way to the conflict between wanting other people to see to my needs and at the same time wishing to be independent' (Vaughan 1986: 24). The dilemma of maintaining a balance between independence and dependence disturbs at every level of our existence. Accepting physical care of our bodies is an obvious struggle. Bauby graphically describes how his perspectives of care could change dramatically from one day to the next.

> One day, for example, I can find it amusing, in my 45th year, to be cleaned up and turned over, to have my bottom wiped and swaddled like a new-born's. I even derive a guilty pleasure from this total lapse into infancy. But the next day, the same procedure seems unbearably sad, and a tear rolls down through the lather a nurse's aide spreads over my cheeks.
>
> (Bauby 1997: 24)

There is powerlessness in being done to and increasing dependency creates a dilemma.

> During my illness I have gained fresh insight into many situations: into the frustration of a small child who lacks the words to communicate his needs; into the anguish of an old person struggling to maintain independence and yet hampered by a slowing body; into the painful emotions of a person coming to terms with his total dependence on other people.
>
> (Richards 1990: 107)

'Hang on a sec . . . ' while carers disappear for a while is doubly frustrating if you are left literally hanging, dangling in a hoist.[3] Swinging helpless in mid-air leaves time to ponder how much personal empowerment has already been given up. Little wonder care may be viewed as a put-down, a cutting down to size. While asking for help may make us better people, we also realise that there is no onus on anyone to give us help. Empowerment is achieved by developing an inner supply of emotional and mental strength to compensate for increasing weakness and impaired communication. Hanging around leaves us time to think—and sometimes to seethe.

Health care professionals report little resistance to care. Patients are understandably grateful for any help on offer. Such gratitude may mask inner turmoil. To know you need looking after, probably for the last time, brings us to a forlorn brink of almost giving up in order to give over to others. It can feel like being written off. We struggle with death looming coupled with the fear of carers walking away. Apprehension may be covered by winning ways: a smile or joke to ease the way. The balance between feeling humbled or humiliated by care is fine indeed. In down moments we find gnawing away inside ambivalence over having to rely on others to fulfil the everyday essentials we wouldn't dream of letting anyone else handle. What is acceptable as routine care in a medical setting may feel intrusive elsewhere, even when we are dying. All too often at an early stage in our dying we miss out on the nourishment of sensuality and sexuality, as if our bodies are given over to a public domain. Yet still we crave intimacy and belonging and long for touch to comfort and affirm us.[8]

Of course there are those who tense up and stubbornly resist being cared for. Sticking with the difficult ones even when they erect barriers is trying but necessary because of safety issues. Neurological dysfunction can result in many types of damage. Failing memory and lack of motivation are among the more easily recognised symptoms. Less obvious but most significant is a glaring lack of insight and sensitivity in patients, which places them in the category of awkward customers.

Who cares . . . and when?

Who can be expected to provide the care needed? Seamless care from cradle to grave sounds brilliant. However, it may only be a sanitised concept that placates health care providers into believing they have done their job and lulls prospective recipients of care into a sense of easy continuum. Can seamless care exist? Patients in need of care can fall between many divides. Generally we assume the most appropriate care will be medical but it could equally well be psychological, social, or spiritual, or a pot pourri offering. Thus a multidisciplinary approach to palliative care is needed, a practice that is informed, pragmatic, and responsive to real patients.

It is becoming increasingly difficult to access care from within the home circle and the friend and neighbour network. The social and economic facts of life mitigate against traditional assumptions of support and care being available at grass roots level. Patients living alone seem most vulnerable, but increasingly, younger patients urge that issues of care be realistically addressed. Some with a strong wish to remain in control at home operate their own health care budget and buy in the care they want. They want to be involved in determining the type of care and carers needed and when. Patients with similar backgrounds might prove more demanding of palliative care.

The timing of care is obvious in emergency situations, a specialty within a medical setting. Life saving is a priority, an unambiguous decision for all but a minority. Hospital patients never fail to express surprise at being attended to swiftly and praise the quality of health care and dedication of the staff. Others, with chronic conditions, nursed at home by family or community carers also endorse high levels of care. However, the balancing of

---

[8] Although touch is open to misunderstanding, medical staff and chaplains frequently comment how reassuring patients find touch to be. I am grateful to Rev. Hilary Johnson and Rev. Elizabeth Jackson for their input.

patients' personal needs and wishes with issues of standardised care and safety can become an arena in which debate, perceived wisdom, and territorial rights juggle for supremacy. This often masks how slowly many domestic emergencies are resolved, especially when lines of communication between disciplines break down and the good of the patient is unclear. Also masked is the burden of care resting upon carers who are such out of the goodness of their hearts. Many reach breaking point and jeopardise health and sanity.

One common hurdle in care-giving is coping with guilt. Inadequate care may be tolerated in order to keep the peace. We feel guilty about getting stuck in no-win predicaments: if we remain at home, we become nuisances and, if removed, we fear the disintegration of the family. This is more likely when the caregivers are family or friends but outside carers too can easily get sucked into a dependency relationship unawares. Guilt affects both those in need of care and carers. Caring can easily become a burden to carers, restricting family activity, and resulting in isolation and entrapment. Anyone unable to offer more care risks feeling inadequate and guilt-laden. Hardly surprising then that escape becomes desirable or depression an option that retains sanity.

One crux of the problem is around boundaries. In a professional setting such as a hospital, residential home, or hospice, safeguards are built in. When providing *quality care* permeates the total ethos of a caring establishment, there is enough safety within caring to invite reciprocity. Both caregivers and care-receivers 'who spontaneously express compassion probably have no idea how much good they do' (de Hennezel 1997: 6). However, boundaries between carer and cared-for are not easily negotiated. Once caring becomes a regular focus of the relationship, the demandingness of care can take over and destroy relationships, an experience of

> . . . grappling with my fears
>
> Of God knows what
>
> Well, I know one that's worse
>
> Than all the rest
>
> My wife's become my nurse.[9]

Facing death

Faced with the process of dying we discover ourselves still very much alive. The inevitability of death need not diminish the process of living. We may remain long incredulous that dying should be our lot. It definitely goes against the grain. So much so that denial of the reality of our condition is a common response. 'As though somebody who is dying is driving around in an old car which he will soon get rid of, and yet keeps on nagging about the new tyres the car needs' (Keiser 1996: 100). In a culture that values productivity, the message is clearly to get on and die. Hanging on to life is messy and disruptive. 'We want the dying to be consistent, a thing we would never demand of those who live on' (Keiser 1996: 100).

Bauby, in one swoop felled from active life into incarceration by locked-in syndrome, discovered the movement of one eyelid his only link with the world outside his head. Through

---

[9] From 'The Worst Fear' by George MacBeth.

this flicker of eye-muscle he dictated his need 'to feel strongly, to love and admire, just as desperately as I need to breathe'. Still young, frozen within, and assaulted by his body state, he determined to remain alert and 'avoid slumping into resigned indifference' and managed to 'maintain a level of resentment and anger, neither too much nor too little, just as a pressure-cooker has a safety-valve to keep it from exploding' (Bauby 1997: 60).

Others who experience the long relentless erosion of chronic illness, with spells of improvement displaced by onslaughts of deterioration, get tired out: the end is all there is to give in to. And even then, despite relentless physical deterioration, the incredulity of reaching death's door. 'I'm not dying, am I?' How do you prepare anyone for the inevitability of death? Especially when he is also profoundly deaf and his eyes dimming—are there words to mouth or looks to share the truth that he is dying indeed? Not all have the opportunity or courage to look death in the eye, knowing they are playing 'a winning loser', but determined to plan a good death. Dying is not a choice but how we face it is. The ultimate in challenges: struggling with living deaths or experiencing dying lives. 'I didn't think I could ever live like this' is a cry from the heart echoed by many. Perhaps if we could look at dying head on, we would be enabled to live better. Not to know we are dying, disempowers us, negates us before we reach the terminus. We might do well to consider how to integrate life into dying rather than denying death its place. Its prospect 'pushes us to enter into the heart and depth' of what living is about (de Hennezel 1997: xi). A place with open doors that welcomes and delights in caring is a true haven.[10] Those in need of palliative care often feel unprotected in a hospital environment, where other patients with different needs prove disruptive and disturbing. Many discover that 'a place dedicated to receiving the dying can be the diametrical opposite of a house of death—that is, a place where life is manifested in all its force.' From such a place the dying send the message: 'Don't pass by life; don't pass by love' (de Hennezel 1997: 10, xiv).

In dreams begin responsibilities

We dream of care that grows out of relationships of respect, in which patients and carers engage in mutual enjoyment of caring, comfort, and kindness. Care is received and given as a natural response to need. Palliative care is more than just nurse skills.[11] It combines sharing, communication, and 'an interchange of love'. Care promises a steady and inexhaustible flow of support at every stage of living and dying. It understands the jangled interface between who the patient really is and the eroding impact of disease. We are not always sure where we and our illnesses begin and end. You respect our will to fight on but gently shore us up and unobtrusively take over the burdens we let fall. The essence of care transcends systems and resides beyond them.

The care we dream of is delivered with reassurance, born of experience, integrity, and compassion. It encourages us to value each new day afresh, especially the day of death. It neither patronises nor cajoles but accepts the status quo with grace and creativity. It knows to maximise but never with pressure.

---

[10] I wish to pay tribute to all such havens. In particular, I want to thank the staff of Beaumond House in Newark, who made me feel as if I belonged.

[11] The inspiration for this section came from Ruth Ann Cannings, who was Jacqueline du Pre's nurse and companion for 13 years until her death.

Such care always keeps a window of communication open. We would ask you to do more than hear when we speak of our needs. We would like you to listen. And, should our voices fail, watch for the way our bodies still communicate. We can learn together day-to-day as we go along. The warm reassurance of your touch means much. The care of our dreams reassures us that we are not burdens. It does not seize control from us ahead of time. Care glides in to ease burdens with graciousness. It gently shows us how to live within our disability, thus releasing you, our carers, to live, too. We need to learn how to accept our different and complementary roles, with no superiority implied. You attend to our needs as they develop. If carers are there to be what patients cannot be, an extension of us in our dependency, that means you are almost giving us your lives. You may also need to teach us by example how to seek nurture and space at a distance from us. To maintain our dignity we must learn this, too, and so discover new dimensions to our living. We value the precious gift of your care and the extra mile you travel.

We dream of care that supports enough to face death calmly once we have learnt 'to savour every moment of being alive' and 'know how to stand still and listen to the soft rustling of existence' (de Hennezel 1997: 00). Above all it reassures us that someone will stay alongside for 'patients need accompanying on that last journey'.[12]

> I, the patient, still exist as a human being,
>
>> not as I would wish to be
>>
>>> but still myself.
>
> I am in a process of change
>
>> — in a shutting down mode —
>>
>> perhaps detaching and floating free,
>>
>> without the vigour and input of what I was
>>
>> and what you knew me to be
>>
>> or the reverse
>>
>> raging in a last ditch stand
>>
>>> to cling on to who I identified myself as.
>
> I am the focus of care,
>
>> centre of stage for a while:
>>
>> either the dying fly in the ointment
>>
>> or the icon.
>
> While I live on in my dying I have needs.
>
>> I do not know how much leeway I can reasonably expect.
>>
>> These are uncharted waters for single craft only.
>>
>> I do not wish to be demanding
>>
>> or use my deteriorating condition to manipulate advantage.
>>
>> I want to end with the integrity I have chosen to live by.

---

[12] Attributed to Dame Cecily Saunders.

I am afraid of the process of dying,
>especially the pain.

I do not know what is ahead.
>Of death I am uncertain
>But so wearied I only care to be at peace.

I have my hopes and fears.

At best I cling to a faith I believe trustworthy.

I am in the hands of my carers
>And already on the way to not being here at all.

Those identifying marks that sum me up are running out:
>they have had their day.

I wish for tenderness of touch,
>love in your voice,
>and compassion for my indignity,
>should I fail to be magnificent in my dying.

Copyright, Cynthia Benz, June 1998

References

Bauby, J-D. (1997). *The Diving-Bell and the Butterfly*. London: Fourth Estate, London.

Benz, C. (1997). Setting the agenda for disease management and patient care in MS. *Update*, vol. 11.

Bowling, A. (1996). The effects of illness on quality of life: findings from a survey of households in Great Britain. *Journal of Epidemiology and Community Health* 50(2): 146–55.

de Hennezel, M. (1997). *Intimate Death—How the Dying Teach Us to Live*. London: Little, Brown.

Frank, A. (1995). *The Wounded Storyteller: Body, Illness, and Ethics*. Chicago, IL: University of Chicago.

Hall, K. (1998). Reflections: Living in a L'Arche community. *Contact* 125: 32.

Jarrett, D. (1997). Palliative care and stroke. *Stroke Matters* 1: 4.

Keizer, B. (1996). *Dancing with Mister D*. London: Transworld Publishers.

MacBeth, G. (1992). *The Patient*. London: Hutchinson.

Mayne, M. (1995). *This Sunrise of Wonder—Letters for the Journey*. London: Fount Paperbacks.

Pattison, S. (1989). *Alive and Kicking*. London: SCM Press.

Richards, J. (1990). *Love Never Ends*. Oxford: Lion Publishing.

Vaughan, I. (1986). *Ivan—Living with Parkinson's Disease*. London: Macmillan.

WHO (1990). *Cancer, Pain Relief and Palliative Care*. Technical Report Series 804. Geneva: World Health Organisation.

Chapter 17

Reforming care through continuous quality improvement

Joanne Lynn

Introduction

Anyone working with those near death in the US at the start of the twenty-first century will recognise the disastrous state of care most patients and families face. Even if most people at the end of life have no overwhelming symptoms and no serious gaps in care, so many people have such bad experiences that everyone fears disaster. Everyone gradually realises that nothing that he or she can do will guarantee that the care system will serve their needs. Few people can look back upon the period of time they or a loved one spent with a serious illness and find that it was meaningful in human terms, or take comfort in the experience of caring for another human being.

This bleak situation persists despite the better strategies we know are possible. Many people have found a safe haven in hospice care, or in the care of a skilled home care or nursing home nurse. Palliative care programmes have shown that virtually all patients with cancer can be kept comfortable. Although much of what is routinely done is not what patients value, providers seem all too sluggish in implementing better plans.

The reform efforts made often fail. In one large study, improved counselling, making outcome probabilities available, and identifying patient preferences were insufficient to change patient experiences (SUPPORT Principal Investigators 1995). Multiple studies of advance directives have failed to show that increased rates of advance directives improve patient outcomes (Teno *et al.* 1997; Schneiderman *et al.* 1992). Rates of serious pain in different populations have stayed discouragingly constant (Committee on Care at the End of Life 1997), and expenses at the end of life have not changed over a score of years (Lubitz *et al.* 1995).

When professionals look at reform, they have mostly considered proceeding by way of formal research, enhanced professional education, and major changes in reimbursement. Formal research is important in defining better drugs or procedures, but it is often surprisingly ineffective in changing practice. Useful observations routinely require a generation to be widely implemented, and few studies directly tackle the questions of health care delivery which stand as barriers to widespread success. Professional education is simply not what prevents good care. What it is essential to know to take care of most cancer pain could be taught in a day. Clearly, the reason that many oncologists admit that they do not know how to handle opioid drugs (Von Roenn *et al.* 1993) cannot really be attributed to a lack of education. It would be too easy to get the facts. Furthermore, no education endeavour on its own has been shown to improve end-of-life care substantially. Thus, the first two strategies rarely accomplish much on their own. The last, altered reimbursement to enhance end-of-life care, rarely can be achieved. Powerful forces act to retain the status quo or to sustain the livelihoods of those who are doing well in the current situation. In the US, only the advent of hospice care under our Medicare programme for the elderly stands out as an example of a reimbursement reform to improve end-of-life care—the only one in over twenty years!

Maybe there is a better way. Seeing the persistent shortcomings of various other strategies, more and more organisations are turning to the techniques of continuous quality improvement (CQI). It is not an easy approach, nor is it foolproof or necessarily reliable. However, it does seem to be better, for most issues in most circumstances, than our former strategies.

Basically, CQI demands persistent effort to keep finding ways to do better tomorrow than you did today. It requires constructing and adhering to a vision of how to provide better care. It requires assembling a team committed to making improvement happen. Then it requires a series of possible changes to be tested, quickly, to try to find the ones that really work; and it requires that steps to make those permanent are taken. It builds a deep understanding of how the system works and what might work to make improvements. It is akin to clinical audit, and involves a similar cyclical process of deciding how things ought to be, of measuring what is actually happening, of implementing improvements, and of measuring whether changes have resulted (Higginson 1993). The chapter will return to a more detailed characterisation of how this CQI process works; first the reader should see what kinds of results it is obtaining.

Results of continuous quality improvement in one national collaborative effort

In July 1997, we started working with 48 separate organisations in a collaborative effort to improve care for the end of life. They included 7 hospices, 30 hospitals, 1 home care agency, 1 site for 'the Program of All Inclusive Care of the Elderly,' and 9 integrated care systems. Each set its own goals, but all helped one another via meetings, conference calls, and e-mail to find ways to improve rapidly. Here are some of their results.

Many teams tackled pain. One hospital based team found, much to their chagrin, that the average cancer patient waited three hours for the first dose of medicine in response to a problem with pain. The reasons were many—all manner of routines, regulations, and low prioritisation. The CQI team started to chip away at the problem—reducing the average response time to one hour, with just a few months' work. Another CQI team found that they could get better medications quicker by authorising an on-the-scene nurse to make adjustments within an agreed range. Many teams found that pain was simply being ignored, and that it was important to require measuring pain as 'a fifth vital sign.'

One hospice team reported virtually annihilating dyspnoea in a hospice population. They started with about half of their patients having frightening shortness of breath at any one time. The team started by prioritising responsiveness, and proceeded to having a physician-endorsed protocol for treatment, having a physician in back-up if the primary attending physician did not respond or the problem persisted, having appropriate opioid drugs in stock (ready to give with a phone call) for housebound patients. The rate of severe dyspnoea lasting more than eight hours by the nurses' assessment fell to nearly zero, after half a year's work.

The leading health care providers of La Crosse, Wisconsin, embarked upon a community-wide effort to improve advance care planning (Hammes and Rooney 1998). In a remarkable collaboration, they instructed elderly persons in senior centres, sick persons as they came to the physician, and ordinary citizens through the mass media. They expanded their vision to include comprehensive advance care planning, aiming to anticipate possible emergencies and to articulate preferences about how the end of life would be lived. In a rare population based analysis, the community reported 85% of over 500 decedents having an advance directive at the time of death—and these were written, on average, more than a year ahead of death. In La Crosse, 98% of decedents had deliberately foregone some procedure to allow death to come. Even more remarkably, virtually all of the advance directives seem to have been followed. How did La Crosse accomplish all this? By having a CQI team with a goal, supporting it through an array of interventions and assessments, and broad implementation of efforts that worked!

Many teams worked on family support. Perhaps it is a mark of just how shabby our usual care is, but virtually every team that worked on family support succeeded in making improvements that mattered. Some initiated bereavement support. Some tackled anger-generating insensitivity in the usual care system. Many hospitals, for example, were sending the final bill to the now-dead patient. Families did not see this with humour—they saw it as one more indication that no one really cared. Other groups worked on ensuring that there was follow-up contact with family after a death. Two provided beepers to family caregivers at home or to families holding vigil in a hospital, allowing family to be absent for a short sleep or to run errands without feeling out-of-touch. One provided a place for families to shower and nap while a loved one was in the hospital. Each of these groups assessed patient and family experience before and after testing changes and can show that the new approaches actually generated improvements.

One team initiated a clever and effective largely volunteer effort. Franciscan Health System in Tacoma, Washington, freed up 50% time for a skilled nurse and 20% time for a chaplain, who then worked with a team of concerned providers to recruit a bevy of local volunteers. Physicians identified those patients who were 'sick enough to die in the next six months'. Volunteers called these patients every few weeks, trying to be a friendly voice and to note things that might be going badly. They notified the nurse, who acted as a community care manager. Patients did better, used more local resources, and came into hospice earlier than a control group in a parallel clinic with no special programme; four-fifths reported being more satisfied with care since the programme began—and the programme paid for itself.

Our teams learned some other quite generalisable things. Most practitioners in the American scene use a 'mental model' of having a (long) phase in the course of eventually fatal illness in which the major effort is to cure or substantially modify the time course of the illness. The mental model goes on to assume a (short) phase of 'dying', in which the person clearly loses ground and during which treatments should be aimed at comfort. The 'trick' is to identify the 'just right' time at which to 'switch from cure to care' (Callahan 1993). Of course, this switch is notoriously difficult to time. Recent evidence shows, for example, that the median person who died of congestive heart failure today had at least a 50–50 chance to live 6 months—yesterday (Lynn *et al.* 1997). Even with colon and lung cancer, the median chance to survive 2 months is over 20% on the day before death, and over 50% one week earlier. So, most people will die shortly after having had an ambiguous prognosis.

When our teams first tried to identify 'dying' patients at whom to target their interventions, most asked physicians to name the 'dying.' Only a few patients were named, and they were, on the whole, very late in the course of their illness. It seemed that physicians had learned to identify people late enough that there were essentially no errors. So, teams came up with what we came to call the 'surprise' question. We asked physicians to identify patients who 'were sick enough that it would not be surprising if he or she died in the next six months'. Interestingly, it doesn't matter whether you ask about six months or a year—the point is that the question encourages physicians to notice that some patients are very sick while making clear that some of them are still expected to live a long time. Using this approach, more patients were identified, far enough before death to make a difference in their lives. Some, of course, should continue to receive aggressive life-sustaining treatment—not 'palliative care only'.

Finally, we learned that no team made substantial strides with professional education endeavours alone, though many focused on it before moving on to other efforts. A few teams also spent considerable time in measurement work, as if they were mounting a major research project rather than a rapid improvement. This approach was almost always an ineffective use of time and energy. The things people care about are actually easy enough to measure, at least enough to be sure that changes are truly improvements.

Assessing CQI

How does one assess such changes? Clearly, these changes are important in the life of their sponsoring organisations. One does not need randomised designs or large numbers to believe that something important is happening when a hospital unit cuts its pain response time by two-thirds, or when a hospice appears to effectively respond to dyspnoea. CQI is valuable in making important, progressive, incremental gains. If the vision of an improved system is strong and achievable, as it often is with end-of-life care, CQI provides a way to make large and sustainable strides in a care system quickly. The growth over the past two decades of quality assurance programmes, including CQI and clinical audit, is at least in part a reflection of the success of such approaches in bringing about real changes in patient and family care (Higginson 1993). This provides further evidence of the value of CQI.

What does CQI find more difficult to achieve? It is hard to generate teams to work across programme lines. Although it seems obvious that a nursing home, hospital, hospice, and home care agency who serve the same patients over time are all part of one care system, that is not at all the way they see it. None of our teams were able to engender co-operation across care programmes. The La Crosse, Wisconsin, effort on advance directives is an illuminating example of rare success.

It is also hard to get the gains made in one place with one team to be replicated or generalised. It is not impossible—good ideas gradually get champions. However, it is striking that there are few places to describe good ideas in this arena. The results are usually too uncontrolled and under-powered statistically to be acceptable in research publications. The results are sometimes even perceived as risky—either because they show just how deficient care was at initiation or because better care might attract costly or otherwise undesired patients.

In response to the paucity of dissemination opportunities, Americans for Better Care of the Dying has engendered a newsletter largely devoted to coverage of early efforts at quality improvement in end-of-life care. ABCD exchange has been available since October 1997, mailed to subscribers in hard copy or for free (and indexed) at http://www.abcd-caring.org. ABCD exchange has been joined by a more formal on-line journal, called *Innovations in End of Life Care* and found at http://www.edc.org/lastacts. Both are referenced in the Growth House information service, at http://www.growthhouse.org, making them widely available to persons in all settings and countries.

Like clinical audit and other related processes (Higginson 1993), CQI is a good way to learn what can be achieved in improving care within the current environment, as shaped by reimbursement patterns as well as professional skills and practices. When done in an array of settings, CQI illuminates which environments encourage which reforms. In our work, we learned a great deal from the presence of public hospitals, veterans hospitals, hospices, poverty-serving home care agencies, managed care organisations, and fee-for-service organisations. Nevertheless, it is unusual that any organisation can fully escape the effects of adverse financing or abjectly untrained professionals. So, the full range of potential reform requires work on multiple fronts.

How to start in CQI

Any provider organisation can improve its practices; improvement may be especially easy in end-of-life care, which has been such a backwater of health care for so long. There are many approaches to CQI, some of which are quite ponderous. The approach we used is a streamlined, rapid cycle approach championed by Nolan (Nolan 1998; Berwick and Nolan 1998). However, it is important to create a climate of welcoming change in the organisation, so a number of early successes are quite helpful. Reformers would do well to think strategically—which improvements can be had quickly, which are visible and seen by leaders to be important, and which ones are risky.

You will need a mission—a clear sense of what is worth working to achieve. That mission might be relatively simple: eliminate overwhelming pain in patients with advanced cancer, for example. The goal might be complex: make care seamless across providers so that patients' transfers are comfortable and so that their care plans do not change along with a change of location or provider.

You will need a team suited to working on this mission. Be sure to include a powerful champion—in the US, that usually means a physician leader or a CEO (chief executive) who cares that the mission succeeds and who will help move obstacles. Be sure to include key 'front-line' providers who know the problem first hand. Part of the success of CQI depends upon the intimate knowledge of people who make the current dysfunctional system work—they often quickly discern a dozen things that could be done better. It also helps to have someone experienced in quality improvement as a facilitator and cheerleader.

You will need to answer three questions in such a way that the responses are all congruent:

♦ What do we want to accomplish?

♦ How will we know if changes amount to improvements (for patients, preferably)?

♦ What changes could be tried?

When your team has answers to these questions, you will undoubtedly have multiple changes that could be tried. You might want to eliminate a wasteful step, or use a different practitioner to do a certain thing for patients, or implement a treatment guideline. You can get ideas from team members, from the professional literature, and from similarly situated teams in other organisations.

How do you pick where to start? So long as you have reason to believe that you can detect improvement—and that each of the changes is likely to lead to improvement—what usually matters most is to get something under way quickly—while people still believe that change is possible and that they can make it happen.

Don Berwick, President of the Institute for Healthcare Improvement, is fond of exhorting teams: 'What can you do by Tuesday?' In fact, you usually don't need to wait until Tuesday! What can you do today or tomorrow? One trick is to start small—try something on a few patients, the patients of a few doctors, or with a few nurses—whatever allows you to test a change. You will know if the change is going to work and adjust your plan before you earn a negative reputation. If the idea works well, you will have some evidence to ease your way into spreading the idea.

Each idea for change should be thoughtfully subjected to 'Plan-Do-Study-Act' cycles:

◆ Make a plan to try out the idea for change and measure its effects;

◆ Implement that plan—'Do';

◆ Study the effects—and learn from them;

◆ Act upon what you have learned—modify the change, extend it to new populations, try another, whatever is appropriate—and make a plan for the next PDSA cycle.

Of course, teams will want to run multiple cycles simultaneously. Cycles can build upon one another. Teams may chart half a dozen measures over time to see if changes keep making improvements and to be sure that their work is adding up. Time series charts are especially helpful in tracing effective interventions, but 'before' and 'after,' or 'control' and 'intervention,' comparisons might be a more efficient method.

This overview is all too brief. Those who are intrigued may want to pursue some training or further reading (Schuster *et al.* 1999). You can find opportunities for both on the web site for the Institute for Health care Improvement at http://www.ihi.org. In co-operation with the Center to Improve Care of the Dying, Growth House is offering an on-line communication service for professionals involved in quality improvement in advanced heart and lung disease (and eventually other related topics) at http://growthhouse.net/~chf-copdnet. Good resources for reading, including the Annals of Internal Medicine series 'Physicians as Leaders in Improving Health Care', are also available.

References

Berwick, D.M. and Nolan, T.W. (1998). Physicians as leaders in improving health care: a new series. *Annals of Internal Medicine* **128**(4): 289–2.

Callahan, D. (1993). *The Troubled Dream of Life: Living with Mortality.* New York: Touchstone/Simon and Shuster.

Committee on Care at the End of Life, Division of Health Care Services, Institute of Medicine. (1997). In Field, M.J. and Cassel, C.K. (eds), *Approaching Death: Improving Care at the End of Life.* Washington, DC: National Academy Press.

Hammes, B.J. and Rooney, B.L. (1998). Death and end-of-life planning in one midwestern community. *Archives of Internal Medicine* **158**(4): 383–90.

Higginson, I. (ed.) (1993). *Clinical Audit in Palliative Care.* Oxford: Radcliffe Medical Press.

Lubitz, J., Beebe, J., and Baker, C. (1995). Longevity and Medicare expenditures *New England Journal of Medicine* **332**(15): 999–1003.

Lynn, J. (1997). Clinical crossroads: an 88-year-old woman facing the end of life. *Journal of the American Medical Association* **277**(20): 1633–40.

Lynn, J., Harrell, F. Jr, Cohn, F., Wagner, D., and Connors, A.F. Jr (1997). Prognoses of seriously ill hospitalised patients on the days before death: implications for patient care and public policy. *New Horizons* **5**: 56–61.

Nolan, T.W. (1998). Understanding medical systems. *Annals of Internal Medicine* **128**(4): 293–8.

Schneiderman, L.J., Kronick, R., and Kaplan, R.M., *et al.* (1992). Effects of offering advance directives on medical treatments and costs. *Annals of Internal Medicine* **117**: 599–606.

Schuster, J.L., Lynn, J., and the Center to Improve Care of the Dying (1999). *Improving Care for the End of Life: A Sourcebook for Managers and Providers.* New York: Oxford University Press (in press).

SUPPORT Principal Investigators, The (1995). A controlled trial to improve care for seriously ill hospitalised patients: The study to understand prognoses and preferences for outcomes and risks of treatments (SUPPORT). *Journal of the American Medical Association* **274**: 1591–8.

Teno. J., Lynn, J., Wenger, N., Phillips, R.S., Murphy, D.P., Connors, A.F. Jr, Desbiens, N., Fulkerson, W., Bellamy, P., and Knaus, W.A. (1997). For the SUPPORT Investigators. Advance directives for seriously ill hospitalised patients: effectiveness with the patient self-determination act and the SUPPORT intervention. *JAGS* **45**: 500–7.

Von Roenn, J.H., Cleeland, C.S., Gonin, R., Hatfield, A.K., and Pandya, K. J. (1993). Physician attitudes and practice in cancer pain management. A survey from the Eastern Cooperative Oncology Group. *Annals of Internal Medicine* **119**(2): 121–6.

Chapter 18

Palliative care for non-cancer patients: a purchaser perspective

John H. James

Introduction

In a publication directed principally to those with a specialist interest in the field of palliative care, it must be stressed at the outset that those who commission or purchase a total range of health care and treatment for a whole population are unlikely to devote much time or energy to considering specific needs for palliative care. From time to time a national policy directive may force the issue up the agenda for a period, or a local champion may emerge, but by and large national policy directives are succeeded by others which compete successfully for resources and attention, while no single local issue can occupy centre stage for long.

Nonetheless since the mid-1980s progress can be seen, from a situation where broadly speaking, palliative care in the UK was the province of a hospice movement largely detached from the NHS mainstream to one where it has a more central place. Clark *et al.* (1997) drew equivocal conclusions from findings that 49% of health authorities had conducted a needs assessment for palliative care and 56% had a strategy, but there is no reason to suppose that these percentages would necessarily have been higher in relation to many other aspects of health care, nor is it wise to assume that the presence or absence of a formal needs assessment or strategy is a guide either to the priority given to an issue or to the quality and adequacy of services provided. My own view is that, regardless of the way in which it is expressed in the visible planning process, all purchasing agencies, whether health authority or general practice based, now have an approach to the purchasing of palliative care which is based on a reasonable degree of empathy with the broad principles on which palliative care provision currently rests. There are, however, reasons, not least financial pressures and the wider issues facing government and society, to be concerned about how well supported palliative care services will be in years ahead.

Purchasing of palliative care 1987–1997

In 1987 the British government directed all health authorities to prepare a plan for palliative care services (HC(87)4). Neale *et al.* (1994) described how this directive was implemented in the Trent region with the publication in 1990 of a Regional Strategic Framework, followed, albeit at no great pace, by the development of strategies in individual districts. It is clear that in some other places the 1987 directive was not so systematically implemented, and that health authorities reviewed palliative care, if they chose to do so, more against the background of the decision in 1990 to introduce separate funding for authorities to spend on hospice care or as a result of having the issue drawn to their attention by local providers or by the National Council for Hospice and Specialist Palliative Care Services (NCHSPCS). The separate funding, which remained earmarked till 1994, was a source of irritation to many authorities, partly their reaction to the requirement for matched funding, partly a perception that the funding encouraged more in-patient provision rather than the home support service perceived to be under-provided.

The introduction of the purchaser–provider split following Working for Patients (Department of Health 1989) began an important process whereby health authorities were obliged to purchase services for populations, rather than, as previously, simply to exercise line management oversight of major units without, in most cases, fixed population coverage. The requirement to contract for explicit services created a focus on the activity that was being purchased and on issues of quality and effectiveness. The parallel development of separately-funded clinical audit offered the prospect of local joint evaluation of effectiveness. However Clark et al. (1997) found in a 1994–95 study that although 97% of hospices were covered by contracts with one or more health authorities, these on the whole lacked specificity.

An additional reason for health authorities to give attention to palliative care arose from the decision that local authorities should become responsible for continuing care, and from the requirement placed on health and local authorities (HSG(95)8) to reach agreement on criteria for their relative responsibilities for each group, including those requiring palliative care. Whereas for some groups agreements were reached that defined an individual as wholly the responsibility of one authority, palliative care was much harder to categorise. My own authority reached agreement on a shared pattern of support whether at home or in a residential or nursing home.

In 1995, the NCHSPCS sent all health authorities guidance on specialist palliative care services. Collectively, therefore, authorities cannot really excuse inactivity or inattention on the grounds of ignorance. They would, however, argue competing priorities.

Purchasing palliative care for non-cancer patients

If palliative care generally is still struggling for a firm toehold in mainstream NHS purchaser thinking, the issue of ensuring that services are accessible for non-cancer patients is necessarily less central still. As a general principle, the view that palliative care should be freely accessible to other groups is not in dispute, but there appears to be limited evidence of how accessible services, particularly residential and respite, have become in the UK to other groups. The evidence available in my own authority will be described in the next section.

Services for people with AIDS or symptomatic HIV represent a separate stream of development, raising distinct issues, and are described in the final section of this chapter.

What has happened in Kensington & Chelsea and Westminster

Kensington & Chelsea and Westminster Health Authority (KCW) reviewed its palliative care purchasing over the period 1993–95. KCW covers an area of 13 square miles in central

London, with a rapidly growing population–376 000 people in 1999. The review took a relatively classical form: needs assessment, review of evidence on effectiveness, analysis of current provision and its use, seminar, focus groups, and preparation of proposals. It also incorporated a survey of general practitioners which brought out very considerable variations in knowledge and interest (Higginson et al. 1994).

The needs assessment phase built directly on the work of Cartwright (1991), utilising her findings of carers' perceptions of the prevalence of symptoms indicative of the likelihood that people who had died of cancer or other conditions would have benefited from palliative care. The 1992 mortality statistics for the district were examined to identify the numbers of deaths, excluding deaths considered unlikely to have had a potential palliative care period. As a result 827 deaths from neoplasms, 1177 from diseases of the circulatory system, 366 from diseases of the respiratory system, and 190 from other diseases (chronic liver disease, diseases of the nervous system and sense organs, endocrine nutritional metabolic, and immunity diseases) were included. Cartwright's findings were then applied to these numbers to calculate the potential prevalence of symptoms (Higginson et al. 1994). Robbins (1997) has questioned this method of extrapolation partly because it is based on carers' perceptions but principally on the grounds that it does not indicate need for specialist palliative care services. In practice the authority has not attempted to utilise the extrapolations to quantify the requirements for specialist palliative care services but rather to reinforce its view that access to these services should be more readily available to non-cancer patients.

The review found that only 1.6% of referrals to the specialist palliative care services in the first three-quarters of 1993–94 were for non-cancer patients, despite the fact that non-cancer patients comprised 68% of the potential beneficiaries. These findings were among issues discussed at a seminar with, inter alia, representatives of the three specialist providers in June 1994. Faced with the question 'Could [a similar level of service] be provided [for non-cancer patients] within existing resources?' the seminar concluded that: there was a 'need to train generic workers to ensure that all staff are aware of good practice guidelines. This would allow a wider group of patients to access high quality palliative care.'

Three years later the Authority conducted a review of the current pattern of utilisation of services by non-cancer patients. In the three in-patient facilities used, the percentages of in-patient admissions for non-cancer patients were 3.2% (1995/96 data) 2.0% and 2.5% respectively (1997/98). This represents a barely perceptible change from the earlier findings, despite the agreement of all three providers to the principles of a more inclusive acceptance policy. Rather more encouraging was 1996/97 data from the local hospital palliative care team who reported 'an increasing number of patients with a non-malignant diagnosis, which accounted for 11% of referrals'.

One possible explanation for this relatively disappointing change might have been shortage of facilities. However the 1994 review found that access to palliative care services in the district was much higher than average. The number of cancer patients likely to use in-patient care in the district was calculated on the basis of a number of studies of national utilisation data (Bennett and Corcoran 1994; Cartwright 1991; Seale 1991; Higginson et al. 1992) as falling in the range 124–207. The actual use was found to be 350. Evidence was also found of higher usage rates among residents living close to the two in-district providers, while there was a suspicion that the absence of a specialist provider in the south of the district, might be being addressed by services provided, but not separately identified, by the local teaching hospital. Nor can restrictions on the availability of resources be an explanation. In 1993–94 the authority had contracts worth £900 000 for hospice and home care teams, plus a further £80 000 for Macmillan and Marie Curie nurses providing specialist care and basic home nursing care respectively. By 1997–98, these figures had risen to £1 216 000 and £180 000 respectively, a significant real terms increase.

A more likely explanation may be inferred from the 1994 review's findings in relation to local general practitioners' knowledge and understanding of palliative care services. Half (49.75%) responded to a postal questionnaire. The general practitioners were referring on average 5 patients a year to specialist palliative care services, generally to those services most local to their patients. Their answers to questions indicated a relatively low level of interest in the services. Four-fifths (79%) had no changes to suggest or problems to identify, 88% did not know of any gaps in the service, and 56% did not know whether there was duplication. Only 5% identified problems securing places for patients who did not have cancer. The general picture which emerges, from those general practitioners who were sufficiently motivated to return the questionnaire, is of a relatively low level of contact with palliative care services generally, usually confined to those most local (Higginson 1999).

A random telephone survey was undertaken of non-respondents. Only 26% of those telephoned were willing to take part. Of these the great majority were unable to identify any of the palliative care services in the area, and two did not know what the term meant.

Overall these findings do not suggest that local general practitioners would be likely to generate a significant change in practice by referring significant numbers of non-cancer patients for palliative care. Nor, clearly, has there been any significant change in the pattern of referrals from local hospitals. Some encouragement can, however, be derived from the fact that both main local teaching hospitals have developed specialist pain care teams which provide a pain management service to staff on any in-patient ward in the hospitals, and that both independently chose to include presentations of these services during quality visits by authority teams in 1997.

This review of what has happened in one health authority clearly demonstrates that reviewing the situation and developing a strategy does not of itself guarantee that complex behaviour changes across many individuals and a number of organisations will follow. In the interim the in-district in-patient services have benefited from significant capital investment and home support services have been greatly extended, but to date the imbalance between cancer and non-cancer patients has only shifted to a small extent.

Wakefield experience

More positive messages about the ability of general practitioners to develop a palliative care agenda generally may be derived from work carried out in Wakefield, Yorkshire, UK, where a total purchasing pilot was established in 1995. The work was described by Michael Vaughan at a Conference on Making Palliative Care Better: Quality Issues in Palliative Care in September 1997, held under the auspices of the Royal Society of Medicine and the NCHSPCS. The process followed by the review was not dissimilar to that in Kensington & Chelsea and Westminster, but there was a markedly higher level of general practice input.

The outcome of the review was a comprehensive description of the services available, identification of problems (particularly duplication, poor co-ordination, and variations in provision and standards), agreement on values and principles, definition of service requirements for a comprehensive 365 days a year service, a set of detailed recommendations with resource investment implications, and an action plan with timetables and responsibility for implementation clearly identified. The process was a model of how to plan services, but with the invaluable addition that the process and outcome are owned by the group whose actions will have most impact on what happens.

The conference paper touched on the issue of access for non-cancer patients, without explicitly identifying a problem. Deaths with palliative care needs for non-malignant conditions were estimated as 2082 of a total of 3054, while one of the four values and principles was that services should be 'available to all who need to irrespective of age and diagnosis'.

The implications of a new government in the UK

The Labour Government which swept to power in the UK in May 1997 made clear that, along with education, the National Health Service was one of its highest priorities. The announcement in early 2000 of unprecedented levels of spending on the National Health Service appears to have elevated health to the position of first priority.

The Labour Government's expectations of the NHS are quite different from those of its predecessor. Although the split between different purchasers and providers has been retained, other features of the internal market have been removed. The emphasis on competition to improve performance locally has been replaced by an emphasis on the need for a service that meets nationally agreed standards. The abolition of general practice fund-holding and the introduction of primary care groups, eventually to be replaced by primary care trusts, responsible both for providing primary and community services and for commissioning secondary care, is of profound significance. For Wakefield, whose total purchasing pilot status may be seen as close to the primary care group model, the change may have been relatively insignificant, and they will have been well placed to carry forward their palliative care service model. In most parts of the country, however, evolution from a situation where the health authority was a main driver of change to a situation requiring a high degree of partnership between a number of agencies to implement national standards, risks a loss of momentum. Structural change, not just the creation of primary care trusts and the abolition of community trusts, but also mergers of health authorities, could be a further distraction in the short term, whatever the longer term benefits.

There is a risk, therefore, that palliative care services in general will be neglected in the immediate future in terms of both serious attention and review. This danger is increased by the government's entirely reasonable wish to see the additional resources it is pumping into the National Health Service reflected in visible improvements in the quality and responsiveness of the service that is provided. It is clear that the public, while still overall wedded to the concept of a service that is comprehensive, publicly funded, and largely free at the point of use, is increasingly less willing to accept the shortcomings which have always been present—poor service, long waits, a lack of appreciation of the patient as a consumer, and very often poor facilities. The difficulty about achieving a modernisation agenda is that not all aspects of the service are measurable, but if improvement is to be demonstrated a measure has to be taken. The focus therefore is on strong performance management of that which can be measured. This agenda is one which will force both organisations and their managers to concentrate on delivery of the tangible at the expense of the intangible.

It will be incumbent on those who wish to see improvement in palliative care services, for whichever groups, to utilise the opportunities which the new approach has given. Of these, the requirement for all health authorities to secure agreement to a health improvement programme (HIMP) represents probably the most powerful, albeit the expectations of HIMPs are probably too high. Another opportunity to advance the topic was presented by the consultation with both NHS staff and the public at large which preceded the publication of the government's National Plan for the NHS. At the time of writing, this is still eagerly awaited.

Palliative care for people with AIDS and HIV

A discussion of the development of palliative care services for people with symptomatic HIV or AIDS must necessarily be preceded by a description of the funding system. In practice, ever since the condition was first identified, funding for treatment and care has been separate from health authorities' main allocations for hospital and community health services.

There were a number of reasons for the separation of funding. First, the Department of Health and the Treasury agreed that funding should be based on the best available estimate of the numbers of cases and the average treatment and care cost per case. Second, it was apparent from the outset that the distribution of cases was so uneven that no amount of adjustment of capitation formulae could adequately compensate. Third, given both the stigma which attached to the condition in the early years and the nature of the illness (in that death so often took the form of opportunistic infections taking advantage of a compromised immune system) it was natural that separate in-patient and hospice facilities developed. These in turn attracted people to move to live within reach of the best-known services, increasing the imbalance of numbers. When the internal market was introduced, AIDS/HIV was exempted because of the confidentiality issue. Services were commissioned by host health authorities regardless of whether users were residents.

In the late 1980s decisions on the use of resources for HIV/AIDS treatment and care largely rested at regional health authority level, and the North West Thames RHA, which had substantially the largest case load at that time, was instrumental in providing funds to support the development of London Lighthouse, which was to become the largest HIV/AIDS hospice in Europe but also one of the most influential organisations in changing public attitudes about HIV and AIDS away from stigmatisation to understanding and sympathy.

London Lighthouse was launched in 1986 and the current building opened in 1988. The Department of Health provided a grant of £1.25 million towards the cost of the building and over the years provided a further £2.75 million in grant aid. Most of London Lighthouse's funding however came directly from the NHS. Until 1994, funding, by then £3.6 million a year, came from North West Thames. In April 1994 the funding was devolved to Kensington & Chelsea and Westminster, which commissioned the services on behalf of other health authorities, A year later, London Lighthouse was given notice that from April 1997 the funds to purchase residential care would be distributed between health authorities on the basis of their usage of the facility, and that funding of remaining services would be disaggregated in April 1998.

The financial regime within which London Lighthouse had operated from 1988 to 1995 had been effectively a block grant covering 80% of its costs allowing considerable discretion as to its use. The balance of funding came mostly from fund-raising and voluntary giving. The style of services which were provided changed to reflect the fact that people were living appreciably longer with AIDS or symptomatic HIV. The emphasis of treatment and care moved from terminal care to respite, day care, and home support. A holistic model developed, and many users were given access to complementary therapies.

The prospective change in the financial regime was an evident threat for three reasons. First London Lighthouse would move from a position in which 80% of its income was from secure NHS funding to one where it was much more at risk. Second, it quickly became apparent that it was a high cost provider relative to others. Third it was always likely that more distant purchasers would seek to redirect resources from London Lighthouse to provide services more locally. The organisation was faced, therefore, with a need dramatically to transform itself if it was to survive. Over the period April 1996 to April 1998, the organisation made substantial cuts in staffing, focusing particularly on management and administration costs, in an endeavour to make itself more competitive.

That it failed in this was influenced by three major external factors. First, in 1996–97, the government reduced funding for AIDS treatment and care by 7.5% reflecting lower numbers of cases than had been projected. Across London, this represented a reduction of over £9 million, and although the health authorities acted collaboratively to minimise the impact of this, they had to find savings both in the statutory and voluntary sectors. Collectively, the bodies funded from AIDS treatment and care allocations had unquestionably done well out of separate funding and standards were distinctly higher than elsewhere. The belt-tightening was painful throughout the system. The grant to London Lighthouse was cut by £270 000. Second in the last half of 1996–97 the advent of combination therapy began to cause cost pressures in the major AIDS treatment centres. The government restored the 7.5% cut in 1997–98, in recognition of the increased costs, but combination therapy costs proved significantly greater than the increased funding, putting major pressure on the AIDS treatment and care budgets of all the main London health authorities. It is estimated that, across London, the costs of drugs, including combination therapy, increased from £14 million in 1995–96 to £38 million in 1997–98. Third, the demand for residential care, the cornerstone of London Lighthouse's income, was falling partly because more effective treatments had been introduced in response to many AIDS opportunistic infections, but principally because of the impact of combination therapy (Hogg *et al.* 1998; Palella *et al.* 1998). The result was that use of London Lighthouse's residential services fell well below contracted levels throughout 1997. The organisation, which had run at a substantial deficit in both of the previous two years, found itself faced with a dramatic loss of projected income for 1998–99. A variety of rescue schemes involving shared use of the facility all came to nothing.

In March 1998 the Council of Management agreed to withdraw from providing residential services, which duly ceased in August that year. As a result a section of the building was leased to meet the costs of restructuring and enable the organisation to continue as a provider of a range of services including day care, home care, and community support from restructured premises. London Lighthouse's Strategic Review of Services, coupled with the subsequent reduction in demand for day care, resulted in their decision to withdraw from providing this service in January 2000 moving instead towards the development of a package of care entitled 'Positive Start', a unique service which comprises skills based training, therapies, support, and workshops. All of these services are also offered individually to clients accessing the Lighthouse 'drop-in' facility. Finally in mid-2000 a merger with the Terence Higgins Trust was proposed.

Small (1998) has suggested that: 'A decision about using residential services other than Lighthouse is based on cost, not on quality or outcome. If simple cost-accounting replaces cost-effectiveness in purchasing, we will see a more general decline in standards.' These observations are only partially justified. London Lighthouse's prices were certainly higher than those offered by its two principal competitors, but purchasers' decisions can only take account of variations in outcomes where the evidence is apparent. No symptomatic distinction can be drawn between different hospices in this field on the basis of outcomes. The only evidence we have had available has been user preference. In this respect 1997–98 saw a sharper decline in KCW residents' use of London Lighthouse residential services than those of the Mildmay, while there was no reduction at all in the use by people with AIDS or symptomatic HIV of St John's Hospice, the only local setting providing palliative care in a non-HIV specific setting.

What then are the lessons to be drawn from the experience of London Lighthouse. First, a high degree of specialisation requires a protected environment to survive. The hospice movement generally has needed to adjust to changes in patients' and carers' expectations, but has always been reasonably certain that demand for palliative care would continue. London Lighthouse as a specialist provider for one condition faced a situation that had only previously happened to tuberculosis sanatoria—that of a sudden and dramatic drop in demand for its services. In the case of tuberculosis there was for many years confidence that the disease had been beaten. In the case of HIV, the evidence for combination therapy, though compelling in the sense that health authorities felt they had no choice but to ensure that the treatment could be offered to all who met the clinical protocol guidelines, is much more equivocal. Experience in the US, where combination therapy became generally available significantly earlier than here, suggests that for many the benefits begin to reduce after two to three years. This experience may not be replicated here since a much higher proportion of Americans will previously have had monotherapy drug regimes, which are known to make combination therapy less effective, but the likelihood is that there will be an overall reduction in benefit. It must be acknowledged too that a proportion, currently thought to be up to 30%, of those eligible for combination therapy will not receive it, most commonly because they cannot tolerate the side effects. Notwithstanding the many who are currently relatively symptom-free because of combination therapy, there will remain a demand for residential care and it is likely to increase from its present low level.

Small (1998) argued that: 'Understandable decisions about short-term financial allocations may mean one loses the accumulated experience of an established unit—a unit that may well be needed in the future.' The dilemma is well expressed, but in practice the answer again revolved around specialisation. London Lighthouse was established at a time when HIV was predominantly associated with gay men. There remain significant numbers of HIV positive gay men, but a growing proportion of the HIV positive population in the London area have acquired the virus through heterosexual sex. Increasingly those newly identified with HIV are members of families, particularly from sub-Saharan Africa. The geographical distribution of case load is also changing, with significant increases in south and east London, while the overall prevalence in Kensington & Chelsea and Westminster has stabilised. For the non-local health authorities, withdrawal from use of London Lighthouse is seen as providing an opportunity to invest in more local services designed from the outset around the needs of families and the cultural requirements of different ethnic groups. London Lighthouse itself correctly identified the change in clientele, and has sought to meet it, but it could not wholly shake off its previous image. Adaptation, as Darwin observed, involves a process of natural selection, painful for those which do not evolve in time.

Conclusion

From a purchaser perspective, palliative care has to be flexible in response to changing demand and changing perceptions of what can be delivered. Development of more inclusive services is desirable on all counts. The skills which evolved in relation to the care and treatment of cancer patients ought to be made available to those affected by other terminal conditions, while the fact that many people with AIDS have chosen to accept treatment and care in non-AIDS specific settings should be seen as a positive sign of the progress that has been made in overcoming the stigma once associated with the condition. From the provider perspective too an inclusive service is undoubtedly one better fitted to adapt to future changes.

References

Bennett, M. and Corcoran, G. (1994). The impact on community palliative care services of a hospital palliative care team. *Palliative Medicine* **8**(3): 237–44.

Cartwright, A. (1991). Change in life and care in the year before death 1969–1987. *Journal of Public Health Medicine* **13**(2): 81–7.

Clark, D., Malson, H., Small, N., Mallett, K., Neale, B., and Heather, P. (1997). Half full or half empty? The impact of health reform on palliative care services in the UK. Policy, ethics, evidence. In Clark, D., Hockley, J., and Ahmedzai, S. (eds), *New Themes in Palliative Care*. Buckingham: Open University Press, pp. 60–74.

Department of Health (1987). *Health Services Development Terminal Care*. London: HC(87)4 Health Circular.

Department of Health (1995). *NHS Responsibilities for Meeting Continuing Health Care Needs*. London: HSG(95)8 Health Services Guidance.

Department of Health (Secretary of State for Health) (1989). *Working for Patients: The Health Service Caring for the 1990s*. London: HMSO, Cm.555.

Department of Health (Secretary of State for Health) (1997). *The New NHS–Modern Dependable*. Cm 3807. London: Department of Health.

Higginson, I. (1997). Palliative and terminal care. In Stevens, A. and Raftery, J. (eds), *Health Care Needs Assessment. Epidemiologically-based Needs Assessment*. Series 2. Oxford: Radcliffe Medical Press.

Higginson, I. (1999). Palliative care services in the community: what do family doctors want. *Journal of Palliative Care* **15**(2): 21–5.

Higginson, I., Bush, R., Jenkins, P., and Collins, M. (1994). *Commissioning Specialist Palliative Care Services*. London: Kensington & Chelsea and Westminster Health Commissioning Agency.

Higginson, I., Wade, A., and McCarthy, M. (1992). Effectiveness of two palliative support teams. *Journal of Public Health Medicine* **14**(1): 50–6.

Hogg, R., Heath, K., Yip, B., Craib, K., O'Shaughnessy, M., Schechter, M., and Montaner, J. (1998). Improved survival among HIV-infected individuals following initiation of antiretroviral therapy. *Journal of the American Medical Association* **279**(6): 450–4.

Neale, B., Clark, D., and Heather, P. (1994). *Palliative Care and the Purchasers: A Study of Recent Developments in the Trent Region*. Occasional Paper 13. Sheffield: Trent Palliative Care Centre.

Palella, F., Delaney, K., Moorman, A., Loveless, M., Fuhrer, J., Satten, G., Aschman, D., and Holmberg, S. (1998). Declining morbidity and mortality among patients with advanced human immunodeficiency virus infection. *New England Journal of Medicine* **338**(13): 853–60.

Robbins, M. (1997). Assessing needs and effectiveness: is palliative care a special case? Policy, ethics, evidence. In Clark, D., Hockley, J., and Ahmedzai, S. *New Themes in Palliative Care*. Buckingham: Open University Press, pp. 13–33.

Seale, C. (1991). Death from cancer and death from other causes: the relevance of the hospice approach. *Palliative Medicine* 5: 12–19.

Small, N. (1998). On the rocks. *Health Services Journal* 2 April: 35.

Chapter 19

Informal carers of dependants with advanced disease

Jonathan Koffman and Penny Snow

Introduction

Over the last two decades there has been a growing body of literature on the practical treatment and management of advanced chronic diseases. Until recently, however, little emphasis has been placed on the family and friends of these patients, and the invaluable contribution they make towards their overall care: a national survey in the UK reported that many informal carers provide assistance to their dependants for more than 80 hours each week (OPCS 1990). Increasing numbers of family members are likely to become informal carers during their lifetime whether or not they feel competent to do so. Social policy has paid heightened attention to the needs of carers in general in many countries. In addition, increasingly research has focused on their needs. Within palliative care this has principally been concerned with informal carers of dependants with cancer. Carers of dependants with advanced chronic diseases other than cancer have, to date, received little attention in the palliative care literature. Yet for many patients and their carers these diseases still remain irrecoverably shattering experiences.

There are a number of reasons why the needs of informal carers of dependants with conditions other than cancer need to be addressed. There is evidence that family members who are unsupported have a particularly difficult time during a patient's illness which can persist for many months and in some instances even years (Davis *et al.* 1996; Travers 1996). This will have a bearing on their physical and psychological health. Importantly, it may also have implications for dealing with their subsequent bereavement. These humanitarian considerations for addressing the needs of informal carers of patients with advanced disease should be sufficient reasons alone. In the UK, the increasing demands on scarce NHS resources, however, represent another cogent argument. The reduction in the number of acute hospital beds and in admissions to what beds are now available, combined with the increasing use of community and day hospital facilities, has made the role of families and friends who care largely indispensable. If, however, families become too exhausted and overwhelmed by the distress of caring for a dependant they may be unable to continue their role and patients will consequently need to be admitted to hospital, or may receive unsatisfactory home care.

This chapter first attempts to define informal care. Then it reviews the sources of stress and satisfaction associated with looking after a dependant in order to understand the milieu of care. According to Orford (1987) many of the issues relating to carers of cancer patients may well be common to other carers irrespective of the disease the patient is suffering. Lastly, it suggests areas where informal carers and their dependants could be better served by health and social care services.

Informal caring

To date, a great deal of attention has been focused on the physical aspects of informal care at the expense of the emotional, social and financial dimensions (Nolan and Grant 1994). A good indication of the degree to which caring is defined with respect to physical and instrumental activity are presented in the following three definitions of 'informal caring':

1 Anyone who looks after or cares for a handicapped person to any extent in their own home, or elsewhere (Equal Opportunities Commission 1982);

2 A person looking after or providing some form of regular service for a sick, handicapped, or elderly person living in their own or another household (Green 1988);

3 A person who takes prime responsibility in the home care of a person who, because of illness or handicap, needs almost continuous care (Social Work Services Development Group 1984).

The last definition is limited in that it only acknowledges informal carers if they are taking prime responsibility and are providing almost continuous care; framing care in this way provides only a partial assessment of need. Several authors have recognised the restricted ways in which caring has been defined and have suggested the need for more comprehensive models. Bulmer (1987) argues that caring concerns issues of help, support and protection. Twigg (1989) suggests that caring includes tasks of a supportive character in addition to social and family responsibilities. Pearline *et al.* (1990) goes further, arguing that 'caring' is best taken as referring to the emotional and affective component, whereas the term 'caregiving' is more appropriate to describe the physical and behavioural aspects. Bowers (1987) argues that much of the carer's role is invisible in that it is not readily apparent to anyone other than the carer; the current task based view of caring means providers remain largely unaware of these latent needs, with obvious consequences for the tailoring of services to individuals' requirements. She therefore suggests that caring should be redefined by its purpose: caring comprises practical tending as well as emotional, social, and psychological aspects, and a general concern for others.

Informal caring: what does it involve?

Informal caring comprises a number of different elements, frequently operating side-by-side. Twigg and Atkin (1994) suggest four although these are by no means exhaustive:

1 *Performing tasks of supportive character that go beyond the normal reciprocities common between adults.* Here caring implies doing things for people that they cannot do for themselves; personal care tasks such as lifting, toilet functions, and washing provide good examples. Twigg argues it is often difficult, however, to distinguish between 'caring' and the patterns of 'personal tending' common within families and gender relations. Many women traditionally perform tasks for their spouses and families that would be classified as caring if provided by men in reverse. Allied to this emphasis on caring tasks is the belief that caring involves actual physical labour, and more often than not hard physical labour,

for example lifting and cleaning. This emphasis arose in part from a desire to dilute romantic notions about caring, to take it away from a preoccupation with love, and to demonstrate how much caring was onerous and burdensome.

2 *Caring involves kinship obligation.* An established body of research has shown that caring almost always takes place within a context of kinship networks (Twigg and Atkin 1994; Finch 1989). The support neighbours and friends offer is limited, and they are rarely involved in intimate or physical care (Wenger 1984; Hills 1991). If friends or neighbours are closely involved, it is usually because some earlier social experience has transformed these relationships.

3 *Caring is closely associated with emotion.* Caring relations, if not explicitly defined by love and affection, are frequently associated with it, although in more complex and ambiguous ways than might be expected. Emotion is significant in other ways too. It is not just that love and other feelings underwrite the obligation to care, but that caring represents a form of emotional labour in its own right (Delphy and Leonard 1992).

4 *Caring can involve co-residence.* Co-residence forms a significant element in the construction of caring although it is not always a vital part of it. Caring can and frequently does take place between households and this is a particular feature where the cared-for person is an elderly parent (Green 1988). Qureshi and Walker (1986) suggest that co-residence is an important factor in defining who within a family ends up a carer, often overriding other factors such as gender and relationship. Sharing a household with the cared-for person can radically affect the experience of caring because it has greater potential for restricting the lives of carers.

Stresses and rewards experienced by informal carers

The stresses and burdens associated with caring for a dependant with a chronic illness are numerous and can comprise physical, emotional, as well as financial costs (see Table 19.1). For many years, and particularly in US based literature, this was the sole focus of much research on caring. In the UK, surveys have revealed that as many as half of those carers who completed the General Health Questionnaire scored within a range indicative of psychiatric morbidity (Travers 1996). Caring imposes its toil in a number of different ways ranging from long periods of isolation because the needs of the cared-for person are constant (Koffman and Taylor 1997), to changes in personality and behavioural changes in dependants (Gilleard *et al.* 1984; Levin *et al.* 1989). Dementia, for example, frequently erodes the relationship between the two parties, the cared-for person may not even recognise the person who looks after him or her and carers may consequently experience an acute sense of loss and bereavement and feel they are living with someone completely different. It is therefore not uncommon for them to experience negative feelings of guilt, pity, impatience, and even repugnance alongside sentiments of love and affection (Lewis and Meridith 1988; Levin *et al.* 1989).

Despite their willingness to look after dependants, many carers are eventually worn down by the constant strain. It has been reported that the greatest improvements in the mental well-being of carers of those with dementia came with the death of the person they looked after (Levin *et al.*1989). This in no way suggests that carers would wish for such an outcome but it does provide an indication that that care is frequently provided in the face of extreme stress.

Table 19.1 Sources of strain and satisfaction experienced by carers looking after dependants

Sources of strain	Sources of reward
Greater vulnerability to physical illness	Expressions of appreciation
Anxiety and depression	Control: feeling of knowing best
Insomnia	Company of the cared-for person
Loneliness and isolation	Improved affinity
Exhaustion	Sense of appreciation
Sense of loss and bereavement	Improved self-esteem as result of caring
Financial implications	Altruism through reciprocity
Relationship tensions	Personal challenge
Role conflicts	Repayment of past services and debts
Preventing admission	

Sources: Davies 1980; Grant and Noble 1993, Heron 1998, Lawton et al 1989, Townsend and Noelkler 1987, Ungerson 1987.

Caring can also impose a considerable strain on the carers' financial resources (Wright 1986). In 1993, the Institute for Actuaries estimated the value of unpaid care in the UK at £33.9 million a year compared to £7 billion for all institutional care and £3.1 billion for all professional home care (Government Actuaries Department 1993). Carers are often unaware of their rights to entitlements, for example attendance allowance. If carers are under the age of retirement, their ability to go to or remain in work can be dramatically affected. In 1993 in the UK, the Department of Health issued a booklet to employers and carers emphasised the need for employers to make their management and personnel practices more amenable to caregivers. The cared-for person's infirmity may also have other serious financial implications including the additional expenditure of extra heating, laundry, and purchasing services.

Despite the high price exacted from informal carers, many, nevertheless, continue to do so and find it a rewarding experience (see Table 19.1). Not surprisingly, evidence suggests that caring is most pleasurable when the cared-for person is considerate, expresses appreciation for what is being done for them, and is concerned for the carer (Heron 1998). This can go a long way towards alleviating the sense of constant hard work that is involved with caring for someone. It helps the carer feel they are making a very positive contribution and that their existence has importance because others have noticed what they do. Furthermore, it has been suggested that caring can result in an improved carer–dependant relationship (Townsend and Noelkler 1987) especially where there is an element of reciprocity. Expressions of appreciation from cared-for persons, family, and friends all contribute to the sense of worth of carers. Carers have an intimate knowledge of the patient gained over a number of years and as such can be pivotal in any decisions that are made, a process which can ease feelings of helplessness. They know the patient emotionally, but also physically. In addition, it appears that one of the greatest rewards for carers is keeping their loved-ones out of an institution (Davies 1980; Ungerson 1987). Lawton *et al.* (1989) used multivariate analysis to identify predictors of caring satisfaction. Sources of satisfaction comprised: enjoyment in the company of the cared-for person; feeling closer to the cared-for person; getting pleasure by giving to the cared-for person; feeling appreciated by the cared-for person; and an improved sense of self-esteem as a result of caring. Others (Grant and Noble 1993) have gone further to describe satisfaction in more detail. Their results provide a hierarchy of satisfactions (although more than one source could be cited) that included the following: altruism as reciprocity, expressions of appreciation, improved affinity, personal challenge, repayment of past services, honouring vows, and honouring religious convictions.

Carers' unspoken negative feelings towards dependants

It is not uncommon for carers to experience overwhelming anger at certain points during their 'caring career' and this will at times be directed towards dependants themselves (Table 19.2). Other feelings may include bitterness and resentment resulting from the many significant sacrifices made, the physical and unpalatable revulsion of having to tend to unpleasant personal care tasks, feelings of impotence to make even the apparent minutiae of care easier to bear, questioning of spiritual faith (particularly painful in those with previous religious convictions), and, lastly, some might harbour secret dreams for the future without their dependant, free of the relentless pressure of perhaps several years of very demanding care.

Table 19.2 Six unspoken negative feelings towards dependants

Unspoken feelings
◆ Anger and frustration
◆ Bitterness and resentment
◆ Impotence to help
◆ Physical revulsion
◆ Questioning one's faith
◆ Secret dreams for the future

Source: Adapted from Doyle 1994.

Dependants with advanced disease: the informal carer's experience

Problems encountered by carers and their dependants during advanced illness include: the specific symptoms dependants experience; the assistance and tending they require on a day-to-day basis; communication issues with health care professionals; and the basic information carers require to make the uncertainty of living alongside a dependant with advanced disease easier to bear. Many problems exist concurrently so it is important that health and social care professionals disaggregate them and prioritise which can be managed immediately to maximum effect. It is also important that they do not lose sight of the overall total cost of caring exacted by the illness.

The characteristics of a dependant with advanced disease will have a strong bearing on the carer's experience. On average cancer patients tend to fall into younger age groups compared to those patients with stroke and heart disease. Non-cancer patients are therefore more likely to have other co-morbidities associated with old age, for example mental confusion and incontinence, all of which may exacerbate their care needs. In addition younger patients with HIV/AIDS, multiple sclerosis, and motor neurone disease may exhibit neurological deficits, resulting in similar symptoms that in turn present considerable challenges.

One of the principal aims of palliative care is the relief of symptoms. Whilst symptoms impact on patients, they also greatly affect their informal carers as well as other family members. Below we describe a number of the main symptoms experienced by patients with advanced disease and explore the available literature for their effects on carers.

Pain

Pain has been described as an overwhelming symptom of cancer that disrupts all dimensions of quality of life in patients. Pain can also become a major concern of carers and many feel utterly helpless or frustrated on behalf of their dependants. In a study to explore the factors that influence cancer pain mangement, Ferrell *et al.* (1991) observed a number of carers wishing they were able to share in the pain or endure it on behalf of their loved ones. Ferrell's research described carers' interpretations of pain as being a 'metaphor for illness' equating it with advanced illness. Pain becomes a tangible indicator mapping the trajectory of the disease's progress and the patient's inevitable decline, the only awaited relief being death, as typified by the following statement.

> It is the worst part. Someone told me that it is God's way of making you relieved when she finally dies. Because it's so horrible seeing her suffer every day. You just wish she would die so she could finally be comfortable.
>
> (Ferrell *et al.* 1991)

Although patients may well under-report pain to avoid distressing their carers, paradoxically it is not unusual for carers to rate pain as more intense and of greater severity than their dependants do (Ferrell *et al.* 1991).

Pain is not the monopoly of cancer patients and their carers, and other disease groups also frequently experience this symptom in varying degrees of severity and associated distress. More than 50% of patients with either motor neurone disease or multiple sclerosis have been reported as suffering pain which has a specific impact on the quality of their mental and social health (Ellershaw 1993; Archibald *et al.* 1993). Addington-Hall *et al.*'s (1995a) analysis of the 'Regional study of care for the dying' (RSCD) revealed that at least half of all stroke patients suffered pain, many for at least six months prior to their death. McCarthy *et al.*'s (1996) further analysis of this data demonstrated that pain was also a common symptom in heart disease. Nearly 80% of patients were reported to have had pain in their last year of life and 63% in their last week of life. Carers described it as having been 'very distressing' in 50% of cases. Interestingly, patients with dementia were also reported as having experienced pain and only slightly less so than patients with cancer (McCarthy *et al.* 1997). In many cases the RSCD reported that adequate pain control was often not achieved. Pain in these patients may be a result of co-morbidities such as arthritis, rather than a direct consequence of the primary disease. This, nevertheless, still has important implications for carers since where pain is reported it is usually experienced for a much longer duration of time. More research is required to explore the meaning carers attach to pain in non-cancer patients.

Incontinence

Incontinence is an aspect of caring that is associated with stigma for both parties in the carer–dependant relationship (Norton 1986). Hicks and Corcoran (1993) reported that a fifth of patients with advanced motor neurone disease admitted to a hospice for respite care experienced incontinence and many more required the use of a urinary catheter. McCarthy *et al.* (1997) reported that 72% of patients with dementia experienced urinary incontinence during their last year of life. A similar frequency has been reported in cancer patients although for a shorter duration of time (Addington-Hall *et al.* 1995b). In addition, 16% of patients with heart disease experienced faecal incontinence (McCarthy *et al.* 1996). These symptoms clearly pose significant practical problems for carers by creating extra laundry from both soiled bed linen and the cared-for person's clothes. Other associated difficulties involve managing catheters, colostomy bags, or incontinence pads.

Anorexia

Anorexia, or loss of appetite, is a troublesome symptom experienced by the majority of cancer patients. Anorexia has important emotional significance, because food and eating are essential for survival. Furthermore, the preparation and serving of food is an expression of love and caring. In line with pain, anorexia in terminally ill cancer patients is frequently used by carers as a barometer to indicate impending death and therefore becomes a source of considerable distress (Holden 1991). Other disease groups similarly experience anorexia: over half of dementia patients in their last year of life were reported by their carers as having experienced loss of appetite (McCarthy *et al.* 1997); 80% of stroke patients, many of whom according to their carers found it very distressing (Addington-Hall 1995a); and nearly a third of patients with advanced motor neurone disease (Hicks and Corcoran 1993). For family members comfort is obtained from providing food to loved ones but when the patients deteriorates this function is subjected to increasing tension. As each attempt to provide palatable food becomes unsuccessful, carers may feel helpless, rejected, and angry (Dixon *et al.* 1985). Holden (1991) suggests that this frustration and anxiety is often even more pronounced in female carers because their dependant's inability to eat impacts on their customary role identity.

Behaviour problems

Behaviour problems have been associated with carer crisis and breakdown (Gilleard *et al.* 1984, Levin 1989). The majority of literature to date has focused on the impact of dementia (Gilhooly 1982; Levin *et al.* 1989). Problems comprise the inability of the cared-for person to converse normally, endless repetition, restlessness, dangerous behaviour (for example, forgetting to turn off a gas cooker), frequent wandering, inability to recognise their carer, disturbed sleep or idiosyncratic sleeping times, and even violence. More specifically, changes in personality are often the cause of stress since they can be associated with a sense of loss and bereavement on behalf of the carer for the previously well person they once knew. In addition, dependants with dementia often do not co-operate in their care, and their inability to respond to their carer can be particularly depressing. Indeed, research carried out by Clipp and George (1993) suggest the carers of dependants with dementia are more adversely affected by their role than cancer carers.

Problems with information and communication with health care professionals

Soothill, Mackay and Webb (1995) point out that since palliative care increasingly takes place in the community, informal carers are becoming important and indispensable partners of professional staff and as such are sharing more of the responsibilities of care, often 24 hours a day. In many instances carers are now assuming responsibility for procedures and treatments that until recently were confined to specialist in-patient care settings. Families assume these responsibilities with little or no education and little emotional support. It is important to bear in mind that health care professionals provide this care alongside other colleagues and the knowledge that the care they provide will be taken over by others in their absence. Carers do not have this luxury and to deliver care successfully they need proper and effective consultation and exchange of information with health care professionals. A recent survey carried out by Carers National Association (1998) reported that carers thought that NHS staff were very poor at providing information. The majority (60%) of carers had never received acknowledgment of their important role, or been informed about the possibilities of contacting other carers through support organisations. The overwhelming majority of carers also reported that information directly relevant to the health service had not been provided. For example, 90% of the respondents were given no advice by health care professionals about lifting and handling techniques that would enable them to care more safely. This concern is poignantly illustrated by an account of a carer writing about his father who had multiple sclerosis:

> Getting John on and off the bed was a massive task, requiring a ceiling-mounted electric hoist. Once on the bed, there followed a series of complex activities to prepare him for his rest involving catheters, ripple mattresses, wrist splints, massage, and the putting on of callipers, requiring brute force to push the knee joints down the until the calliper locked the knee joint straight–and all, if you got it right, timed perfectly to avoid bringing on a chronic, body-shaking muscle spasm that would then put you back to square one. Nobody taught me how to do all this. . . . Should we have been doing this skilled mixture of primary nursing and physiotherapy at all, considering we didn't know what we were doing? None of the district nurses, or doctors raised any objections. But then who else was going to do it?

> (Berbiers 1996)

Whilst many carers of dependants with cancer experience poor communication and obtain unsatisfactory information, carers of dependants from other patient groups appear to be fairing as badly. The RSCD revealed that nearly 40% of respondents of dependants with dementia felt they were unable to obtain all the information they wanted compared to over 50% of cancer patients (McCarthy et al. 1997). Carers of dependants with heart disease encountered similar problems with more than half wanting more information (McCarthy et al. 1997). The consequent uncertainty about a dependant's condition may compromise the carer's psychological resources.

What do informal carers need?

At the beginning of this chapter we suggested that many of the problems experienced by cancer patients are common to patients in other disease groups. What is apparent, however, is that a number of these specific problems may well be experienced for longer periods of time with serious implications for the physical and psychological health of the carers. Furthermore, carers often become so immersed in their problems that they have difficulty even thinking about let alone identifying what their specific needs are (Koffman and Taylor 1997). This is significant given that most informal carers do not willingly choose their role, so it is therefore important that their problems and losses are not discounted simply because they have not raised them as issues. All problems experienced by carers, either in isolation of in combination, should be sensitively sought out, acknowledged, and, where at all possible, addressed.

One of the most important ways in which the experience of caring can be turned into something more positive is for the carer to feel that they are entitled to breaks away from the person they are looking after. This can take the form of respite care, one of the few strategies aimed directly at the carer. Respite care has been broadly defined as 'temporary care to permit caregivers to relinquish their duties, stress and responsibilities for a time-limited period in order to maintain their physical and emotional strength' (Miller 1986). In practice, however, this may be difficult emotionally, as it is not always easy for carers to remove themselves from the situation. Carers need to be encouraged to believe that they are 'allowed' a life outside the caring domain. It is not just that they have a life that they have to get on with, i.e. paid employment, or looking after children, but they have time for themselves to try to reflect on what is happening to them. For many carers who are living with the dependant home becomes their workplace—and they need to get away from work. Berbiers (1996) writes: 'I hadn't slept for weeks. After a while you get used to the exhausted, skewed, blurred, edgy, the reality it creates. The sleeplessness was because John (my father) hardly ever slept.'

Perhaps one of the most important factors for carers is that as their dependants' conditions gradually deteriorate and their workload increases, they are given permission by the professionals involved to say 'no' and are helped to understand that they should not feel guilty about this. Carers who feel supported, understood, and that they are a person in their own right who cannot always be all things to all people, probably experience caring more positively than they would if there was no one with whom they can talk. In Table 19.3 we have listed a number of the needs carers of cancer patients have described (Hampe 1975). We believe they generalise equally well to other patient groups we have outlined during the course of this chapter.

Table 19.3 Needs of informal carers of dependants with advanced disease

Needs of carers
◆ To be with the dying patient
◆ To be helpful to the dying patient
◆ To receive assurance of the dying person's comfort
◆ To be informed of the dying person's condition
◆ To be informed of the impending death
◆ To ventilate emotions
◆ To receive comfort and support from other family members
◆ To receive acceptance, support, and comfort from health care professionals

Source: Hampe 1975.

How can services respond?

Although the policy on informal carers has become better developed in recent years, there is still some way to go before practice catches up with it. In England and Wales, The Carers (Recognition and Services) Act of 1995 was an important landmark in recognising the role and contribution of carers. The Act enshrined the statutory right of carers to an assessment of their ability to care, and placed a duty on local authorities to take account of such assessments when deciding what services they should provide. Its implementation to date has been patchy with fewer than 20% of known carers requesting an assessment (Carers National Association 1997). The need for co-ordinated efforts to ensure more carers are aware of their rights and how these rights relate to their own situation should be highlighted. However, it is not only local authorities that play an important part to play in supporting carers. Other services are also very important, and the role of the NHS is especially significant. General practitioners in particular are often the health care professionals carers are most likely to come into contact with, and they have the potential to make a real difference to carers' lives.

At the time of writing the policy and practice environment which is evolving as a result of the 1997 White Paper, *The NHS: Modern—Dependable*, has the potential to be of great value to both patients with advanced disease and their carers. The White Paper places particular emphasis on public involvement and consultation and a greater recognition of the role of primary care which must endeavour to be accessible and responsive to need to local needs. Furthermore, the performance of the NHS will be judged against a new national framework which will include assessment against the experiences of patients and carers alike.

The problems of fragmentation of health and social care provision are well documented and the government is currently exploring new and innovative ways of encouraging closer working between these two sectors. It is essential that carers experience seamless care and are not sent from one to the other in order to protect budgets.

Conclusion

Although many patients with advanced diseases spend at least some time in hospital, the majority of their last year of life will be spent at home, a situation that would prove impossible without the support from informal carers. Although the balance of research in palliative care to date has favoured carers of dependants with cancer, we argue, based on research available on other patient groups, that the experience of caring is by no means less eventful or stressful. On the contrary, in many instances their problems may be even more severe or wearing since the duration of care is frequently longer and unpredictable, inter-dispersed with frequent periods of great uncertainty. The challenge for palliative care in the future will be to develop adequate, appropriate and cost-effective support to address the many issues carers and the dependants experience. Not investing more in their specific needs has the potential of costing these service providers dearly as delicate care networks have great potential to become compromised.

References

Addington-Hall, J., Lay, M., Altmann, D., and McCarthy, M. (1995a). Symptom control, communication with health professionals, and hospice care of stroke patients in the last year of life as reported by surviving family, friends, and officials, *Stroke* **26**: 2242–8.

Addington-Hall, J. and McCarthy, M. (1995b). Dying from cancer: results from a national population-based investigation, *Palliative Medicine* **9**: 295–305.

Archibald, C.J., McGrath, P.J., Rivto, P.G., *et al.* (1993). Pain prevalence, severity, and impact in a clinical sample of multiple sclerosis patients, *Pain* **58**: 89–93.

Berbiers, N. (1996). A carer's tale, *Community Care* **28**: 24–6.

Bowers, B. (1987). Inter-generational care-giving: adult caregivers and their adult parents, *Advances in Nursing Science* **9**: 20–1.

Bulmer, M. (1987). *The Social Basis of Community Care*. London: Allen and Unwin.

Carers National Association (1997). *Still Battling? The Carers Act One Year On*. London: Carers National Association.

Carers National Association (1998). *Ignored and Invisible? Carers' Experience of the NHS*. London: Carers National Association.

Clipp, E. and George, L. (1993). Dementia and cancer: a comparison of spouse caregivers, *Gerontologist* **33**(4): 534–41.

Davies, A. (1980). Disability, homecare, and the care-taking role in family life, *Journal of Advanced Nursing* **5**: 475–84.

Davis, B., Cowley, S., and Ryland, R. (1996). The effects of terminal illnesses on patients and their carers, *Journal of Advanced Nursing* **23**: 512–20.

Delphy, C. and Leonard, D. (1992). *Familiar Exploitation: a new analysis of marriage in contemporary western societies*. Cambridge: Polity Press.

Dixon, C.E., Emery, A.W., and Hurley, R.S. (1985). Nutrition in cancer patients with a limited life expectancy. *American Journal of Hospice Care* **2**: 27–33.

Doyle, D. (1994). *Caring for the Dying*. Oxford: Oxford University Press.

Ebrahim, S. (1990). *Clinical Epidemiology of Stroke*. Oxford: Oxford University Press.

Ellershaw, J. (1993). Motor neurone disease (part 1). *Palliative Care Today* **2**: 25–6.

Equal Opportunities Commission (1982). *Who Cares for the Carers? Opportunities for Those Caring for the Elderly and Handicapped*. Manchester: Equal Opportunities Commission.

Ferrell, B., Rhiner, M., Cohen, M., and Grant, M. (1991). Pain as a metaphor for illness part 1: impact of cancer pain on family caregivers. *Oncology Nursing Forum* **18**: 1303–9.

Finch, J. (1989). *Family Obligations and Social Change*. Cambridge: Polity Press.

Gilhooly, M. (1982). Social aspects of senile dementia. In Taylor, R. and Gilmore, A. (eds), *Current Trends in Gerontology: Proceedings of the 1980 Conference of the British Society of Gerontology*. Aldershot: Gower.

Gilleard, C., Belford, H., Gilleard, E., Whitlick, J.E., Gledhill, K. (1984). Emotional distress amongst the supporters of the elderly infirm. *British Journal of Psychiatry* **145**: 172–177.

Government Actuaries Department (1992). *National Population Projections: Great Britain*. London: HMSO.

Grant, G. and Noble, M. (1993). Informal carers: sources and concomitants of satisfaction, *Health and Social Care in the Community* **1**: 147–159.

Green, H. (1988). *Informal Carers, General Household Survey 1985 Series*. London: OPCS, Social Survey Division, GHS No. 15 (16).

Hampe, S. (1975). Needs of a grieving spouse in a hospital setting, *Nursing Research* **25**: 113–19.

Heron, C. (1998). *Working with Carers*. London: Jessica Kingsley Publishers.

Hicks, F. and Corcoran, G. (1993). Should hospices offer respite admissions to patients with motor neurone disease? *Palliative Medicine* **7**: 145–50.

Hills, D. (1991). *Carer Support on the Community: Evaluation of the Department of Health Initiative; Demonstration Districts for Informal Carers 1986–1989*. London: HMSO.

Holden, C.M. (1991). Anorexia in the terminally ill cancer patient: the emotional impact on the patient and the family, *Hospice Journal* **7**: 73–84.

Koffman, J. and Taylor, S.J. (1997). The needs of caregivers, *Elderly Care* **6**: 16–19.

Lawton, M., Kleban, M., and Moss, M. (1989). Measuring caregiving appraisal, *Journal of Gerontology* **44**(3): 61–71.

Levin, E., Sinclair, I., and Gorbach P. (1989). *Families, Services and Confusion in Old Age.* Aldershot: Gower.

Lewis, J. and Meridith, B. (1988). *Daughters who Care: Daughters Caring for Mothers at Home.* London: Routledge and Kegan Paul.

McCarthy, M., Addington-Hall, J., and Altmann, D. (1996). Dying from heart disease, *Journal of the Royal College of Physicians* **30**: 325–8.

McCarthy, M., Addington-Hall, J., and Altmann D. (1997). The experience of dying with dementia: a retrospective study, *International Journal of Geriatric Psychiatry* **12**: 404–9.

Miller, D. (1986). The realities of respite care for families, clients and sponsors, *Gerontologist* **25**: 467–70.

Nolan, M., Grant, G., Caldock, K., and Keady, J. (1994). *A Framework for Assessing the Needs of Family Carers: A Multidisciplinary Guide.* University of Surrey: BASE Publications.

Norton, C. (1986). Continence promoting research , *Nursing Times* 9 April.

Office of Population Censuses and Surveys (1990), *General Household Survey.* London: HMSO.

Orford, J. (ed.) (1987). *Coping with Disorder in the Family.* London: Croom Helm.

Pearline, L., Mullan, J., Semple, S., and Skaff, M. (1990). Caregiving and the stress process: an overview of concepts and their measures, *Gerontologist* **30**(5): 583–94.

Qureshi, H. and Walker, A. (1986). Caring for the elderly people: the family and the state. In Phillipson, C. and Walker, A. (eds), *Ageing and Social Policy: a critical assessment.* Aldershot: Gower.

Social Work Services Development Group (1984). *Supporting the Informal Carers: Fifty Styles of Caring—Models of Practice for Planners and Practitioners.* London: DHSS.

Soothill, K., Mackay, L., and Webb, C. (1995). *Interprofessional Relations in Health Care.* London: Edward Arnold.

Townsend, A. and Noelkler, L. (1987). The impact of family relationships on perceived caregiving effectiveness. In Brubaker, T. (ed.), *Aging Family and Health: Long-term Care.* California: Sage.

Travers, A. (1996). Carers. *British Medical Journal* **313**: 482–6.

Twigg, J. (1989). Not taking the strain. *Community Care* **77**: 16–19.

Twigg, J. and Atkin, K. (1994). *Carers Perceived: Policy and Practice in Informal Care.* Buckingham: Open University Press.

Ungerson, C. (1987). *Policy is Personal: Sex, Gender and Personal Care.* London: Tavistock.

Wenger, C. (1984). *The Supportive Network: Coping with Old Age.* London: Allen and Unwin.

Wright, F. (1986). *Left to Care Alone.* Aldershot: Gower.

Chapter 20

Specialist palliative care for non-cancer patients: the ethical arguments

Katherine Wasson and Rob George

Introduction

Death, when spoken of at all, often appears in the same breath as cancer, and is equated with pain, suffering, and a lack of dignity. It is not surprising, therefore, that care of the dying and its roots in the charity sector and the hospice movement have focused historically on care of patients with cancer (Saunders 1993; Doyle *et al.* 1993). Thanks to this, specialist palliative care is now a core requirement in the Policy Framework for Commissioning Cancer Services in the UK (Calman and Hine 1995). It is an indivisible part of best practice in managing cancer and it is clinically indefensible to deny cancer patients access to specialist services.

Whilst some services are actively engaging 'genericism' and diseases other than cancer, it is not the norm, although the question of access to specialist services for all terminally and chronically ill patients has been raised recently both by the specialty (George and Sykes 1997) and the government (HSC 1998; Calman and Hine 1995). However, sufficient doubt remains about the role or responsibility of the specialty and the hospice movement in other chronic and fatal diseases to merit specific ethical reflection.

Ethics offer frameworks in which to make decisions and guide us in what we ought to do in given circumstances: the business of what is right and what is wrong. The relationships between ethics, individuals and a society are complex and changeable. Currently, a high value is placed on the individual and the language of equality and rights is the norm. Ethical reflection is meant to identify issues, give clarification, and a chance to explore and analyse the moral landscape and perspective around a particular problem (Boyd, Higgs and Pinching 1997).

The question

The question we explore here is whether there are good reasons for specialist palliative care being restricted to cancer patients. We do this by analysing the aims, duties, and responsibilities of palliative care, issues of justice in relation to non-cancer patients, and the moral implications of drawing a distinction between cancer and other disease groupings. The answer is rather important. If we fail to find clinical, practical, and defensible moral distinctions between cancer and other fatal diseases, we are left with a much more disturbing question: what it may mean for society if cancer is set apart from other diseases.

We begin our investigation into the extension of specialist palliative care to all patients by looking at the clinical aims and distinctions of the specialty.

The clinical aims of specialist palliative care

All practitioners should aim to maximise the health of their patients. However, the approaches of palliative care differ fundamentally from those of curative medical care. Curative care is focused on disease: symptoms are explored and used as markers of under-lying pathology. The treatments, strategies, services, and resources necessary are, therefore, totally dependent upon pathology. For example, the services for neurosurgery are quite different from those for renal disease, and rightly so. Conversely, palliation is concerned with the suffering caused by disease, not necessarily the disease alone. Our 'diagnostic activity' focuses on the roots of distress across the whole of a person's physical, mental, psychosocial and spiritual domain. A person's primary pathology forms only a small part of the analysis.

The matters that arise with chronicity or the dying process—pain and symptom control, psychosocial need, issues around the family, and so on—are independent of diagnosis. Because a disease is not curable, then care is directed at its consequences not the primary pathology: specialist palliative care is the care of patients with symptomatic or incurable ill-ness, not incurable cancer. This is reflected in the definition given by The World Health Organisation (WHO):

> [palliative care] is the active total care of patients whose disease is not responsive to curative treatment. Control of pain, of other symptoms, and of psychological, social and spiritual prob-lems is paramount.

(WHO 1990)

In order to examine this 'generic' definition of specialist palliative care in more detail, let us consider the primary aims or duties of care set by the specialty. These involve obligations to relieve pain, symptoms, and suffering; to optimise quality of life; to take into account the uniqueness of individuals, their values, and views, and to uphold the dignity of all involved in the dying process (NCHSPCS 1995; Randall and Downie 1996). This leads to our first series of questions: are cancers unique or different from other fatal diseases in these ele-ments of clinical practice?

- *Cancer is not the only cause of pain and symptoms.* As the other chapters in this book have demonstrated, patients with chronic and terminal diseases other than cancer experience pain and distressing symptoms. Cancer does not have the monopoly on suffering.

- *The issues of whole person care and dignity are not different in the care of cancer.* Certainly, one could have claimed some years ago that cancer was almost universally fatal in the short to medium term, and the disease was relentless, distressing, and undignified. How-ever, today there are diseases with a much more certain claim on incurability, disability, and helplessness. Progressive heart, lung, renal, or liver diseases, motor neurone disease, and other neuro-degenerations such as multiple sclerosis or Alzheimer's disease all have an equal claim on these aims with cancer.

- *Recognising dignity and integrity also includes that of the health care professionals.* Care and responsibility for one's patients is enshrined in all the professional codes of conduct and it is indefensible to fail to act in a patient's best interest.[1] This is irrespective of disease, personality, social class, religion and so on. It must also be indefensible, by undermining one's duty to care, to restrict specialist palliative care on any of these bases. Our own data clearly show that GP's and community nurses would benefit from specialist support in a diversity of cases and do not see why they cannot have it (George and Robinson 1996).

To answer our first question: with regard to the aims of specialist palliative care, cancers are not unique or different from other fatal diseases and there appears to be no clinical evidence or reason to confine specialist palliative care to cancer patients. If there is no justifiable clinical evidence, then we must ask whether there are other reasons to limit specialist palliative care? We turn now to the ethical questions.

Ethical issues

General responsibilities and duties in the chronic sick and dying

These are to provide care, to protect the patient's best interests, respect patient autonomy, to do no harm, and to do good. They are linked, may conflict, and often lead to complex and difficult situations, especially when we look at some specific responsibilities relevant to this debate. We deal with each in turn.

To protect the patient's best interest

To act in someone's best interest is a specific and particular thing and goes beyond medical issues. In coming to a decision, our charge is to find, within appropriate ethical and professional parameters, a balance that maximises benefit, however that is defined. Clearly with a competent patient, this means to facilitate them in their choices and to respect their autonomy. Options must be presented even-handedly and we should assist patients in evaluating benefit and burden, aspects of disease progression, uncertainty, etc. With respect to the terminally ill, for example, best interests may include advocacy on their behalf in decisions about place of care, time wasting in unnecessary clinical review, hospital visits, investigations or treatment, and so on.

Duty to care

As caring professionals, we have a fundamental duty to provide care for our patients. It forms part of our professional integrity. Where there is pain, suffering, problems of letting go, and the integrity and dignity of patients and families, the assistance of a specialist in palliative care is, we would argue, clearly needed. One may draw best interest and duty to care together by saying that if a specialist opinion is in the patient's best interest, then it should be sought. Diagnosis carries little persuasion for front-line, general clinical practitioners as a reason not to help.

---

[1] In this respect, of course, a patient cannot demand a treatment as a doctor or nurse cannot be forced to act against their clinical judgement simply on the basis of a patient's request.

To do no harm

The third general element of care is for all professionals to do no harm to their patients: the key duty of non-maleficence[2] (Munson 1988: 33–5) which contrasts with the positive duty of beneficence, or doing good (Beauchamp and Childress 1994). Within palliative care these duties can be seen, for example, in good pain and symptom control, helping with the inevitability of death, but never hastening it intentionally.

Ethical dilemmas arise regarding these responsibilities not least because evaluations of interest in the dying are determined more by questions of quality, which are evaluative, rather than pathology or curability, which tend to be empirical. Second, the role of palliative care, as we have seen from the preceding section, includes 'family'[3] in the holistic care of a patient. The interests of the family may be very different from those of the patient. Judgements will therefore vary according to what is being assessed and by whom. As examples, we may believe it is in the patient's best interests to take all the drugs prescribed for pain relief and symptom control, an oncologist may feel that chemotherapy is a priority, while the patient disagrees because of side effects and wants neither. Further conflicts may arise within the family about the patient's choice to be at home, to refuse social support or nursing care, and so on. These in turn will impact any professional involved if they are unable to fulfil a duty to care.

Specific responsibilities in caring for dying patients

We have covered some general examples where conflicts in interest arise. However, managing patients through the transition from curative to palliative treatments may be seen as a specific responsibility of specialist practice. This is particularly relevant in balancing the benefits and burdens of care, when, in order to benefit, harm may initially be necessary. Sometimes, it is almost impossible not to do some harm in order to achieve some good for a patient. Chemotherapy and radiotherapy are good examples of harm preceding good. Initial harm to a patient is virtually unavoidable, but may be followed by control of pain or further disease spread. Steroids may be seen as examples of drugs given for short-term good whilst anticipating possible long-term harm. These dilemmas are, of course, not confined exclusively to medical care. For example, the specialist practitioner can facilitate confrontation between a patient and his partner, knowing initially that it will be emotionally painful and distressing, but may benefit their relationship. In the spiritual domain, an orthodox religious view may suggest that suffering is seen to have a purpose, or can be given meaning when the outcome is a 'greater good'.

The balances between avoiding/causing harm and benefit requires judgement, partnership, and a clear view of one's intentions. It can be very difficult and certainly justifies the presence of specialist palliative care in diseases where there are toxic treatments or unpredictable elements to clinical decision-making. Cancer care is clearly one, but so is any discipline that deals with technical and invasive measures in treating or palliating disease.

---

2 Non-maleficence can be seen as a negative duty in the sense of limiting harm to patients while beneficence can be seen as a positive duty in the sense of being an obligation to do good. It is conventionally argued that the obligation to restrain harm exceeds that to do good. See footnote 1 as an example.

3 By family we mean both biological and social family, whether conventionally defined or not.

In summary, our various ethical responsibilities include the fundamental duty to care and protect the patient's best interests, the negative duty of non-maleficence, and the positive duty of beneficence. These responsibilities do not focus solely on cancer. The needs and obligations they demand are generic and related to the conflicts and dilemmas of changing the focus of therapeutic strategy, facilitating communication, and ensuring that among competing interests, the best is achieved for one's patient.

The answer to our second question, whether there is an ethical justification to limiting specialist palliative care to cancer, is therefore also negative:

1 It is emerging that specialist palliative care by definition is beyond diagnosis much as our patients are beyond cure.

2 It is unethical based on our general and specific responsibilities. Some specialists in palliative care now realise that their specific knowledge and expertise needs to be applied in wider areas of medicine (NCHSPCS 1998).

3 We have argued that there appear to be no clear distinctions in the clinical or psychosocial needs of patients with cancer or other diseases once they are beyond cure.

4 The aims or responsibilities of the specialty do not warrant cancer's apparent exclusive status

As these arguments have failed to support discrimination in favour of cancer, we must now ask the explicit question: is it an injustice to limit specialist palliative care to any disease category?

Issues of justice

Patients do not present to specialist palliative care unless they are chronically or terminally ill. Despite this, they may well require substantial resources in psychosocial care, home support, and medication. Fortunately in the UK, we do not have to ask or justify whether dying patients merit decent care. Calman and Hine (1995) have done that for us. At the beginning of the new millenium, we merely have to ask whether it is just for patients with cancer to have decent care when patients with other diseases are dying without that sort of help. In examining justice, we look at its three elements: fairness, equality, and equity before considering the arguments around resource allocation.

Fairness: entitlement and what one deserves

Fairness provides a uniform standard by which people are treated the same. Part of this fairness can be related to what a person deserves. Justice as desert, or merit, entails giving people their due (MacIntyre 1988; MacIntyre 1984; Aristotle 1980). Fairness also can be based on entitlement. For example, all UK citizens are entitled to free health care. Like desert, entitlement considers a person's capacities and contributions to society. It also considers the resources already used on a particular patient.

From our point of view, can we say that people deserve specialist palliative care because they have cancer or because they are suffering? Which is fair? Viewing justice primarily as fairness highlights difficulties between cancer and non-cancer patients. What criteria constitute cancer patients deserving or being entitled to receive palliative care services, while non-cancer patients are not?

One reason for this current situation is that specialist palliative care started with cancer patients (Saunders 1993). This in itself is perfectly reasonable. At the outset of a new initiative it is good practice to establish or 'pilot' a project in a single group and a standard process in health service research. Cancer patients were an identifiable group with suffering and pain. The hospice movement identified and highlighted that and has demonstrated that these problems are manageable. One may say that the piloting is now over, as the point has been made and the solution established. The historical development of the specialty—of itself—now no longer provides a sufficient moral basis for confining it to cancer; in fact, one could argue quite the reverse. By demonstrating that specialist palliative care is of benefit in cancer, there is arguably a moral obligation to look for the same needs in all symptomatic and incurable diseases. Should they be found, unless cancer falls into a different moral category, the ethical obligation would seem to call for care to be extended. The work in cancer, and the recommendations of Calman and Hine (1995) have shown that people with cancer should not be left to suffer. Both have established a precedent. Hence, the current situation is not fair to suffering non-cancer patients. We pick this up again in our concluding reflections. This brings us to the second element of justice: equality.

Equality

Justice involves not only fairness, but also equality. Equality requires that similar cases are treated in similar ways. Take an example: two terminally ill patients of the same age and general health have similar symptoms of pain, breathlessness, constipation, and anxiety. One has lung cancer, while the other has respiratory disease. The former is likely to receive specialist palliative care while the latter is not.

According to equality, both these patients should have access to the same quality of input from specialist palliative care professionals. In contrast, inequality would allow similar cases to be treated in different ways. Given both patients have the same physical symptoms, not to mention similar emotional and psychological needs, it is not morally justifiable within the principle of equality to deny the patient with respiratory disease the expertise and benefits of specialist palliative care. To do so would be to treat these patients unequally.

Opposing inequality is important to prevent inappropriate discrimination among and between cases (Wasson 1997). This might be based on the patient's diagnosis or race, class, sex, personality, family dynamic, and location in the country. Equality ensures such discrimination is not permitted and provides a basic, minimum level of consistency, below which treatment of any patient should not fall. For example, it is unacceptable that a recognised and proven treatment is only available in certain areas of the country because a health authority feels it to be too expensive or an inappropriate use of resource. At the time of writing, this debate is active in the media, as a patient's chance of getting adequate treatment for certain malignancies is determined by their address. This is an inequality.

Ideas of fairness and equality are fine, but what does the same or equal mean and where does appropriateness come in? Principles of justice must also consider what is appropriate or inappropriate in a given case. This is called equity.

Equity

In considering justice as fairness and equality, there should be some recognition that it may not always be appropriate to treat similar cases in exactly the same way. For example, two patients may have similar symptoms from different diseases, such as cancer and heart disease. Pain control in both may be achieved with drugs, but radiotherapy turns out to be the best treatment for the cancer patient and coronary artery surgery for the patient with heart disease. It would be fair and equal to offer both the choice of radiotherapy or surgery, but entirely inappropriate.

Equity, then, allows for justified differences in treatment of specific individuals in specific situations. Downie and Telfer (1980) argue justified differences in equity are based on variations in need, where like cases are treated similarly and unlike cases are distinguished for 'morally appropriate reasons'. This notion of appropriateness requires the use of judgement. Such judgement may be linked to professional, legal, or personal standards—in our case, clinically and morally defensible minimum standards.

Equity allows health care professionals to treat similar cases differently, but only for justified reasons. For example, ways of delivering treatments or the exact details of a regime may take into account individual factors that have an impact on the balance between the benefit and harm of a particular treatment. We may justifiably manage an elderly and excessively frail patient differently from a young patient with the same pathology.

However, equity does not permit minimum standards and levels of palliative (or any other) care to be compromised, particularly for morally unjustified reasons. We would submit for example that it is inequitable and unjustified to provide different standards of pain relief and symptom control for cancer and non-cancer patients on the basis of diagnosis (NCHSPCS 1998).

Two key diagnoses highlight questions of justice in palliative care for non-cancer patients. The first, and oldest, is motor neurone disease, which has been included in specialist palliative care almost since the beginning of the hospice movement (O'Brien et al. 1992). The second diagnosis is HIV/AIDS. Both are particularly unpleasant diseases that very obviously merit attention and these patients have been able to obtain specialist palliative care (George and Spittle 1998; George and Jennings 1996). It has now become more acceptable to utilise the expertise of palliative care professionals in dealing with the complex symptoms arising from HIV and AIDS (Sim and Moss 1991; Sweeney et al.1991; Kelleher et al. 1997), as well as provide psychological, social, and spiritual support (Foley et al. 1995; Barnes et al. 1993). Part of this success in HIV may be due to the patient population consisting of young dying people who are often highly informed, articulate, and assertive (George and Jennings 1993). These patients have demonstrated the need for and benefits of translating palliative care expertise into a non-cancer area. If palliative care is provided for this group of non-cancer patients, then why should other non-cancer groups such as those with heart disease, renal failure, and respiratory disease, continue to be excluded or have inconsistent access to specialist support and care?

Through examining the principles of fairness, equality, and equity, we have argued that it is not morally justifiable to discriminate against non-cancer patients and deny them the expertise and benefits of specialist palliative care:

* it is not just or justifiable to discriminate between patients on the basis of diagnosis, the historical focus of the specialty or levels of assertiveness;
* justice requires there to be a general availability of specialist palliative care that provides for all terminally and chronically ill people.

An obvious response to our general statement about justice is that this is all fine in principle, but the resources simply are not there. In contrast to cancer, the status and progression of chronic illnesses and the prognosis of patients with other diseases can be difficult to assess and often pose long-term difficulties with symptom management. Whilst the pain and other symptoms could be managed with palliative care expertise (NCHSPCS 1998), are the differences in pattern or the potential impact on resource use a justified reason for excluding any diagnoses? Some people consider it to be so. Are there any other justifiable reasons for the current inconsistencies in the provision of specialist palliative care for all?

The problem of resources: 'distributive justice'

Difficulties regarding resource allocation

Difficulties over resource fall into two categories, money and manpower. Money is usually seen as the solution. However, what is actually needed in most situations is to look at new ways of solving old problems. For example, altering patterns of practice may solve both problems with a minimum of additional finance. Changes in attitude may be needed. Alternatively, new skills may be acquired or passed on to other practitioners. We briefly examine the resource question under two headings: financial and educational.

Financial resource

Inadequate resource is a common excuse given for limiting specialist palliative care. In fact, even current provision for cancer depends upon sustained charitable giving. It is argued that specialist palliative care is time- and energy-intensive and this level of resource consumption is difficult to sustain, far less increase, in the National Health Service (NHS) given its limited resources. However, one cannot leave the argument there. We need to face the fact that prioritisation and the use of resources within specialist palliative care is necessary. We need new ways to solve the problem.

Alternative approaches to optimise resources

One response to such objections argues that there are different types of palliative care input. The hypothesis is that intensive and expensive specialist palliative care is not required in all cases. Specialist knowledge can be used strategically to benefit the patient and still be cost-effective. This finds an early voice in the three levels of palliative care given in the general UK definitions as the palliative care approach, palliative interventions, and specialist palliative care. What is needed now is a further division of the specialist category.

There are specialist teams and practitioners based in hospices, hospitals, and the community who provide palliative care. George and Sykes (1997) argue that input from these professionals can be given on three different levels. First, there is consultative input that is focused and brief. This type of consultation is short term and has clearly defined end points. Such contact might entail a phone call from a general practitioner or a few visits by palliative care specialists to address specific symptoms or pain control issues. Second, there is full multidisciplinary palliative care input, that is conventional specialist palliative care based on psychosocial and holistic need. This level of service is provided for patients who are reaching the end of life in the short to medium term. It is a complete service addressing physical, emotional, psychosocial, and spiritual issues, and providing on-going support and input from a range of palliative care professionals. Third, there is terminal care. This level of palliative care is provided in the final days of a patient's life and may be quite intensive. Terminal care often involves concentrated support for primary health care or in-patient clinicians who require quick, effective symptom control, assistance, or ethical advice in dealing with the patient's changing needs, as well as communication and pastoral issues involving the family.

The immediate logic of this approach is that it brings specialist palliative care into line with other specialties, namely that the fact, level, and nature of advice or involvement is based on need and not diagnosis. Second, we then can operate as genuine specialists, namely those who are involved when there is a need that genuinely merits expert help. This has educational implications both into the specialty and out from the specialty.

Education resource

The foregoing discussion presupposes two things. First that specialists in palliative care have sufficient skill to work with all diagnoses (assuming that these skills are transferable). Second, that general clinicians have enough basic skills in the palliative care approach to deal with straightforward issues and to make referrals that are appropriate and genuinely in need of specialist help.

A barrier to specialist palliative care for all?

One reason given to defend the inconsistent application of specialist palliative care beyond cancer is that symptom management is different in other diseases or illnesses and that the skills required are new to the specialty. Even if this is accurate, it is not a justifiable reason to exclude non-cancer patients from the benefits of palliative care. This reason constitutes a problem of knowledge, not clinical distinctions, ethics, or justice. It highlights the need for continuous development of expertise to cope with the need to apply palliative care to a variety of conditions other than cancer (NCHSPCS 1998). This is the perfectly legitimate and generally accepted responsibility of any serious specialty to develop and educate its members.

A solution for specialist palliative care for all?

In addition to the development of specific expertise in using palliative care for non-cancer conditions, there needs to be a more general level of palliative care knowledge among clinicians. To increase the general awareness and use of palliative care a better level of training in the specialty should be required for all doctors and nurses. The impetus for incorporating such training might stem from a wider awareness of the fruits of the specialty. The knowledge and benefits of palliative care should be more widely discussed and passed on to other areas of medicine and nursing (House of Lords 1994).

The application of a palliative care approach and knowledge should be a standard part of what it means to be a good doctor or nurse. Both increased general training and greater awareness of the benefits of specialist palliative care could lead to more appropriate use of specialist teams and their clinicians for *all* terminally and chronically ill patients.

Summary

In this section, we have asked whether the principles of justice or the practicalities of limited resources offer defences for limiting specialist palliative care to cancer.

1 Justice as fairness, equality, and equity requires that palliative care be extended to non-cancer patients.

2 Neither an argument based on limited resources nor lack of specific knowledge or expertise is justifiable in limiting specialist palliative care to cancer. What it may require is a different approach.

Further reflections

In our analysis of whether there are good reasons for specialist palliative care being restricted to cancer patients, we have looked at clinical distinctions, our general and specific ethical obligations to patients, the broader questions of justice, and the difficulties that may arise around resources. In none have we found justifiable reasons to deny patients specialist palliative care should they need it.

Health care professions or government may wish to decide that once a disease is not curable, then there is restricted access to resources. Currently, this is indefensible based on the recommendations of Calman and Hine (1995) and recent NHS Health Executive directives. Were this to be the case, then all of society would need to be involved in the debate, and must be clear about the implications and assumptions of such a choice. We need finally to reflect on these implications from both sides of the 'fence', namely to continue positive discrimination towards cancer patients or to embrace the disadvantaged dying.

On one side, if we accept the case for specialist palliative care for all in extending full access to patients in need, the first challenge for specialist clinicians is to develop further clinical expertise and knowledge. A second is that a general level of training in the palliative care approach and knowledge of the benefits of specialist palliative care be taught to all relevant caring professionals. Both approaches will contribute to specialist services being more practically accessible outside the remit of cancer. This level of generic palliative care experience and knowledge would allow specialist palliative care to concentrate on the difficult cases that genuinely merit specialist input. Furthermore, this expansion of palliative care knowledge and expertise, and the consequent improvement in care, can take place without the support of substantial further resources. Fundamentally our question to the specialty now is to ask, not whether, but *how* we are to treat the chronically sick and dying. One key challenge is to take our place and responsibility as a fully developed specialty that manages patients according to their needs. As we have said, specialist palliative care is beyond diagnosis, much as our patients are beyond cure.

Looking from the vantage of history, the hospice movement has become a superlative of society's conscience. It has recognised, piloted, and funded the pioneering work on care of the dying in this country and has a valid stake in future developments. However, with that, and the movement's success in advocating for those dying with cancer, must surely come the new challenge to advocate for the remaining disadvantaged dying patients.

Much funding for hospices has come from charities. Charity has the right and freedom to specify its use, but specialist palliative care has moved beyond being a charitable extra to being a core requirement for cancer care. We would suggest that charities might respond to the needs of the disadvantaged dying by being inclusive and moving their ground to demonstrate and advocate for the dignity of the suffering individual. Pain is pain; suffering is suffering; its character and intensity is independent of diagnosis, but very much to do with being human. Donors may wish to confine their giving to cancer, but perhaps it should be required of people that they specify this or else their funds will be assumed to have no ties. We would encourage any constitutional change necessary to permit giving for the dying not just those dying with cancer.

Clearly, the government must also grasp this nettle. It is now committed to providing palliative care for cancer patients (Calman and Hine 1995), and suggests that this is appropriate to all dying patients (HSC 1998). It ought now to make explicit the unacceptability of providing specialist palliative care for one main group and not others, and attach financial inducements and standards to this practice.

If we continue to look on this debate from the cancer side of the fence, one conclusion becomes clear: that people dying of cancer are more 'worthy'. If this is the case, we, as caring professionals, should ensure that people are informed about health care entitlements. Where dying well, with minimum suffering and maximum pain and symptom management is important to a patient, they should be encouraged to develop cancer. How ironic that the justification for smoking and defaulting from breast or cervical screening would be the insurance that at least one's death would be well managed.

References

Aristotle (1980). *Nichomachean Ethics*. Book V. Translated by David Ross. Oxford University Press.

Barnes, R., Barratt, C., Weintraub, S., Holowacz, G., Chan, M., and LeBlanc, E. (1993). Hospital response to psycho-social needs of AIDS in-patients. *Journal of Palliative Care* 9: 22–8.

Beauchamp, T.L. and Childress, J.F. (1994). *Principles in Biomedical Ethics* (4th edn). Oxford University Press, pp. 35–7.

Boyd, K.M., Higgs, R., and Pinching, A.J. (eds) (1997). *The New Dictionary of Medical Ethics*. London: BMA.

Calman, K. and Hine, D. (1995). A framework for commissioning cancer services. A report by the expert advisory group on cancer to the chief medical officers of England and Wales. London: Department of Health.

Downie, R. and Telfer, E. (1980). *Caring and Curing: A Philosophy of Medicine and Social Work*. New York and London: Methuen.

Doyle, D., Hanks, G.W.C., and MacDonald, N. (eds) (1993). *The Oxford Textbook of Palliative Medicine*. Oxford University Press.

Foley, F.J., Flannery, J., Graydon, D., Flintoft, G., and Cook, D. (1995). AIDS palliative care—challenging the palliative paradigm. *Journal of Palliative Care* 11: 19–22.

George, R.J.D. and Jennings, A-L. (1993). Palliative care. *Postgraduate Medical Journal* 69: 429–49.

George, R.J.D. and Jennings A-L. (1996). Palliative care of HIV disease and AIDS. *Progress in Palliative Care* 4: 44–7.

George, R.J.D. and Robinson, V.R. (1996). *Camden and Islington Palliative Care Team Review*. London: Palliative Care Centre.

George, R.J.D. and Spittle, M.F. (1998). AIDS and the young dying. In Karim, A.B.M.F., Kuitert, H.M., Newling, D.W.W., and Wortman, V. (eds), *Death: Medical, Spiritual and Social Care of the Dying*. Amsterdam: V. U. University Press pp. 55–73.

George, R.J.D. and Sykes, J. (1997). Beyond cancer. In Clark, D., Hockley, J., and Ahmedzai, S. (eds), *New Themes in Palliative Care*. Buckingham: Open University.

Health Service Circular (1998): 115.

House of Lords. (1994). Report of the Select Committee on Medical Ethics. London: HMSO.

Kelleher, P., Cox, S., and McKeogh, M. (1997). HIV infection: the spectrum of symptoms and disease in male and female patients attending a London hospice. *Palliative Medicine* 11: 152–8.

MacIntyre, A. (1984). *After Virtue: Study in Moral Theory.* Notre Dame: Notre Dame University Press, p. 192.

MacIntyre, A. (1988). *Whose Justice? Which Rationality?* Notre Dame: Notre Dame University Press, p. 104.

Munson, R. (ed.) (1988). *Intervention and Reflection: Basic Issues in Medical Ethics.* 3rd edn. Belmont: Wadsworth Publishing.

National Council for Hospice and Specialist Palliative Care Services (1995). *Specialist Palliative Care. A Statement of Definitions.* Occasional Paper 8. London: NCHSPCS.

National Council for Hospice and Specialist Palliative Care Services and Scottish Partnership Agency for Palliative and Cancer Care (1998). *Reaching Out: Specialist Palliative Care for Adults with Non-malignant Diseases.* Occasional Paper 14. London: NCHSPCS.

O'Brien, T., Kelly, M., and Saunders, C. (1992). Motor Neurone Disease: a hospice perspective. *British Medical Journal* 304: 471–3.

Randall, F. and Downie, R.S. (1996). *Palliative Care Ethics: A Good Companion.* Oxford University Press, pp. 18–20.

Saunders, C. (1993). Foreword. In Doyle, D., Hanks, G.W.C. and MacDonald, N. (eds), *The Oxford Textbook of Palliative Medicine.* Oxford University Press.

Sim, R. and Moss, V. (1991). *Terminal Care for People with AIDS.* London: Edward Arnold.

Sweeney, J., Peters, B.S., and Main, J. (1991). Clinical care and management: *AIDS Care* 3: 457–60.

Wasson, K. (1997). The ethics of care or the ethics of justice? A middle way. Ph.D. dissertation. The Whitefield Institute, Oxford and the Open University.

World Health Organisation (1990). *Cancer Pain Relief and Palliative Care.* Technical report series 804. Geneva: World Health Organisation.

Chapter 21

Cultural issues in palliative care for non-cancer patients

Peter W. Speck

Introduction

Most studies of cultural influences in palliative care have related mainly to people coming to terms with a cancer-related diagnosis. Some of the work undertaken can be applied to non-cancer patients but more research is needed specifically with non-cancer patients. In this chapter we shall examine what we mean by culture and ethnicity, the experience of becoming ill, and the way in which that may be culturally determined (Foster and Anderson 1978; Baer *et al.* 1986; Lupton 1996). The importance of being aware of ethnocentricity will then be explored together with two aspects of care where some research has been undertaken: pain and communication. Finally the chapter will look at staff needs and training, managerial issues, and suggestions for further research in this area of care.

The main aspects of palliative care have been defined by The National Council for Hospice and Specialist Palliative Care Services (NCHSPCS) in the UK as: a holistic approach with a focus on quality of life, including symptom control. The focus of care is defined in terms of the person who is dying and those who matter to him/her. Autonomy of choice, and both open and sensitive communication between the various professionals involved in providing that care are also key components of *specialist* palliative care. Within a general health care setting this approach is consistent with that in the NHS Patient's Charter Standard (UK) which emphasises the importance of 'respect for the privacy, dignity, religious and cultural needs' of those receiving care.

A *culture* can be understood as a shared set of beliefs, values, behaviour patterns, rituals, and symbols, of which religion can be a crucial part. These serve to influence how we live our lives and understand our experience of the world, both internally and externally, and form the basis for an individual's sense of identity. The term '*ethnic group*' usually refers to a group of people who have the same cultural, racial and linguistic backgrounds even though they may be geographically separated. Thus members will have the same permanent genetic ancestry, have adapted their behaviour and attitudes through assimilation into a variety of geographical settings and perhaps modified their language forms, but still experience a psychological need to retain a strong group identity and sense of belonging (ethnicity). For example, the Jewish people originated in the same part of the Middle East, and, although widely dispersed, still retain their Jewish identity even if they do not all practice their faith or attend synagogue. Growing up and being educated within the cultural group serves to shape the person's identity which is internalised and provides a valuable inner reference point when moving from one cultural group to another. If this identity is not reasonably secure the individual can feel threatened by other cultural groups and respond in either a submissive or aggressive way. The onset of illness can be a trigger for checking the experience against the person's internalised 'map' or reference set in order to understand what is happening within the body.

The experience of illness

When a person becomes ill they enter into a process of exploration and negotiation concerning the symptoms and experience of disease within their body and its possible meaning, both now and in the future. This process begins within the person as they decide whether the symptoms are worth reporting to someone else, drawing upon their knowledge of illness and previous experience of their own body to decide on the next step. Frequently, if they decide they are 'ill', they will discuss this with a family member and the accepted norms of the family and/or culture will be influential in deciding whether this is a situation where they should 'self treat' or refer for outside help.

How and where they access that outside help will be culturally determined, in that the evaluation of symptoms by others will decide the options open to them by way of treatment or other responses. The value system, codes of practice and set of explanations people use to interpret the world will have been provided by the culture within which they find themselves. For those who have moved from their country of origin, there may be an additional experience of feeling 'dislocated' within the cultural setting in which they are now located which may also have different practices and explanations. Thus a woman who arrives by plane from rural Bangladesh to join her family in England may be transferred to a British hospital because of suspected illness. Not only is she separated from the family she hoped to join, where the cultural norms of home would have provided some buffer against the very different culture of the surrounding community, but she has been precipitated into an unfamiliar, if not alien, western bio-medical setting. The resultant problem is often not just one of spoken language but of a different understanding of symptoms and different remedies, rules and standards which can result in the person experiencing a crisis of identity in addition to the effects of the illness itself.

Ethnocentricity

Because the cultural group we belong to influences our view of the world and helps shape our identity, we tend to assume that this world view is the 'natural' or right one, both practically and morally. This is known as *ethnocentricity*. Cultures are dynamic and so, when confronted by another culture, we may find that its different values and assumptions conflict with or threaten our own, causing us to respond defensively in order to protect ourselves from any possible undermining of our own identity and power. This can lead to stereotyping, or debunking, as a way of minimising the perceived personal threat from something seen as 'different'. Ethnic and cultural identity are very personal and it is always best to enquire from the individual as to how they would define their ethnic group or cultural background. However, because of the experience of stereotyping, many people find this an especially sensitive area. In a medical setting it is not only people by whom we may feel threatened, we can also be affected when evaluating the effectiveness of new treatment approaches which are valued by people in different cultural settings. Various complementary treatment approaches have had great difficulty in being accepted as 'complementary' in a biomedical western setting. This includes the Chinese medical techniques of acupuncture and Qigong (a breathing exercise for progressive muscular relaxation) which many Chinese people see as important ways of restoring the energy balance and augmenting the autoimmune system. Patients are sometimes puzzled by the unwillingness of a western doctor to prescribe a similar remedy to one that they would have received in their original home setting. Health care professionals, as a result of their training in the western biomedical model, enter and create their own cultural setting which people often find difficult to understand when they access it as vulnerable patients. If we are not aware that we are adopting an ethnocentric view, we can find ourselves measuring the other culture's approach against our own in a patronising or disparaging way, rather than entering into an open-ended dialogue from which both can learn.

Each person who seeks health care for themselves or their family may have an individual ethnic identity and therefore, a culturally-determined way of understanding what is wrong with them which may differ from that of the health care professional. Thus the consultation needs to take into account, therefore, the fact that the health carer belongs to a cultural group, as does the prospective patient. Effective communication and a willingness to listen to and learn from the patient are essential if the needs of the sick person are to be properly assessed. In the field of palliative care, where many people are either experiencing a life-threatening illness or a chronic illness with difficult symptomatology, this is especially important.

Pain

Pain has always been central to many of the symptoms for which people seek relief or palliation. But pain is interpreted, expressed and given meaning by the individual who experiences it within their particular cultural setting.

Zoboroski (1969) assessed some of the cultural influences on responses to pain among four groups of people, all resident in the United States: Italians, Jews, Irish and 'Old Americans'. He found that Italian and Jewish people tended to manifest similar behaviour. They talked freely about pain, complained, groaned, and cried. They were not ashamed of emotion and expected sympathy, understanding and help from others. The 'Old Americans' tried to avoid being a nuisance, were matter of fact and focused. There were very few verbal or physical expressions of pain, but they did tend to withdraw socially. Within the Irish group most were reluctant to discuss pain and felt they were not expected to share feelings or troubles with other people. Older people were more prone to show pain than to hide it and pain tolerance decreased with age, irrespective of cultural grouping, with men being more tolerant than women. Much of the pain behaviour, he concluded, was learnt from various models in the family and culture, with a key factor being the giving or withholding of approval for the expression of feelings by significant people.

Greenwald (1991) has argued that although several investigators had reported a link between ethnic background and expression of pain, such links were highly problematical. Few studies of pain and ethnicity had used quantitative measures of pain combined with multivariate methods of data analysis and most had focused on populations characterised by highly distinct ethnic groups. Therefore, Greenwald interviewed 536 persons recently treated for forms of cancer known to cause significant pain. Pain was assessed using standard, well-validated instruments.

The study took place in an area with a low proportion of recent immigrants to the US and only small concentrations of distinct ethnic minorities. No statistically significant relationships were observed between ethnic identity and measures of pain sensation. However, pain described in affective terms according to the McGill Pain Questionnaire did vary among ethnicities. Greenwald concluded that cultures associated with specific ethnic identities still condition individual expression of pain despite the high degree of assimilation that has occurred among ethnic groups in the US. We should not, therefore, assume that any group will assimilate and lose the impact of their own cultural influences even after several generations. In fact, 'crisis theory' teaches that, when our equilibrium is disturbed by a crisis, we first of all try to restore our equilibrium by going back to previous ways of coping. However well assimilated we may be within a new culture, in a crisis, we will still revert initially to our primary cultural ways of coping before rejecting those which are unhelpful and seeking new coping strategies.

Bates *et al.* (1993) reported on a study of 372 patients with chronic pain, from six ethnic groups, who attended for treatment at a multidisciplinary pain-management centre. They found that ethno-cultural affiliation was important to chronic pain perception and variation of response. In this study population, the best predictors of pain intensity variation were ethnic group affiliation and locus of control (LOC) style (ethnic group identity also being a predictor of LOC style). It appeared that variations in pain intensity might be affected by differences in attitudes, beliefs and emotional and psychological states associated with the different ethnic groups. Although it is likely that intense pain affects attitudes and emotions, it is also very likely that attitudes and emotions influence reported perceptions of pain intensity. Pain intensity variation in this study population was not significantly associated with diagnosis, present medication types, or types of past treatments or surgeries for pain.

Juarez *et al.* (1998) used qualitative research methods to look at cultural influences on cancer pain management in Hispanic (Mexican and Central American) patients. Responses suggest that culture, family beliefs, and religion contribute significantly to management and expression of pain by the patient and caregiver. In addition, this group showed that pain may be approached with stoicism; therefore, lack of verbal or behavioural expression of pain does not indicate a lack of pain itself. Patients also demonstrated a reliance on folk beliefs and non-drug interventions. The most common reason cited for non-compliance with pharmacological treatment was an inability to understand instructions. They concluded that there was a need, when providing care, to be non-judgmental, sensitive, and respectful.

To improve compliance, this work suggests that the multidisciplinary team should

- incorporate the patients' folk health care practices and beliefs into the plan of care when possible;
- involve family members and friends in the patient's care, identifying one key family contact;
- ensure that instructions for medications are available in Spanish and understood by the patient and caregiver.

This study of Hispanic patients highlights a second important issue in offering palliative care to cancer and non-cancer patients from differing cultural backgrounds, that of communication.

Communication

The UK definition of specialist palliative care emphasises the importance of open and sensitive communication. From the time of entering the GP's surgery or being admitted to hospital, the inability to communicate can lead to a worry that the patient will not receive a proper assessment of need and therefore not receive the help required. This worry can quickly become a fear if miscommunication persists. The use of interpreters can help but is not a panacea. Patients may feel embarrassed to discuss certain symptoms with some family members present, especially if a young child has been requested to translate. In addition to an age difference, gender or non-medical background can create barriers. Language cards in the person's own language may not help if the person does not read their own language or reads only a dialect of the text depicted. The family hierarchy can also be influential in some cultures, resulting in the patient not speaking until the key member of the family gives permission or indicates approval of the treatment or of the consultation. This is well illustrated in a brief report by Clarke *et al.* (1991) regarding a 38-year-old Korean lady living in Cardiff (Wales) whose husband refused to allow her to receive medication, although she was in pain from what seemed to be secondary deposits from breast cancer and advanced pulmonary tuberculosis. She was admitted to a hospice unit eventually, where she ultimately died. In spite of attempts to use interpreters, communication remained a major problem, coupled with the controlling influence of the husband. The authors state:

> The cultural barriers of language were both verbal and, to a large extent, nonverbal behavioural differences. Within her culture, the wife viewed herself as totally obedient to the husband, although her nonverbal signals suggested that she would have readily accepted more help had she felt free to do so. The presumptive diagnosis of tuberculosis allowed us to provide a limited degree of symptom control. The medical and nursing staff who were with the family at the time of her death were deeply affected by the distress of the children and their own sense of helplessness.

This situation also illustrates the difficulty of knowing whether one is dealing with an identifiable cultural response to illness or a particular family's idiosyncratic response to crisis. An Indian man died at our London hospital one weekend. The family would not accept that he was dead, even though the doctor, nurse manager, and chaplain explained how death is certified in the UK and why we knew he was dead. Eventually the body had to be transferred to the mortuary and the family accompanied the staff and stayed with the body, insisting that the man was only asleep. They were waiting for the man's brother to come from the Holy Temple of Amritsar with holy water which would revive the 'sleeping' man. We contacted a local Sikh priest who spoke with them and later said: 'You have got a difficult family. It is clear that the man is dead. I suggest you wait for the man's brother to come and then discuss it with him.' On the brother's arrival he pronounced the man dead! He later explained that, in India, a corpse turns black within hours of death. Because our mortuary was cold this did not happen and the man's skin colour changed little. Therefore, the family were convinced he was not dead, because the signs of death were absent. No book of explanations about Sikhism and attitudes to death could have prepared us for this event; it needed intervention from the right person at the right time and patience from the medical staff.

There may also be an issue around what can be communicated and to whom. In China, for instance, death still remains a taboo for many and talking about death is thought to hasten it. Families will therefore frequently avoid such discussion to protect the patient, yet spend hours preparing intricate soups and other food which symbolically speak of their care and concern. In Japan, a study showed that 18% of patients who died of cancer had been told their diagnosis. The diagnosis is often shared with the family but not the patient. In the same study 98% of the families, usually spouses, had been told of the diagnosis. One consequence of the Japanese patients' ignorance of their diagnoses is that they frequently receive aggressive treatment right up to the end of life. In addition, 80% of the dying do not ask questions (Ishikawa 1992).

Other studies have looked at 'truth telling' and what people wish to know. Studies in Spain (Centeno-Cortes and Olarte 1994), Italy (Toscani *et al.* 1991) and Hong Kong (Fielding and Hung 1996) showed that age and gender were as much a factor as culture, although the researchers did not reflect on how their own cultural backgrounds and views on 'truth telling' may have influenced how they designed the research and how they spoke with the participants.

In a later study, De Trill and Kovalcik (1997) focused on the child with cancer. They stress that the cultural life of a community will be very important in determining the value given to children, the measures taken to care for their health, and a family's responses to an ill child. Health care professionals should be sensitive to culturally defined health beliefs and practices, since they may explain behaviours such as non-adherence to prescribed therapies, as well as the degree and quality of parents' involvement in patient care, and the family's relationship with health care staff. Assessments of health beliefs and practices, family composition, religious rites, and beliefs about the causes of illness should be undertaken for each family. This will help the design of treatment plans that are in keeping with a family's cultural background.

The authors make the very important point that we should try to identify the individual as well as culturally defined characteristics of the family. This will protect against any tendency towards cultural stereotyping that may occur in the context of behaviours that are not well understood in a particular health care setting. But how competent do professionals feel to make sensitive assessments and to deliver cross-cultural care?

Delivering cross-cultural care

In Australia, McNamara *et al.* (1997) attempted to assess the perceived competence of 191 Australian palliative care professionals to deliver cross-cultural care. The results identified clear areas where staff felt less competent to deliver appropriate care and where additional training and resources were needed. Given that there are over 100 cultural variations in Australia, this is not easily resolved. Some workers had had negative (de-skilling) experiences of working with some ethnic groups and the researchers identified that teaching was probably more effective than simply encouraging multicultural exposure. Language was clearly an issue and guidelines to the most effective use of interpreters or language cards were required. Information concerning particular beliefs about dying, death and bereavement, and as 'truth telling' issues for the various cultural groups was another need. There were dangers of grouping or stereotyping individuals because of variations in beliefs among individuals or families who seem to have the same cultural background. In the Australian study resources considered helpful for cross-cultural care included:

People	Professionals with the same cultural background
	Volunteers with the same cultural background
	Family members
	Ethnic liaison workers
Education	Lectures, books, visual aids, and interactive workshops run by/including ethnic community representatives
Language aids	Medical terms translated, communication boards, brochures for patients, and personal/telephone interpreting service

One important lesson from the results is that, in order to provide a culturally sensitive service, we have to address managerial, resource, and training needs.

Training and development for palliative care staff

The present skill level of palliative care team members will need to be assessed and the relevant training/resource needs identified. Staff will need specific training in the cultural norms of those groups most likely to enter into a palliative care programme, preferably provided in collaboration with members of those communities. As shown by the Australian study, having interpreters available is one thing, knowing how to use them properly is another. Staff may require training in how to brief an interpreter and how to offer debriefing if the interpreter has found the session distressing. It is also helpful to forge links with the leaders or other contacts within the different communities and establish whether the providers of spiritual care have already undertaken some of this work already. The chaplaincy and spiritual care departments of many hospitals have frequently already done some of this liaison work, in order to provide for the spiritual needs of other patients in the health care setting. They will already have knowledge of any religious taboos concerning talking about death or how people wish to prepare for it. They will also have experience of providing or facilitating rituals and religious ceremonies for those who wish to continue to express their faith while hospitalised. They should also be a resource to staff and families on ethical issues such as post-mortem examinations or dietary laws and fasting.

Managerial issues

Each palliative care service needs to make an assessment of its particular catchment area and likely patient population. This will entail developing knowledge of the local ethnic groups and monitoring their use of the service.

The documentation of patients may need to be re-examined to ensure that it prompts sensitively for details regarding the patient's religious or other beliefs, values, practices, dietary requirements and available choices, and family relationships or hierarchy. Managerially it is important to ensure that the appropriate policies are in place (according to the country's own employment laws) regarding equal opportunities for staff recruitment, and policies concerning anti-discrimination are in the NHS Patients' Charter in the UK, and mission statements.

Research issues

While there is some research now being undertaken into cultural influences in palliative care, most relates to cancer symptoms or problems. Apart from one or two studies on chronic pain, most studies on illness behaviour and responses have been general in approach. Therefore, it is currently a matter of trying to apply insights from these general studies to the more specific area of palliative care for non-cancer patients. However, some work is beginning and DeTrill and Kovalcik (1997) reported on the need for research studies in which health behaviours are correlated with culturally defined values and practices.

The International Psycho-Oncology Society, through its National Representation Committee, is currently investigating oncology practices around the world. Nearly 30 countries are participating in this attempt to identify cultural variations in truth-telling, palliative care, pain control, and use of alternative medicine in oncology. This is especially important because of the joint effort that is required to share professional experiences and to enhance efficient communication among oncologists internationally. However, there is also a need for multi-professional studies to be undertaken as all professions contributing to specialist palliative care services need to be reflecting on the multicultural dimension of the care they offer. Another area for research might be the accessibility and acceptability of palliative care programmes to people from a variety of cultural backgrounds.

Many of the quality of life and outcome scales that are in use in the field of palliative care may also need to be reviewed to ensure that they are equally meaningful when used in cross-cultural studies. In 1996 Goh and colleagues in Singapore looked at the issue of measuring quality of life in different cultures and whether such measures could be translated satisfactorily for use in China and Malaya. These measures are usually given to patients so that they can self-assess their physical, psychological and social functioning as well as the effect of any distressing symptoms. The fact that the measures then give a patient-centred view of health outcome makes them especially valuable in planning a holistic approach to care. Most of these questionnaires have originated in the West and have been developed in English. Because translation always involves interpretation, it is difficult to know if the final version in another language still retains its meaning. Goh *et al.* (1996) have therefore utilised a stepwise process of translation and back translation with field trials at each stage, in order to see if the translated questions correlate well with the English counterpart. So far the results they report are positive, but their work highlights the difficulties that can be encountered in cross-cultural work and in the development of valid tools for research and care.

Conclusion

Whatever structures or training are in place, the main experts in this area of care are the patient and the family. It is very important, therefore, to always try to obtain information from the patient concerning their experience of illness and how this is understood within the context of their culture, religion, race, gender, sexuality, and so on. Culture only becomes meaningful when it is interpreted in the context of the patient's own story, family history, structure and status. The danger in training staff in short overviews of different cultural patterns is that these overviews can be used as simplistic predictors of belief and behaviour which quickly stereotype the patient and result in insensitive care. Several books already exist which describe the main faith traditions and their relevant practices in time of illness or death (Rees 1997; Speck 1989; Fuller and Toon 1988).

Training must enable us to examine how we feel about difference, how we respond to it, and how we can overcome any tendency to ignore difference which leads to fragmented care. Kelly (1992) when talking about the problems of coping with chronic illness identified four aspects of care:

• the technical and practical management of the condition,

• the management of thoughts and feelings,

• the management of interpersonal relations,

• interpreting and making sense of the condition.

In seeking to provide palliative care for people with non-cancer conditions these four aspects are relevant. It is in relation to the fourth aspect, of interpreting and making sense of the condition, that culture has a vital part to play.

Yasmin Gunaratnam (1998), in a talk on multicultural service provision at a UK hospice concluded by saying: 'In the tradition of hospice care there is a need to strive for open and empowering services, which can resist the pressures to find handy and manageable solutions to address the complexities of lived experiences.' I believe that it is the interplay between how you and I each make sense of and interpret the chronic condition that is the challenge of cross-cultural care. If we can listen and learn together, in an open way, then there will be a good chance of that care being of good quality.

References

Baer, H.A., Singer, M., and Johnsen, J.H. (1986). Toward a critical medical anthropology. *Social Science and Medicine* **23**: 95–8.

Bates, M.S., Edwards, W.T., and Anderson, K.O. (1993). Ethnocultural influences on variation in chronic pain perception. *Pain* **52**: 101–12.

Centeno-Cortes, C. and Olarte, J.M. (1994). Questioning diagnosis disclosure in terminal cancer patients: a prospective study evaluating patients' responses. *Palliative Medicine* **8**: 39–44.

Clarke, M., Finlay, I., and Campbell, I. (1991). Cultural boundaries in care. *Palliative Medicine* **5**: 63–5.

de Trill, M. and Kovalcik, R. (1997). The child with cancer. Influence of culture on truth-telling and patient care. *Annals of the New York Academy of Sciences* **809**: 197–210.

Fielding, R. and Hung, J. (1996). Preferences for information and involvement in decisions during cancer care among a Hong Kong Chinese population. *Psycho-oncology* **5**: 321–9.

Foster, G.M. and Anderson, B.G. (1978). *Medical Anthropology*. New York: John Wiley.

Fuller, J.H.S. and Toon, P.D. (1988). *Medical Practice in a Multicultural Society*. Oxford: Heinemann.

Goh, C.R. *et al.* (1996). Measuring quality of life in different cultures: translation of the Functional Living Index for Cancer (FLIC) into Chinese and Malay in Singapore. *Annals of the Academy of Medicine, Singapore* **25**(3): 323–34.

Greenwald, H.P. (1991). Interethnic differences in pain perceptions. *Pain* **44**(2): 157–63.

Gunaratnam, Y. (1998). Re-thinking multi-cultural service provision. *Hospice Bulletin* **6**(2): 16.

Ishikawa, Y. (1992). *Cancer Death in Middle Age*. Report of the Statistics Bureau of the Ministry of Health and Welfare of Japan.

Juarez, G., Ferrell, B., and Borneman, T. (1998). Influence of culture on cancer pain management in hispanic patients. *Cancer Pract* **6**(5): 262–9.

Kelly, M.P. (1992). *Colitis*. London: Tavistock/Routledge.

Lupton, D. (1996). *Medicine as Culture: Illness, Disease and the Body in Western Societies*. London: Sage.

McNamara, B. *et al.* (1997). Palliative care in a multicultural society: perceptions of health care professionals. *Palliative Medicine* 11: 359–67.

Rees, D. (1997). *Death and Bereavement: The Psychological, Religious and Cultural Interfaces*. London: Whurr.

Speck, P. (1989). Cultural and religious aspects of dying. In Sherr, L. (ed.), *Death, Dying and Bereavement*. Oxford: Blackwell. pp. 36–47.

Toscani, F. and Cantoni, L. *et al.* (1991). Death and dying: perceptions and attitudes in Italy. *Palliative Medicine* 5: 334–43.

Zoboroski, M. (1969). Cultural components in response to pain. *People in Pain*. San Francisco:Jossey-Bass.

Chapter 22

Clinical implications

Irene J. Higginson

Introduction

This chapter seeks to draw together the main clinical implications from this body of work on the care of patients with non-cancer. Rather than deal with each particular condition (individual chapters deal with this) the sections below concentrate on common issues. In some instances where there are marked differences between diseases these are highlighted.

Assessment and diagnosis

Accurate and appropriate assessment is the cornerstone of good management in progressive illness and terminal care. It is important to determine the likely cause of the symptom or problem, and to assess its significance to the patient and family, in order to determine treatment. Many people with progressive diseases other than cancer are older and have multiple health problems, and so determining which problem is most important and which the patient and family would like dealt with first becomes a priority. Diagnosis can be made more difficult when patients are frail or find it difficult or uncomfortable to move. Unnecessary or excessive tests, if uncomfortable, can increase rather than reduce suffering. Clinicians should elicit a history and determine signs and symptoms before progression to more invasive tests. They should ask themselves—would the results of the test make a difference to my treatment? If the answer is 'yes', then the test is needed, but if the answer is 'no', then it is not.

Not all symptoms may be due to the main disease. For example, weakness or debility may be caused by secondary effects of the illness, by side effects of treatment, or by unrelated, concurrent illness (see Table 22.1).

Table 22.1 Interaction of symptoms

- Symptoms are concurrent but unrelated in aetiology
- Symptoms are concurrent and related to the same pathological process
- Symptoms are concurrent and the second symptom is directly or indirectly a consequence of a pathological process initiated by the first symptom
- Symptoms are concurrent and one symptom is a consequence or side effect of therapy directed against the other symptom

Source: (Ingham and Portenoy, 1996)

Attention to detail, reassessment, and the development of treatments and interventions that are individualised to patients' needs are the cornerstones of successful management in palliative care. Assessment can be aided by using standardised audit schedules.

Appropriate treatment and appropriate death

All patients must die eventually. Part of the skill of medicine is to decide when attempts to sustain life are essentially futile. In palliative care the main aim of treatment is not to pro-long life, but to make the life which remains as comfortable and as meaningful as possible. The decision must be made as to what is the most appropriate treatment, given the patient's biological prospect, and personal and social wishes. One of the main difficulties faced by doctors caring for patients with non-malignant progressive diseases is the uncertainty around prognosis. While some diseases, such as motor neurone disease, show a steady period of progression, others show a more varying course (see Chapters 2 and 3). The difficulty with these conditions , for example heart failure or chronic progressive respiratory disease, is that patients and their clinicians need to plan for two potential eventualities:the patient dying soon, or living for a long period. Future research may provide more guidance to patients and their clinicians about the likely prognosis of different conditions. In the meantime, patients and the clinicians advising them about the treatment, or making decisions if patients are unable to do so, need to weigh the potential benefits, in terms of symptom relief and quality of life, of different treatments against any adverse effects in the long or shorter term.

Information and communication

Effective symptom control is impossible without effective communication. The most pow-erful drugs will be of little value if health care professionals do not accurately understand the patient's problems and priorities. Every chapter in this book, no matter what the condi-tion, has alluded to research findings concerning un-met information and communication needs of both patients and their families.

There are many barriers to good communication. Contemporary society has been going through a phase of virtual denial of death which has influenced individual patients and their families as well as the health care system. There is a lack of experience of death in the fam-ily—a lot of adults may not witnessed a previous death. There are higher expectations of health and life, which are often reported in the media. There is the changing role of religion and of materialistic values. These societal attitudes vary between countries and cultures, but, to work effectively, a clinician must be aware of them. Patients and their family members often have fears about dying (see below). In addition, professionals have fears about being blamed, about dealing with areas in which they have not been taught, about admitting that they do not know, for example, the prognosis, and about expressing emotions. A doctor or nurse may have fears about their own illness or death.

The following general discussion of communication issues should be balanced with the patients' and families' cultural background (see Chapter 21).

Listening skills

The physical context of an interview sends important messages to the patient, even before verbal communication begins. Introductions are needed so the patient knows who you are and what you do. Although difficult to obtain in institutions, privacy is important if a patient's dignity is to be maintained and if they are to take in what you say.

Sitting down is an almost universal rule. Simple measures, such as ensuring that the patient has been able to get dressed after being examined in order to restore a sense of personal modesty, and moving physical objects out of the way so that they are not between you and the patient, are important. It is also important to be seated at a comfortable distance from the patient. This distance (the body buffer zone) will vary from culture to culture. Some authors suggest that touching the patient—for example, on the hand or arm—can be beneficial, although this varies from patient to patient and in general is an interview skill that requires great care.

As a dialogue begins, the professional should show that they are in 'listening mode'. This can be achieved by letting the patient speak, waiting for them to stop, encouraging them to talk, and by tolerating short silences. Repetition and reiteration by using key words is often highly valuable. Similarly reflection, the re-statement of the patients' main points, is also a helpful technique.

Specific communication in palliative care

Breaking bad news

There are many occasions when new medical information needs to be discussed. This occurs at the first assessment and is common later on. Buckman (Buckman 1988; Buckman 1998; Maguire and Faulkner 1988) has outlined a six-step protocol for breaking bad news (see Table 22.2). It is beyond the scope of this chapter to describe in detail the process of breaking bad news. There are many texts and guides on the subject.

Therapeutic dialogue

A supportive dialogue during any stage of palliative care is often regarded as an exceptionally valuable resource. It can be the most important ingredient in a patient's care. The central principle is that the patient should perceive that his or her emotions have been heard and acknowledged.

Starting and withdrawing treatments

As treatments become more complex and patients and their families are faced with an increasing array of different options, the process of discussing treatment choices with patients and families is of growing importance. This is made more complex by the fact that many patients are ill, and doctors and nurses themselves often feel that it is important that they offer a positive outlook on treatment options—in some instances so that

Table 22.2 Six step protocol for breaking bad news

1 Getting the physical context right
2 Finding out how much the patient knows
3 Finding out how much the patient wants to know
4 Sharing information
5 Responding to the patient's feelings
6 Planning and follow through

they can maximise the potential benefits of any placebo effect. One first important principle in discussing the commencement or withdrawal of treatments with patients and families, is to determine the extent to which patients themselves desire full information, and the opportunity to make decisions, or whether they wish either family members or professionals to deal with these issues. Individual wishes vary but, increasingly in our cultures, patients want a greater role in the process of decision-making. The second task of the doctor, having listened to the patient's wishes, is to try to explain the different treatment options and the potential trade-off. It is important to try to avoid jargon and to explain things simply.

Dealing with uncertainty

This is a particular problem among patients with progressive non-cancer conditions, where it is often not clear how long the condition will last, or what the course of progression will be. Common uncertainties include the level of treatment, its likely benefits, how long before death comes, what the intervening period will be like and how death will come. Living with uncertainty often creates great anxiety, and patients, their carers, and professionals may feel the need for concrete statements on some of these issues. In the face of uncertainty, health professionals may think it best to say little, if anything, about the possibility of, for example, the patient dying suddenly or of treatment finishing. This ignores the knowledge patients have of their own bodies and the knowledge they, therefore, acquire about how well they are doing. It also ignores the fact that patients and families increasingly access information through the media and Internet. There is little known about the best mechanisms of communication in non-cancer patients. However, among cancer patients, Maguire and Faulkner suggest that professionals should acknowledge their uncertainties and the difficulties this will cause. They propose a scheme of responses which checks if the enquirer would like to know what signs may herald further deterioration. They also encourage positive use of present time, a willingness to monitor the situation regularly, and a readiness to respond to any emergency. This gives the security of feeling that someone with more experience recognises the problem and can be called on if there are particular worries or difficulties (Maguire and Faulkner 1988).

Planning to live and planning to die

For some the strategy of 'hoping for the best and planning for the worst' is helpful. The approach sometimes taken in cancer care of thinking through with the patient or carer what the situation would be if the best happened and what they would need to consider if the worst happened may be helpful here, although further work is needed to understand its value in non-cancer care. However, in these instances it may enable patients and their families to take a variety of considerations into account without necessarily focusing too heavily on one scenario or the other.

Such a strategy assumes particular importance with patients who show a fluctuating trajectory of illness, as is common in severe heart failure, some neurological conditions, and some other illnesses (see Chapters 3, 4 & 13). In contrast to the research in breaking bad news or establishing a therapeutic dialogue, much less is known about this aspect of communication. Work is needed to better understand patient and family concerns and wishes, and to determine the best mechanisms of communication when dealing with these levels of uncertainty, as well as in planning to live and planning to die.

Communicating with the family and with other professionals

In palliative care, the patient and their family or those important to them are regarded as the unit of care. However, this does not mean that carers should be given information before patients. The carer who buttonholes the professional at the front door or in the hospital corridor and firmly says 'she mustn't be told' is not uncommon in cancer care and can be found in other progressive conditions. If the strategy of discussing with the patient at the start of care how communication should be handled has been followed, the professional should have some idea of the patients wishes and to what extent they wish the carer to be involved, so that they can react accordingly. If not, then the ethical issue of who has the right to this information comes to the fore. However, even if the professional wishes to assert the primacy of the patient's right to know, a stark statement of this principle is likely to be counter-productive. The fears, anxieties, and concerns of the carer need to be explored and their more intimate knowledge of the person drawn out. Asking 'what would worry you particularly about her knowing?' gives an opportunity for this and shows that the listener values the carer's opinions. It may also be helpful to discuss with the carer the strain that the situation is placing on them and ways in which services and the professionals may help. Most carers with such anxieties will then accept a reassurance that the doctor or nurse will undertake not to initiate any discussion on the outcome of illness, but that if the patient raises the issue the professional will respond truthfully in order to maintain and deserve that person's trust. In instances where patients are unconscious or unable to respond to verbal communication, support of the carers and communication with the carers, as well as continued communication with the patient, are important.

One of the common concerns of individuals in hospitals and in the community is that of receiving mixed messages from different professionals. It is important that all of the team involved in the care of the patient and family are kept fully informed of the important decisions and wishes of the patient and their family or carer. If people are at home and different services are visiting, the carer or patient can sometimes feel that they have a full-time job co-ordinating these visits. It is important in these instances to identify a key worker for that patient and family who helps to take on some of the role of co-ordination and advocacy, so that the patient and the carer receive the services and benefits to which they are entitled. Similarly, in hospitals patients and carers may ask for information from different nurses, depending on who is with the patient at any one time. There may also be different teams involved. This may be particularly likely with palliative care patients, who may be seeing members of the hospital palliative care team as well as their own doctors. When the circumstances and condition of the patient change rapidly, it is especially important that all members of the team are kept rapidly informed of relevant changes, possibly in the treatment plans, or in the patient's condition, or their wishes.

Management of three common symptoms

One major challenge of palliative care in non-malignant disease is that patients tend to be older than cancer patients and, therefore, often have several different conditions. Symptom management needs to bear this in mind. It is not possible to cover all symptoms, so three common ones are considered here.

Breathlessness

Breathlessness is one of the most common and most distressing symptoms found in non-cancer palliative care. Breathlessness (or dyspnoea) means difficult, distressing breathing. As the individual chapters show, it is particularly common in chronic respiratory disease (see Chapter 2), in heart disease (see Chapter 3) and in neurodegenerative conditions, where the ability to breathe is lessened because of muscular weakness (see Chapter 4). In any condition there may be breathlessness due to infection, anaemia, metabolic changes, anxiety, or depression (Simon *et al.* 1990). There are two important components to breathlessness—the first is the increased effort needed to breathe, and the second is the subjective distress associated with it. Early work on pain suggested that pain has physical, emotional, social, and spiritual components (Twycross 1989). A similar model is useful for breathlessness where the distress of breathlessness may also have physical, emotional, social, and spiritual components.

New research is trying to understand how the different descriptors of breathlessness and the different timing, relieving, and precipitating factors, along with associated symptoms, may help to establish the major causes of breathlessness (Table 22.3).

Many of the therapies for breathlessness are described in the sections on the individual conditions in this book. These include, for example, oxygen and bronchodilators in chronic obstructive pulmonary disease (see Chapter 2), which should be used as the first-line treatment for the specific condition. In addition, antibiotics may be relevant, if required, to relieve breathlessness from pneumonia. Opioids have been used for some years in breathlessness related to cancer. They reduce the sensitivity of the respiratory centre and peripheral

Table 22.3 Common causes of breathlessness

Respiratory	Primary lung cancer
	Lung or pleural metastases
	Pleural effusions
	Lung collapse or consolidation
	Pneumonia
	Chronic obstructive airways disease
	Asthma
	Pulmonary fibrosis
Gastrointestinal	Ascites
Cardiovascular	Pulmonary embolus
	Heart failure
	Anaemia
	Ischaemic heart disease
Metabolic	Uraemia
	Exercise
	Muscular/neurological
	Muscle weakness
	Fatigue
Psychogenic	Anxiety
	Depression
	Hyperventilation syndrome

chemoreceptors, leading to a reduced rate and depth of ventilation. They decrease anxiety, stop pain associated with ventilation (such as pleurisy), reduce the occurrence of heart failure, and, as analgesics, may reduce any hyperventilation due to underlying chronic pain (Heyse-Moore 1993). However, they may sometimes cause bronchoconstriction by release of histamine from mast cells in the lung, while at the same time blocking bronchoconstriction from vagal stimulation. Thus, the effects of opioids on ventilation are complex and sometimes paradoxical. They are widely used in palliative care for the subjective relief of breathlessness, and fears about respiratory depression causing respiratory failure or pneumonia have not been found to be valid among cancer patients (Heyse-Moore 1993). Thus, breathless patients taking opioids do not necessarily die quickly and may actually improve their mobility (Bruera *et al.* 1993a). In a small study, patients with chronic obstructive airways disease who also had high dose morphine were not found to have respiratory failure (Walsh 1984). There is debate about whether nebulised opioids are of more benefit or not than oral opioids (Davis 1995; Farncombe *et al.* 1994). Similarly, there is debate as to whether breathlessness is best helped by the regular use of opioids or whether intermittent dosage is more helpful (Cohen *et al.* 1991). Psychotropics, atropinics (to reduce bronchial secretions), local anaesthetic inhalation, corticosteroids, oxygen, and the use of prostaglandin inhibitors have also been considered in breathlessness (Bruera *et al.* 1992; Bruera *et al.* 1993b; Congleton and Mures 1995; Mann and Sproule 1986; Mitchell-Heggs *et al.* 1980; Weir *et al.* 1990; Woodcock *et al.* 1981). General supportive procedures to assist the patient and family—such as bedside fans (Schwartzstein *et al.* 1987), or perhaps muscle relaxation exercises, guided imagery, or supportive counselling—are probably also helpful. Pulmonary rehabilitation, including a multi-professional programme of physiotherapy, education, and exercise may also be valuable (see Chapter 2). There may be value in developing the nurse-led clinics, as tested in cancer care, to help individuals to deal with their breathlessness (Bredin *et al.* 1999). The effective control of breathlessness remains a major challenge for palliative care in the future, even among cancer patients (Heyse-Moore *et al.* 1991). More than 10 years ago breathlessness was highlighted as remaining uncontrolled, whereas pain was better controlled (Higginson and McCarthy 1989; Reuben and Mor 1986). Some improvements have occurred in the intervening years, but these are limited. A programme of research, similar to that already undertaken in order to understand and control pain, is now needed for breathlessness, which, like pain, is frequently feared by patients and their families.

Fatigue and weakness

Fatigue is among the most prevalent symptoms reported by patients with progressive illness, including cancer. Despite this, there are no generally accepted definitions of fatigue. The experience is often characterised by a spectrum of problems that include muscular weakness, lethargy, sleepiness, mood disturbance, and difficulty in concentrating (Bruera 1997). Closely related to fatigue is weakness or asthenia. *Asthenos* (Greek) means absence or loss of strength. Asthenia includes three different main symptoms:

1 fatigue or lassitude defined by easy tiring and decreased ability to maintain performance;

2 generalised weakness defined as the anticipatory sensation of difficulty in initiating a certain activity;

3 mental fatigue defined as the presence of impaired mental concentration, and loss of both memory and emotional ability.

Fatigue and weakness have traditionally been associated with cancer, particularly in association with cancer cachexia, and approximately 90% of individuals with cancer have been found to suffer from asthenia (Neuenschwander and Bruera 1998).

There are multiple causes of fatigue and asthenia and these causes may well interrelate (see Table 22.4). Fatigue and weakness are frequently overlooked as important symptoms for the patient and family and are known to be difficult to treat well in cancer. In this book, many of the discussions of illnesses where fatigue might be relevant do not include a specific discussion of this symptom, perhaps because it is so difficult to treat well. There is little research in the management of fatigue in progressive illnesses other than cancer. In cancer care, general and non-pharmacological measures include correcting any known cause (such as adaptation of lifestyle) and, more recently, testing some of the interventions used in chronic fatigue syndrome (such as modified exercise and cognitive behavioural therapy). Pharmacological measures include the use of corticosteroids and, as a few small studies in the US have shown, of amphetamines (Beller *et al.* 1997; Bruera *et al.* 1996; Fainsinger 1996; Farr 1990; Neuenschwander and Bruera 1998).

Work is needed to develop valid and reliable tools for the assessment and staging of the intensity and association of these symptoms. There needs to be work to understand the likely causes and to test potential treatments, particularly in correcting nutritional deficiencies, and in the areas of activity and rest. The role of drugs, such as corticosteroids, megestrol acetate, and anabolic steroids, should be better established.

Pain

It used to be believed that pain was not a problem in progressive illnesses other than cancer. This is now known to be untrue. As many of the chapters in this book show, pain is a common symptom in many progressive, non-malignant conditions, and during terminal care.

Table 22.4 Common causes of weakness and fatigue

+ Infection (recurrent acute infection or chronic infection)
+ Anaemia
+ Chronic hypoxia
+ Neurological disorders (autonomic dysfunction, myasthenia syndrome, Parkinsonian, demylenisation)
+ Psychogenic causes
+ Metabolic and electrolyte disorders
+ Endocrine disorders (thyroidopathy, Addison's disease, diabetes mellitus, etc.)
+ Dehydration
+ Malnutrition
+ Insomnia
+ Over-exertion (chronic/acute)
+ Pharmacological toxicity (narcotics, sedatives, alcohol, chemotherapy, etc.)
+ Cachexia (due to HIV/AIDS, cancer, or other progressive illness)
+ Chronic pain
+ Release of cytokines in cancer and in other chronic conditions

Unfortunately, current knowledge about the frequency, pathophysiology, and clinical course of pain syndromes in non-cancer patients is limited compared to that in cancer patients. Chapter 6 (as well as individual disease based chapters) outlines the characteristics and patterns of pain in different non-cancer patients, and discusses potential pharmacological interventions. Most authors concur in recommending non-opioid analgesics as a first step for patients with mild to moderate pain (see Chapter 6) (Takeda 1986; Ventafridda *et al.* 1987). Many patients may also require opioid analgesics following the general recommendations usually made for the treatment of cancer pain (Walker *et al.* 1988; Walsh *et al.* 1992). Unfortunately, there is a very small number of controlled trials on the role of opioids for non-malignant pain. In addition, it appears that palliative, non-cancer patients have a higher frequency of neuropathic pain syndromes than do cancer patients (see Chapter 6). Commonly used adjuvant analgesic drugs for these conditions include tricyclic antidepressants (McQuay *et al.* 1996; Portenoy 1993), seratonin re-uptake inhibitors, anticonvulsants (McQuay *et al.* 1995), and, in certain circumstances, oral local anaesthetics, Gabapentin, corticosteroids, baclofen, ketamine, and clonidine (see Chapter 6) (Higginson and Edmonds 2000).

Non-pharmacological interventions that raise the pain threshold (the greatest level of pain that a subject is willing to tolerate) are also important (see Table 22.5).

Emotional needs

Reaction to change in role

Psychological and emotional problems are common in progressive illness. In-depth discussion is often needed to identify the cause or causes of the problems and sometimes these can be quite different from what one would expect. There are many potential interwoven factors, including concern over the change in role, functioning, family, finances, spiritual needs, guilt, anger, fear of dying, and unrelieved physical symptoms. It often helps to identify and discuss the problems, which may differ according to the condition. For example, with stroke

Table 22.5 Factors that raise or lower the pain tolerance threshold

Threshold lowered	Threshold raised
Sleeplessness	Sleep
Fatigue	Understanding
Anxiety	Companionship
Fear	Relaxation
Anger	A feeling of being heard
Sadness	Reduction in anxiety
Isolation	Creative activity
Depression	Elevation of mood
Boredom	Relief of other symptoms
Abandonment	Analgesics
Discomfort	Anxiolytics
Spiritual fears	Antidepressants

the changes in physical function occur suddenly, so initially the patient may be in shock. There may be a process of grieving for their former self. There may be fears about a future stroke, suddenly becoming a burden to others, and about the future in general. In the case of more slowly-progressive illnesses, these and other problems can arise. A patient with motor neurone disease may have major concerns regarding future care, the disability, and symptoms they will face. Individuals may be influenced by the manner of progression or death of family members and friends.

Individuals may employ a number of different defence mechanisms and coping strategies, such as regression, denial, rationalisation, intellectualisation, projection, displacement, introjection, repression, withdrawal, and avoidance. Understanding these can help staff to explain and empathise with an individual's behaviour. Such mechanisms are normal—it is only when they are in excess that problems occur.

The stress of a prolonged illness, or the shock of a recent diagnosis, can predispose a person to psychological problems.

Fear and anxiety

Individuals may have fears about their prognosis and, in particular, may have difficulty dealing with the uncertainty expressed over their illness. There may be fears or anger about the fact that they are still experiencing the illness and that it cannot be cured. Individuals may also have fears and anxiety about dying, about the mode of death, or about what will happen to their family members (Hanratty 1989; Miller and Walsh 1991).

In-depth discussion is often needed over a period of time, and any causes for anxiety (such as poor symptom control) should be dealt with. Some individuals find comfort from living each day for what pleasures and joys it holds, and by looking forward to close positive events. It is well worth considering using non-drug techniques such as relaxation, exercises in breathing control, and massage. Occasionally, drug treatment is needed (Payne and Massie 2000).

Depression

The chapters in this book indicate that depression is found in a fairly small, but significant, minority of patients with progressive non-malignant illness. It often goes undetected, partly because individuals do not readily volunteer the symptoms, partly because staff do not readily screen for depression, and partly because it is often difficult to decide where natural sadness ends and depression begins. Too often it is assumed that depression in a progressive illness is to be expected or is untreatable. Depression should be distinguished from adjustment disorders, which are more common and more fluctuating. Depression causes considerable suffering for the patient and their family and should be rigorously treated. It is usually characterised by a gradual onset of the following symptoms and signs: depressed mood or irritability, loss of interest and enjoyment, agitation, or retardation, self-neglect or self-mutilation, diurnal mood swings, early-morning wakening, change in behaviour, and a cognitive triad of self as worthless, the outside world meaningless, and the future as hopeless (Wilson *et al.* 2000).

Often the physical symptoms of depression, such as weight loss, anorexia, fatigue, and constipation, cannot be used for diagnosis in progressive illness, because they are already present as a result of the condition. The management should include withdrawal of any drugs likely to cause depression, provision of emotional and psychological support, and the use of antidepressant drugs (Cody 1990).

Social needs

Finances

Illness often places a strain on an individual's financial circumstances. Chronic illness in itself can lead to a cycle where an individual's capacity to work and function is reduced, leading to a reduction in income and, in some countries, a reduced eligibility for health insurance, which often in turn leads to further ill health. Similarly, a carer may find that they have to spend increasing time in the caring role, reducing their capacity to work, and thus their income. Changes in weight and appearance may mean that an individual needs to buy new clothes, and functional disability may often mean that home adaptations are needed. In addition, individuals may be concerned about the future finances for their family.

These issues can lead to psychological and emotional problems. Financial issues do need to be discussed with patients and families and, where appropriate, application for any available benefits should be facilitated.

Home support

Much of the care in the last year of life occurs at home, but there has been an increasing trend towards hospitalisation of the dying in many countries. In the oldest age groups, there is an increased reliance on residential and nursing homes. Most individuals want to be cared for and, if possible, to die either at home or in a home-like environment (Higginson and Sen-Gupta 2000). Chapter 14 discussed the fact that maintaining a normal life for as long as possible, and being in familiar surroundings cared for by a relative and supported by health professionals well known to them, have been found to be aspects of home care valued by patients and families. Achieving this care requires both the availability of services in the community and suitable home circumstances. Research in cancer has found that home care is much more difficult to achieve in deprived areas (Higginson *et al.* 1997). Such research needs to be repeated for non-cancer patients. In addition, home care is more difficult among the oldest age groups and for those individuals who do not have a carer living at home (Higginson *et al.* 1998).

Environment

Early texts on palliative care and terminal illness placed a great emphasis on the importance of environment and the imaginative use of architectural space (Saunders 1978). This highlighted the importance of space for families, windows for patients to look from, opportunities for them to move around, room for staff to work easily and to relax, and 'transition spaces' for those who are anxious to take time off or to brace themselves for a meeting. It is difficult to achieve this environment in a busy hospital ward and countries have approached this problem in different ways. In the UK the move has been particularly towards freestanding hospice units, although currently, as outlined in Chapter 15, these have concentrated on cancer patients and a small number of other groups. This model has been followed in many countries, but in some the approach has been to adapt a hospital ward to provide the environment of a more traditional hospice unit. Neither of these developments helps the majority of patients who find themselves on general hospital wards. A greater attention to the environment is generally needed in hospital settings. Palliative care in nursing homes is discussed in detail in Chapter 12.

Spiritual and existential needs

Palliative care integrates physical, emotional, social ,and spiritual aspects. It is helpful to distinguish spiritual from religious. The spiritual or existential dimension is the deepest and is concerned with ultimate concerns, a search for meaning and values. It is a highly individual response and strongly influenced by culture. Assessing the spiritual needs of those who are at the end of life relies greatly on a relationship being formed between the patient and those caring for him or her. For some that relationship may be formed with a priest or relevant religious leader, but for others it is formed with a volunteer, a doctor or nurse, a family friend, or a fellow patient. What is important is that the individual is able to choose who they talk to and share with, and that help is available if needed. Quite a few texts provide greater guidance on the assessment of spiritual aspects of care in cancer, which apply equally to non-cancer patients (Lunn 1993; Speck 1998).

Dignity

Palliative care is concerned with maintaining as good a quality of life as possible, given the complex and disabling problems that the individual and their family face. This involves a sense of dignity—not an easy thing to define, but acknowledged as important by everyone. It is an essential human state and many individuals wish to die as they have lived. For some this might mean being able to wear particular clothing, undertake some simple daily activities once taken for granted, or use a lavatory rather than a commode. For others dignity means being addressed with respect, receiving nursing and social care, being in a reasonable environment, or returning, even in a limited way, to activities they once enjoyed.

Achieving good control of symptoms and alleviating fears, anxieties and psychological problems are important steps towards achieving dignity, but the factors above also need to come into play.

Family and carers

The care of the family is an integral part of care in progressive illness. As many of the individual chapters show, it is easy for health professionals to miss meeting the family, particularly when patients are in hospital. Little is known about the psychological impact on family members, as most research has focused on family members at the bereavement stage. However, in progressive illness, family members can experience heightened symptoms of depression and anxiety, psychosomatic symptoms, restriction of role and activities, strain in relationships, and poor physical health. Some research has reported spouses as experiencing the same level of distress as patients. A longitudinal study suggested that a substantial group of carers experience distress one year after diagnosis and that mental health status declines for 30% of them (Ell *et al.* 1988). In a more recent study, 32% of family members were rated as having severe anxiety at referral to six specialist palliative home care teams, and anxiety remained severe for 26% during the patients' last week of life (Hodgson *et al.* 1997). Therefore, it is not only during bereavement that family members need support. Interventions designed specifically for family members are scarce and have rarely been evaluated. More work is needed in this area, specifically in non-cancer groups. However, family members need support, communication, and information, and may have specific fears and concerns that require support. The previous functioning of the family may be important and there may be particular family concerns that require attention (see Chapter 19).

Bereavement and grief affect both feelings and behaviour. Reactions vary, but can be physical, such as muscular tension, decreased resistance to illness, fatigue and weakness, sleep disturbances, increased blood pressure, and loss of appetite and weight change; emotional, such as numbness, sadness, helplessness, despair, confusion, guilt, anger, and bitterness; and behavioural, such as poor concentration, blaming others, preoccupation, seeking solitude, withdrawal from friends and activities, forgetfulness, and tearfulness.

Bereavement has a major impact, therefore, on morbidity and subsequent mortality—both ill health and death rates are higher after a recent bereavement. Several risk assessment schedules are available to help identify those individuals who are more likely to have a poor outcome during bereavement (Relf 1999). These include an untimely, unexpected, or disturbing death, a dependent relationship, little perceived support by the bereaved individual, presence of denial and anger, presence of concurrent stressful life events, previous severe losses, and a concurrent physical or psychological illness that may be exacerbated by the loss.

Multi-professional care

Those who may be included in a multi-professional team are doctors of different specialties, nurses, social workers, home care workers, chaplains, therapists, and psychologists or psychiatrists. The team aims to:

+ achieve accurate and speedy assessment and diagnosis of the problems;
+ plan and implement effective, integrated treatment and care;
+ communicate effectively internally and with the patient and patient's family, as well as with all other professionals and agencies involved in the care of the individual;
+ audit and review its activities and outcomes.

It may be that specialists in palliative care are needed to give advice, support, or expertise in the care of patients and families, or that other individuals are needed. Many patients with non-progressive disease are in the older age groups and have multiple health problems. They may need the approach of a specialist in the health care of elderly people who is accustomed to dealing with many different diseases. Some studies have evaluated specialist palliative care, including care for patients with non-cancer as well as cancer. In these studies, the specialist co-ordinated approach resulted in similar or improved outcomes in terms of patient satisfaction, the patient being cared for where they wished, family satisfaction, and better control of family anxiety and the patient's pain and other symptoms. The studies examining cost showed a tendency for a reduction in hospital in-patient days, more time spent at home, and equal or lower costs (Hearn and Higginson 1998).

Audit, education and research

Clinical audit and quality assurance are a crucial part of practice if the care of patients in this under-researched field is to be better understood and improved in future. A wide range of different approaches to audit and quality assurance is available (see Chapter 17). These can include an audit of key indicators using, for example, systematic assessment systems such as the support team assessment system, the palliative outcome scale or the Edmonton symptom assessment system; an audit of particular topics or symptoms, such as breathlessness—or audits of particular components of care (Hearn and Higginson 1997; Hearn *et al.*

1999; Higginson 1993). One advantage of auditing key indicators or outcomes is that it enables specific and sometimes neglected variables to be monitored as part of routine care. These are important in aiding assessment.

The prevalence of progressive illness and its increase in the future will mean that education programmes at undergraduate and postgraduate levels are increasingly important. Because of the need to provide care in multi-professional teams, methods of multi-professional education, particularly at postgraduate level, need to be explored further in the future. Some methods of education can be adapted from those already established in cancer care.

The research challenges in this field are enormous and wide ranging. However, a few of the key aspects that will be important in clinical practice are:

◆ development of a better understanding of the natural history of symptoms and problems in non-cancer palliative care;

◆ establishment of a better understanding of the mechanisms of difficult-to-control symptoms, particularly breathlessness, fatigue and depression, and the evaluation of treatments to alleviate these symptoms;

◆ evaluation of new and improved ways to offer support to family members and carers;

◆ evaluation of demonstration projects to test models for the improvement of care for patients with different progressive illnesses; ideally this would include a comparison of different approaches.

Conclusion

Palliative care in non-malignant illness should be an important part of health and social care. The patient and their family should be regarded as the unit of care. The term family is taken in its broad sense and encompasses close relatives, a partner and close friends. Palliative care is concerned with physical, emotional, social and spiritual problems for patients and families. It focuses on the quality of life and on support of the family and those close to the patient. Appropriate and rigorous assessment, giving of information, communication, management of symptoms, psychological, social, spiritual, and family concerns are essential, as is improving dignity for patients and families. This will often involve a multi-professional team, the audit of care, and appropriate education. There is a great need for further research.

References

Beller, E., Tattersall, M., Lumley, T., *et al.* (1997). Improved quality of life with megestrol acetate in patients with endocrine-insensitive advanced cancer: a randomised placebo-controlled trial. *Annals of Oncology* **8**: 277–83.

Bredin, M., Corner, J., Krishnasamy, M., Plant, H., Bailey, C., and A'Hern, R. (1999). Multicentre randomised controlled trial of nursing intervention for breathlessness in patients with lung cancer. *British Medical Journal* **318**: 901–4.

Bruera, E. (1997). ABC of palliative care: anorexia, cachexia and nutrition. *British Medical Journal* **315**: 1219–22.

Bruera, E., MacEachern, T., Ripamonti, C., Hanson, J. (1993a). Subcutaneous morphine for dyspnoea in cancer patients. *Archives of Internal Medicine* **119**: 906–7.

Bruera, E. de Stoutz, N., Velasco-Leiva, A., *et al.* (1993b). The effects of oxygen on the intensity of dyspnoea in hypoxemic terminal cancer patients. *Lancet* **343**: 13–14.

Bruera, E., Ernst, S., Hagen, N., Spachynski, K., Belzile, M., and Hanson, J. (1996). Symptomatic effects of megestrol acetate (MA): a double-blind crossover study. *Proceedings of the American Society for Clinical Oncology* **1716**: 531–1.

Bruera, E., Schoeller, T., and MacEachern, T. (1992). Symptomatic benefit of supplemental oxygen in hypoxemic patients with terminal cancer: the use of the N of 1 randomized controlled trial. *Journal of Pain and Symptom Management* **7**: 365–8.

Buckman, R. (1988). *I Don't Know What to Say: How to Help and Support Someone Who is Dying.* London: Papermac.

Buckman, R. (1998). Communication in palliative care: a practical guide. In Doyle, D., Hanks G.W.C., and McDonald, N. (eds.), *Oxford Textbook of Palliative Medicine* (2nd edn), Oxford: Oxford University Press, pp. 141–56.

Cody, M. (1990). Depression and the use of antidepressants in patients with cancer. *Palliative Medicine* **4**: 271–8.

Cohen, M.H., Anderson, A.J., Krasnow, S.H., *et al.* (1991). Continuous intravenous infusion of morphine for severe dyspnea. *Southern Medical Journal* **84**: 229–34.

Congleton, J. and Mures, M.F. (1995). The incidence of airflow obstruction in bronchial carcinoma, its relation to breathlessness and response to bronchodilator therapy. *Respiratory Medicine* **89**: 291–6.

Davis, C. (1995). The role of nebulised drugs in palliating respiratory symptoms. *European Journal of Palliative Care* **2**: 9–15.

Ell, K., Nishimoto, R., Mantell, J., and Hamovitch, M. (1988). Longitudinal analysis of psychological adaptation among family members of patients with cancer. *Journal of Psychosomatic Research* **32**: 429–38.

Fainsinger, R.L. (1996). Pharmacological approach to cancer anorexia and cachexia. In Bruera, E. and Higginson, I. (eds.), *Cachexia-anorexia in Cancer Patients.* Oxford: Oxford Medical Publications, Oxford University Press, pp. 128–40

Farncombe, M., Chater, S., and Gillin, A. (1994). The use of nebulised opioids for breathlessness: a chart review. *Palliative Medicine* **8**: 306–12.

Farr, W. (1990). The use of corticosteroids for symptom management in terminally ill patients. *Am J Hosp Care* **1**: 41–6.

Hanratty, J. (1989). *Palliative Care of the Terminally Ill.* Oxford: Radcliffe Medical Press.

Hearn, J. and Higginson, I.J. (1997). Outcome measures in palliative care for advanced cancer patients: a review. *Journal of Public Health Medicine* **19**: 193–9.

Hearn, J. and Higginson I.J. (1998). Do specialist palliative care teams improve outcomes for cancer patients? A systematic literature review. *Palliative Medicine* **12**: 317–32.

Hearn, J. and Higginson, I.J. on behalf of the Palliative Care Audit Project Advisory Group (1999). Development and validation of a core outcome measure for palliative care—The Palliative Care Outcome Scale. *Quality in Healthcare* **8**: 219–27.

Heyse-Moore, L.H. (1993). Respiratory symptoms. In Saunders, C. and Sykes, N. (eds.), *The Management of Terminal Malignant Disease* (3rd edn). London: Edward Arnold, pp. 76–85.

Heyse-Moore, L.H., Ross, V., and Mulles, M. (1991). How much of a problem is dyspnoea in advanced cancer? *Palliative Medicine* **5**: 20–6.

Higginson, I.J. (1993). *Clinical Audit in Palliative Care.* Oxford: Radcliffe Medical Press.

Higginson, I.J., Astin, P., Dolan, S., and Jarman, B. (1997). Which cancer patients die at home? Effects of social deprivation and patient characteristics in England. London: Department of Palliative Care and Policy. Internal Report.

Higginson, I.J., Astin, P., and Dolan, S. (1998). Where do cancer patients die? Ten-year trends in the place of death of cancer patients in England. *Palliative Medicine* **12**: 353–63.

Higginson, I.J. and Edmonds, P. (2000). Effectiveness and efficiency in the management of cancer pain: current dilemmas in clinical practice. In Hillier, R., Finlay, I., and Miles, A., (eds), *The Effective Management of Cancer Pain*. London: Aesculapius Press, pp. 3–14.

Higginson, I.J. and McCarthy, M. (1989). Measuring symptoms in terminal cancer: are pain and dyspnoea controlled? *Journal of the Royal Society of Medicine* **82**: 1761–4.

Higginson, I.J. and Sen-Gupta, G. (2000). Place of care in advanced cancer: a qualitative systematic review of patient preferences. *Journal of Palliative Medicine* **3**: 287–300.

Hodgson, C., Higginson, I.J., McDonnell, M., and Butters, E. (1997). Family anxiety in advanced cancer: a multicentre prospective study in Ireland. *British Journal of Cancer* **76**: 1211–14.

Ingham, J. and Portenoy, R. (1996). Cachexia in context: the interaction among anorexia, pain and other symptoms. In Bruera, E. and Higginson, I.J. (eds), *Cachexia-anorexia in Cancer Patients*. Oxford: Oxford University Press, pp. 158–71.

Lunn, L. (1993). Spiritual concerns in palliation. In Saunders, C.M. and Sykes, N. (eds.), *The Management of Terminal Malignant Disease*. London: Edward Arnold.

Maguire, P. and Faulkner, A. (1988). Communicate with cancer patients: 2 Handling uncertainty, collusion and denial. *British Medical Journal* **297**: 972–4.

Mann, G.C.W. and Sproule, B.J. (1986). Effect of aprazolam on exercise and dyspnea in patients with chronic obstructive pulmonary disease. *Chest* **90**: 832–6.

McQuay, H., Carroll, D., Jadad, A.R., Wiffen, P., and Moore, A. (1995). Anticonvulsant drugs for management of pain: a systematic review. *British Medical Journal* **311**: 1047–52.

McQuay, H.J., Tramer, M., Nye, B.A., Carroll, D., Wiffen, P.J., and Moore, R.A. (1996). A systematic review of antidepressants in neuropathic pain. *Pain* **68**: 17–27.

Miller, R.D. and Walsh, T. (1991). Psychosocial aspects of palliative care in advanced cancer. *Journal of Pain and Symptom Management* **6**: 24–9.

Mitchell-Heggs, P. Murphy, K., Minty, K., *et al.* (1980). Diazepam in the treatment of dyspnoea in the pink puffer syndrome. *Quarterly Journal of Medicine* **69**: 9–20.

Neuenschwander, H. and Bruera, E. (1998). Asthenia. In Doyle, D., Hanks, G.W.C., and MacDonald, N. (eds), *Oxford Textbook of Palliative Medicine* (2nd edn). Oxford: Oxford University Press, pp. 573–81.

Payne, D.K. and Massie, M.J. (2000). Anxiety in palliative care. In Chochinov, H.M. and Breitbart, W. (eds), *Handbook of Psychiatry in Palliative Medicine*. Oxford, New York: Oxford University Press, pp. 63–74.

Portenoy, R.K. (1993). Adjuvant analgesics in pain management. In Doyle, D., Hanks, G.W.C., and MacDonald, N. (eds), *Oxford Textbook of Palliative Medicine*. Oxford: Oxford University Press, pp. 229–44.

Relf, M. (1999). Bereavement. In Twycross, R. (ed.), *Introducing Palliative Care*. Oxford: Radcliffe Medical Press, pp. 45–54.

Reuben, D.B. and Mor, V. (1986). Dyspnea in terminally ill cancer patients. *Chest* **89** 234–6.

Saunders, C. (1978). *The Management of Terminal Disease*. London: Edward Arnold.

Schwartzstein, R.M., Lahive, K., Pope, A., *et al.* (1987). Cold facial stimulation reduces breathlessness induced in normal subjects. *American Review of Respiratory Disease* **136**: 58–61.

Simon, P.M., Schwartzstein, R.M., Weiss, J.W., *et al.* (1990). Distinguishable types of dyspnea in patients with shortness of breath. *American Review of Respiratory Disease* **142**: 1009–14.

Speck, P. (1998). Spiritual issues in palliative care. In Doyle, D., Hanks, G.W.C., and MacDonald, N. (eds.), *Oxford Textbook of Palliative Medicine* (2nd edn). Oxford: Oxford University Press, pp. 805–16.

Takeda, F. (1986). Results of field-testing in Japan of the WHO draft interim guidelines of relief of cancer pain. *Pain Clinic* **1**: 83–9.

Twycross, R.G. (1989). Cancer pain—a global perspective. In Twycross, R.G. (ed.), *The Edinburgh Symposium on Pain and Medical Education*. London: Royal Society of Medicine Services, pp. 3–16.

Ventafridda, V., Tamburini, M., Caraceni, A., De Conno, F., and Naldi, F. (1987). A validation study of the WHO method for cancer pain relief. *Cancer* **59**: 850–6.

Walker, V.A., Hoskin, P.J., Hanks, G.W., and White, I.D. (1988). Evaluation of WHO analgesic guidelines for cancer pain in a hospital-based palliative care unit. *Journal of Pain and Symptom Management* **3**: 145–9.

Walsh, T.D. (1984). Opioids and respiratory function in advanced cancer. *Recent Results in Cancer Research*. **89**: 115–17.

Walsh, T.D., McDonald, N., Bruera, E., Shepherd, K.V., Michaud, M., and Zanes, R. (1992). A controlled study of sustained-release morphine sulphate tablets in chronic pain from advanced cancer. *American Journal of Clinical Oncology (CCT)* **15**: 268–72.

Weir, D.C., Gove, R.I., Robertson, A.S., *et al.* (1990). Corticosteroids trials in non-asthmatic chronic airflow obstruction: a comparison of oral prednisolone and inhaled beclomethasone diproprionate. *Thorax* **45**: 112–17.

Wilson, K.G., Chochinov, H.M., de Faye, B.J., and Breitbart, W. (2000). Diagnosis and management of depression in palliative care. In Chochinov, H.M. and Breitbart, W. (eds), *Handbook of Psychiatry in Palliative Medicine*, New York: Oxford University Press, pp. 25–49.

Woodcock, A.A., Gross, E.R., and Geddes, D.M. (1981). Drug treatment of breathlessness: contrasting effects of diazepam and promethazine in pink puffers. *British Medical Journal* **283**: 343–6.

Chapter 23

Discussion

Julia Addington-Hall and Irene Higginson

In this book, clinicians from a range of specialties have outlined what they consider to be the palliative care needs of their patients. Some have been concerned primarily with patients who have a distinct period of hours, days, or weeks during which death is certain and not far off. This category includes patients for whom a sudden catastrophic event has moved them abruptly from (at least relative) health to the terminal phase of life, such as patients who have had a severe stroke or a massive heart attack. It also includes patients who have lived for weeks, months, or years with a potentially fatal condition which is no longer treatable and for whom death is now inevitable in the short- (e.g. end-stage renal disease post-dialysis) or longer- (e.g. cancer) term. Other authors have written about patients who do not have such a distinct terminal phase to their illness, if they have one at all—patients who experience a gradual or unpredictable decline and who may therefore not be recognised as dying. Dementia patients, patients with chronic lung diseases, or chronic heart failure are examples in this category. Regardless of the dying trajectory, the authors have identified a role for palliative care in addressing the needs of patients and families.

Some have seen a role for direct service provision by hospices and palliative care services, whilst others have placed more emphasis on ensuring that those who currently care for these patients provide good care, informed by the philosophy and practice of palliative care. The patient and family problems which warrant palliative care differ between diseases, but there is consensus that palliative care is needed by non-cancer patients. Indeed, Wasson and George argue persuasively that it is unethical to limit palliative care to cancer patients. Greater access to palliative care for non-cancer patients is also clearly the wish of Cynthia Benz, who has provided a patient's perspective on the issues discussed in this book. It is, we believe, now clear that palliative care is needed by non-cancer patients. The best way of providing this is less clear.

Hospice and palliative care services for cancer patients have developed in a multitude of different forms; from just a handful of in-patient units in 1967 there are now independent in-patient units and dedicated hospital wards, home care teams providing a variety of services, hospital teams, day hospices, day care centres, and 'hospice-at-home' services (see Introduction). In addition to services caring primarily for cancer patients, there are hospice and specialist palliative care services specifically for HIV/AIDs patients and (primarily in the US) for dementia patients. Many services are staffed primarily by nurses, while others are multi-professional; doctors specialising in palliative medicine have a growing role. Some services focus almost entirely on educating and supporting other health professionals, while others provide care directly to patients and families. Many services care primarily for patients in the last weeks and days of life, yet others have an increasing role throughout the 'cancer journey'. The growth of the hospice movement has been marked by diversity. Palliative care provision for non-cancer patients will also take diverse forms, with service configurations and emphases varying according to the disease, the wishes of patients and families, and the health care system. Extending palliative care to non-cancer patients will require the same qualities of imagination and creativity, of willingness to change and to experiment, and, above all, of willingness to listen to patients and families and respond accordingly, which have been hallmarks of the international hospice movement over the past 30 years.

Many palliative care specialists in the UK and, to a lesser extent, elsewhere have backgrounds in oncology. They do not have, and cannot be expected to have, an in-depth understanding of all the diseases discussed in this book or of the complex ways in which these can interact in older patients. Extending palliative care to non-cancer patients will not necessarily mean a great expansion in the number of patients cared for in hospices or in other specialist palliative care services. It has been argued that for many patients, occasional or one-off access to specialist palliative knowledge and advice will be the most that it needed; others may require short-term access to specialist palliative care services, whilst a minority with particularly complex needs will require access to a full range of hospice and palliative care services (George & Sykes 1997; Addington-Hall 1998). The majority of non-cancer patients with palliative care needs will continue to have these needs met within their current health care setting, if at all. Effective partnerships are therefore required between health and social care professionals currently caring for these patients and palliative care experts. No one discipline or specialty will have the answers. Education, whether formal or informal, will need to be two-way, as will access to consultancy services and advice.

The question of how best to extend palliative care to non-cancer patients highlights a number of critical issues which have implications for hospice and palliative care in general, as well as for non-cancer palliative care in particular. These include changes in the age structure of industrialised countries which will impact on both the demand for palliative care and the availability of informal carers to provide care, and the growing heterogeneity in palliative care provision which raises questions about the fundamental values of hospice and palliative care. These are discussed below.

The ageing society

World-wide populations are ageing. In the UK, more than 16% of the population is aged 65 years or over, compared to only 12% in 1965. By 2020, this will increase to 21.5% (Ebrahim & Kalache 1996). In 1995 more than 2.3 million people were aged 80 or over—this will increase to 3.75 million over the next 20 years. More and more people die from chronic rather than acute diseases. As Table 23.1 shows the main causes of mortality are heart disease, cerebrovascular disorders, chronic respiratory disease, and the cancers.

Health care is, therefore, increasingly concerned with achieving the best possible quality of life for patients and for their families (WHO Expert Committee 1990). Uncontrolled symptoms or severe patient and family distress while a patient has a progressive illness, or is at the end of life, diminishes the patient's quality of life and impairs the carer's or family members' subsequent resolution of their grief (Saunders & Sykes 1993).

Table 23.1 Main causes of death in 1990 and predicted for 2020, in developed countries

Disorder	Ranking 1990	2020	Change in ranking
Within top 14 now/or top 10 for 2020			
Ischaemic heart disease	1	1	
Cerebrovascular disease (including stroke)	2	2	
Lower respiratory infections	3	4	−1
Diarrhoeal disorders	4	11	−7
Perinatal disorders	5	16	−11
Chronic obstructive pulmonary disease	6	3	+3
Tuberculosis	7	7	
Measles	8	27	−19
Road traffic accidents	9	6	+3
Trachea, bronchus, and lung cancers	10	5	+5
Malaria	11	29	−18
Self-inflicted injuries	12	10	+2
Cirrhosis of the liver	13	12	+1
Stomach cancer	14	8	+6
HIV	30	9	+21

Source: Murray and Lopez 1997.

The ageing population means not only will chronic and progressive disease become more common, but also that care will need to take place in the context of a more widely scattered family, with increasing numbers of older people living alone. There are likely to be fewer available informal carers, who themselves will be reaching older age (Chapter 19).

Implications for health care costs

The last year of life already places a heavy toll on health care costs. It is often regarded as more expensive, in terms of spending, than any other time of life. Based on random samples of deaths, Cartwright and Seale estimated that in England people who were in the last year of life took up approximately 22% of hospital bed-days (Seale & Cartwright 1994). In the US, end of life expenditure through Medicare consumes 10–12% of the total health budget and 27% of the Medicare budget (Lubitz & Riley 1993). A study of older people showed that health care expenditure for those in the last year of life was 276% higher than for people of similar age (Experton *et al.* 1996). Health care costs are therefore likely to rise as the population ages.

What does it mean for palliative care—is it ageist?

It has been argued that the distinctive philosophy of hospice and palliative care is less suited to non-cancer than to cancer patients, and that this is primarily due to the fact that non-cancer patients are on average older than cancer patients (Seale 1991). According to this view, the hospice philosophy promotes a particularly heroic approach to death, in which 'dramatic moments of truth are reached and confronted . . . intensely stressing physical suffering is controlled . . . where death and dying is attended by an audience of grieving relatives'. This approach, it is suggested, is most relevant to younger cancer patients, and elderly people without cancer need a different approach '. . . albeit one that, as in good hospice care, respects people's autonomy and dignity'. The view that age is the critical difference between cancer and non-cancer patients is challenged by evidence that non-cancer and cancer patients in the last year of life differ significantly at all ages with, for example, different patterns of dependency and of symptomatology (Addington-Hall & Karlsen 2000). It also overlooks the fact that although cancer is responsible for a greater proportion of deaths before the age of 65, more people aged 65 or above die from cancer than younger people: in 1999, 37% (32 462) of people aged under 65 died from cancer in England and Wales, compared to 22% (100 984) of people older than this. The cause of death, rather than age, appears to be the principal difference between cancer and non-cancer patients. However, the question of whether the hospice philosophy is relevant to older patients, particularly older non-cancer patients, is relevant to the debate on extending palliative care to non-cancer patients, particularly given the demographic changes outlined above.

Older cancer patients do not access hospice and specialist palliative care services in the proportions that would be expected. There is growing evidence of an age bias in hospice admissions (Addington-Hall, Altmann & McCarthy 1998; Gray & Forster 1997) and use of community specialist palliative care nurses (Addington-Hall & Altmann, 2000) in the UK, and in the use of hospice services in Australia (Hunt & McCaul 1996). Patients over the age of 65 made up 60% of new hospice admissions and 65% of new home care patients in the UK in 1994/5, but 75% of people who died from cancer. The reasons why older cancer patients are under-represented are unclear. It may reflect a belief among referrers, hospice personnel, or patients themselves, that older people are less in need of hospice care. It may be believed that older people are less likely to have grieving relatives who need support (but this ignores the distress of life-long partners), that symptoms are likely to have been more long-lasting but less distressing (for which the evidence is limited), that facing death becomes easier with age (again, a largely untested belief), because physical restrictions are likely to be due to the ageing process, rather than solely to cancer, and/or because of related difficulties in determining prognosis (Catt et al. in press). Research is needed to investigate whether these beliefs are a reflection of prejudice towards older people rather than of true variations in need amongst dying cancer patients of different ages.

The exclusion of non-cancer patients from hospice and palliative care services to date may, at least in part, be part of a wider exclusion of older people. Older people may be seen as less 'worthy' recipients of palliative care. Such views are consistent with the ageism apparent in Western societies, and may help explain growing evidence of poor pain control in older people (Bernabei et al. 1998). Awareness of the ageism common in society and of the effects this can have on the attitudes of health professionals, patients, and families will be needed if equitable and appropriate palliative care services are to be developed for non-cancer patients.

Partnerships between care of the elderly teams and nursing home staff on the one hand and hospice and palliative care providers on the other will be an essential component of ensuring that the palliative care needs of older people are met, regardless of their cause (or causes). Health care of older people is closely related to palliative care in that it also looks beyond the disease process to consider the wider impact on patients and families, and it subscribes to a holistic view of need. In the UK, however, few physicians in health care of older people have become involved in palliative care. Links between hospice and geriatric medicine are closer in the US, where a larger proportion of hospice admissions have a non-cancer diagnosis. Developing closer links will be an essential component of meeting the palliative care needs of non-cancer patients and their families. In England and Wales, 41% of stroke deaths, 78% of deaths from dementia, 26% of deaths from IHD, and 22% of those from chronic lung diseases are of people aged 85 or above; 37%, 19%, 37%, and 41% respectively are of people aged 75 to 84. Palliative care for non-cancer patients is therefore inextricably linked to the provision of health and social care for older people.

What is palliative care?

Extending palliative care to non-cancer patients raises fundamental questions about the nature and purpose of palliative care. In what ways, if at all, is palliative care different from other forms of health care? What are the essential, defining characteristics of palliative care? What role will it play in the care of non-cancer patients?

Pain and symptom control, to enable patients to live until death

Palliative care places great emphasis on pain and symptom control. Unlike much of modern medicine which is concerned with diagnosing and treating the underlying pathology, palliative care is focused on the impact the disease has on the patient—on the pain and distressing symptoms which they experience. It recognises, at least in theory, that pain control does not just require physical solutions but that pain and distress also have psychological, social, and spiritual components. It is by definition holistic and person centred. Traditionally palliative care has particularly focused on pain and symptom control for patients who have received maximal curative or life-sustaining therapy, and for whom death is now certain. The boundaries of palliative care therefore change as medical science advances, as demonstrated by introduction of effective therapies for AIDS/HIV (Chapter 11). However, some palliative care specialists see a role for palliative care expertise in pain and symptom control alongside active treatment for cancer or other diseases, especially where the treatment itself is associated with severe side effects (Chapters 5, 11).

Palliative care could, therefore, be defined as being primarily concerned with pain and symptom control, where patients may have had maximal therapy, or no therapy at all, or alongside therapy. As this book has demonstrated, there is plenty of scope for better pain and symptom control in non-cancer patients, and this definition therefore gives palliative care a clear role outside cancer. The difficulties inherent in judging prognosis in many non-cancer patients (Fox, Laudrum-McNiff, Zhong et al. 1999), and doctors' general reluctance to do so (Christakis 1999), means that models that focus solely on patients who are beyond active treatment will exclude most non-cancer patients. They are also inappropriate models for diseases such as AIDS/HIV or severe heart failure where continued active therapy is an important component of symptom control. The inclusion of patients who are still receiving treatment is one way around this problem.

It is fundamental to palliative care to see pain and symptom control problems as barriers to patients living full lives until they die, and to develop and use effective physical, psychological, and spiritual techniques to alleviate these problems. Palliative care specialists are therefore uniquely placed to provide pain and symptom control. A model of service provision which saw this as uniquely the role of palliative care specialists could, however, lead to two health care teams being involved in the patient's care, one concentrating on the bodily system or systems directly affected by the disease, and the other on providing holistic, patient centred care to deal with the effects on the patient of both the disease and its treatment. This would fragment patient care and make unsustainable demands on resources. It would enable other health professionals to relinquish responsibility for the well-being of the person, rather than the body, under their care, to the dismay of some (but not all) doctors and nurses currently caring for these patients. It also contradicts the original vision of the hospice movement, which was to develop expertise which could then be integrated into mainstream health care, so that all patients who need it receive good palliative care, regardless of health care setting. Despite the continued difficulties in raising the standards of palliative care within conventional health care settings, this remains an important goal.

Pain and symptom control are important components of palliative care provision for non-cancer patients. As in cancer, however, the emphasis must be on enabling the doctors, nurses, and other health professionals who currently care for these patients to understand the importance of reducing the distress caused by uncontrolled symptoms, to know how to go about doing this, and to be able to apply this in their work setting. As many palliative care specialists have little or no experience outside cancer palliative care, they will need to work closely with, for example, cardiologists, stroke physicians, or old age psychiatrists to enable them to develop an understanding of the diseases and their treatments, so that, together, they can investigate and test ways of alleviating pain and symptom distress in these patients.

Death and dying

In addition to expertise in pain and symptom control, palliative care specialists have experience in dealing with death and dying, and the complex, varied effects of these on everyone involved—patients, families, and staff. Many doctors and nurses are neither comfortable with nor skilled at discussing death and dying with patients and families (Christakis 1999). This is, or should be, a core skill of doctors and nurses who chose to specialise in hospice and palliative care. Palliative care is based on a philosophical position in which death is neither a failure nor taboo, and where existential concerns and suffering are not avoided. Paradoxically, alongside the recognition and focus on death runs an emphasis on living fully, until death comes.

Along with pain and symptom control, death and dying are central to palliative care. Apart from these, palliative care shares many of its values with other branches of health care. For example, nursing, family practice, and geriatric medicine also place emphasis on the need for holistic care, and acknowledge the importance of patients' families and social networks. The growing quality of life movement also has much in common with palliative care. Extending palliative care to non-cancer patients will require recognition of the common ground with other health care providers, as well as a clear vision and understanding of what palliative care can uniquely offer.

Palliative care should be embedded in most, if not all, areas of health care. Specialists in palliative care need to be advocates for quality of life, rather than just life prolongation, to offer advice and support for colleagues trying to provide good, holistic care in health care settings geared more towards cure than care, and to promote excellent pain and symptom control. But to do this effectively, and to sustain the unique role of palliative care as a movement promoting life in the midst of death, palliative care will continue to need specialist centres of excellence. In these, the core values of palliative care can be sustained and developed, specialists in palliative care can be refreshed and supported, and, in partnership with others, the knowledge base of palliative care can be extended. Some of this, at least, will need to be outside established health care structures to enable the focus on death and dying to be maintained and developed in the face of what continues to be a death-defying society.

A continued role for specialist services?

Specialist centres are needed as 'beacons', as examples of what is possible, and as centres of education and research. Who should these centres of excellence care for? At present, in the UK most care almost exclusively for cancer patients, with the exception of specialist AIDS/HIV hospices. In the US, hospice care is more diverse, although the focus is still on cancer. Many of the chapters in this book provide evidence that the philosophy of promoting life whilst acknowledging death is applicable outside of cancer. It is relevant, for example, to patients with severe heart failure or AIDS/HIV who live with considerable uncertainty about their future, as it is to patients and their families following a severe stroke or the withdrawal of dialysis who need to be enabled to make the best of the limited time available. There is, therefore, no rationale on this basis for restricting hospice and palliative care to cancer patients.

However, one of the original reasons for focusing on the care of terminally ill cancer patients was to enable rapid progress to be made in developing expertise in the care of these patients. Patients with terminal cancer, severe heart failure, dementia, and end-stage kidney failure may all have needs for pain and symptom control, better quality of life, and help in dealing with the likelihood or certainty of death, but these needs are diverse. Rapid progress in extending palliative care to non-cancer patients is likely to require services to focus on particular patient groups. The relative inexperience of many specialists in palliative care outside of cancer and the consequent need to develop services and initiatives in partnership with the health professionals currently caring for these patients may make this inevitable. Examples of successful developments of palliative care initiatives specifically for non-cancer patients can be found throughout the book (although a purchaser of health care cautions against the development of disease-specific services (Chapter 18)). These services need to have the same tripartite goals as Dame Cicely Saunders did when St Christopher's Hospice opened in 1967; to provide direct patient care, to educate others, and to undertake research to provide a secure evidence base. The growing emphasis on quality of life, on holistic care, and, in the US in particular, on end-of-life care means that unless hospice and palliative care specialists are willing to form partnerships to develop their expertise in and services for non-cancer patients, those currently caring for these patients may 'go it alone', with the consequent risks of fragmentation, of 're-inventing the wheel'—and ultimately of the marginalisation of palliative care specialists.

Priorities for research

The palliative care needs of non-cancer patients and the effectiveness of palliative care interventions and services have received little research attention. Research and evaluation must play a larger role in the development of palliative care for non-cancer patients than they have in palliative care in general. There are too many deficits in our knowledge of hospices and palliative care services: what models of care work best, in what conditions, for whom, and under what circumstances (Bonsaquet & Salisbury 1999). It is important to recognise that, outside some neurological conditions, AIDS/HIV and (to a lesser extent) dementia, there is no evidence that patients with non-cancer benefit from palliative care—or that they find it acceptable. Priorities for research include the extent to which attitudes towards the palliative care needs of older people reflect true differences in need as opposed to ageism, evaluation of different approaches to providing palliative care for older people, demonstration projects of both extending existing palliative care services to non-cancer patients and of developing disease-specific services, and research into effective methods of improving palliative care in mainstream health care settings. Many of the authors in this book have usefully highlighted research priorities for their particular disease group or setting, and clinical research priorities have been summarised in Chapter 22.

Conclusion

In this book, we have heard of the needs of patients at the end of life, and of their families. We have begun to grapple with the complexities and challenges of addressing the palliative care needs of patients and families whose clinical problems and dying trajectory appear to have little in common with those of cancer patients, with whom most palliative care specialists are familiar, and we have learnt from the experiences of those who have begun to address these needs in hospitals, family practice, nursing homes, and hospices. As the hospice movement reaches maturity, it is timely to acknowledge that achieving good palliative care for terminally ill cancer patients is the first step on the road towards ensuring that people continue to live well, in the face of death: it is not the destination. Much still remains to be done in cancer. However, this book reflects a wider acknowledgement that it is time to start the journey beyond cancer in earnest, and to ensure that *all* patients, whether cancer or non-cancer, who die receive excellent care and that their families are supported—regardless of their diagnoses or the settings in which they receive care.

References

Addington-Hall, J.M. (1998). *Reaching Out: Specialist Palliative Care for Adults with Non-malignant Disease*. London: National Council for Hospices and Specialist Palliative Care Services.

Addington-Hall, J.M., Altmann, D., McCarthy, M. (1998). Who gets hospice in-patient care? Social Science and Medicine **46**:1011–16.

Addington-Hall, J.M. and Altmann, D. (2000). Which terminally ill cancer patients receive care from community specialist palliative care nurses? *Journal of Advanced Nursing*, **32**: 799–806.

Addington-Hall, J.M. and Karlsen, S. (1999). Age is not the crucial factor in determining how the palliative care needs of people who die from cancer differ from those of people who die from other causes. *Journal of Palliative Care* **15**:13–19.

Bernabei, R., Gambassi, G., Lapane, K. *et al.* (1998). Management of pain in elderly patients with cancer. *Journal of the American Medical Association*. **279**:1877–82.

Bosanquet, N. and Salisbury, C. (1999). *Providing a Palliative Care Service: Towards an Evidence Base*. London: Oxford University Press.

Catt, S., Blanchard, M., King, M., Addington-Hall, J.M. Age-related inequalities in access to palliative care: ageism or true variation in needs? Submitted.

Christakis, N.A. (1999). *Death Foretold: Prophecy and Prognosis in Medical Care*. Chicago, IL: University of Chicago Press.

Ebrahim, S., and Kalache, A. (1996). *Epidemiology in Old Age*. London: BMJ Publications.

Experton, B., Ozminkowski, R.J., Branch, L.G., and Li, Z. (1996). A comparison by payor/provider type of the cost of dying among frail older adults. *Journal of the American Geriatric Society*. **44**:1098–1107.

Fox, E., Landrum-McNiff, K., Zhong Z. *et al.* (1999). Evaluation of prognostic criteria for determining hospice eligibility in patients with advanced lung, heart or liver disease. *Journal of the American Medical Association*. **282**:1638–45.

George, R. and Sykes, J. (1997). Beyond Cancer? In Clark, D., Hockley, J., and Ahmedzai, S. (eds.), *Beyond Cancer? New Themes in Palliative Care*. Buckingham: Open University Press.

Gray, J.D., Forster, D.P. (1997). Factors associated with utilisation of specialist palliative care services: a population-based study. *Journal of Public Health Medicine*. **19**:464–9.

Hunt, R. and McCaul, K. (1996). A population-based study of the coverage of cancer patients by hospice services. *Palliative Medicine*. **10**:5–12.

Lubitz, J. and Riley, G.F. (1993). Trends in Medicare payments in the last year of life. *New England Journal of Medicine*. **328**:1092–96.

Murray, C.J., and Lopez, A.D. (1997). Alternative projections of mortality and disability by cause 1990–2020: Global Burden of Disease Study. *Lancet* **349**: 1498–504.

Saunders, C. and Sykes, N. (1993). *The Management of Terminal Malignant Disease*. London: Edward Arnold.

Seale, C. (1991). Death from cancer and death from other causes: the relevance of the hospice approach. *Palliative Medicine*. **5**:12–19.

Seale, C. and Cartwright, A. (1994). *The Year Before Death*. Aldershot: Avebury Press.

WHO Expert Committee (1990). *Cancer Pain Relief and Palliative Care*. Geneva: WHO.

Index